Advances and Updates in Internal Medicine

Guest Editor

KEMBA MARSHALL, DVM, Dipl. ABVP–Avian

VETERINARY CLINICS OF NORTH AMERICA: EXOTIC ANIMAL PRACTICE

www.vetexotic.theclinics.com

Consulting Editor
AGNES E. RUPLEY, DVM, Dipl. ABVP–Avian

September 2010 • Volume 13 • Number 3

SAUNDERS an imprint of ELSEVIER, Inc.

W.B. SAUNDERS COMPANY

A Division of Elsevier Inc.

1600 John F. Kennedy Boulevard • Suite 1800 • Philadelphia, Pennsylvania 19103-2899

http://www.vetexotic.theclinics.com

VETERINARY CLINICS OF NORTH AMERICA: EXOTIC ANIMAL PRACTICE Volume 13, Number 3
September 2010 ISSN 1094-9194, ISBN-13: 978-1-4377-2503-2

Editor: John Vassallo; j.vassallo@elsevier.com
Developmental Editor: Donald Mumford

Veterinary Clinics of North America: Exotic Animal Practice (ISSN 1094-9194) is published in January, May, and September by Elsevier, Inc., 360 Park Avenue South, New York, NY 10010-1710. Subscription prices are $198.00 per year for US individuals, $329.00 per year for US institutions, $103.00 per year for US students and residents, $234.00 per year for Canadian individuals, $388.00 per year for Canadian institutions, $264.00 per year for international individuals, $388.00 per year for international institutions and $132.00 per year for Canadian and foreign students/residents. To receive student/resident rate, orders must be accompanied by name of affiliated institution, date of term, and the *signature* of program/residency coordinator on institution letterhead. Orders will be billed at individual rate until proof of status is received. Foreign air speed delivery is included in all *Clinics* subscription prices. All prices are subject to change without notice. **POSTMASTER:** Send address changes to *Veterinary Clinics of North America: Exotic Animal Practice*, Elsevier Health Sciences Division, Subscription Customer Service, 3251 Riverport Lane, Maryland Heights, MO 63043. **Customer Service: Telephone:** 1-800-654-2452 (U.S. and Canada); **1-314-447-8871** (outside U.S. and Canada). **Fax: 1-314-447-8029.** E-mail: **journalscustomerservice-usa@elsevier.com** (for print support); **journalsonlinesupport-usa@elsevier.com** (for online support).

Reprints. For copies of 100 or more of articles in this publication, please contact the Commercial Reprints Department, Elsevier Inc., 360 Park Avenue South, New York, New York 10010-1710. Tel.: (212)-633-3813; Fax: (212)-633-1935; E-mail: reprints@elsevier.com.

Veterinary Clinics of North America: Exotic Animal Practice is covered in *MEDLINE/PubMed (Index Medicus)*.

Printed and bound by CPI Group (UK) Ltd, Croydon, CR0 4YY

Transferred to Digital Print 2012

Contributors

CONSULTING EDITOR

AGNES E. RUPLEY, DVM
Diplomate, American Board of Veterinary Practitioners-Avian Practice; and Director
and Chief Veterinarian, All Pets Medical and Laser Surgical Center, College Station, Texas

GUEST EDITOR

KEMBA MARSHALL, DVM
Diplomate, American Board of Veterinary Practitioners-Avian Practice; PetSmart Store
Support Group, Phoenix, Arizona

AUTHORS

ARMANDO G. BURGOS-RODRÍGUEZ, DVM
Diplomate, American Board of Veterinary Practitioners-Avian Practice; Avian and Exotic
Veterinarian, Clínica Veterinaria San Agustín, Rio Piedras, Puerto Rico

SUE CHEN, DVM
Diplomate, American Board of Veterinary Practitioners-Avian Practice; Gulf Coast
Avian & Exotics, Gulf Coast Veterinary Specialists, Houston, Texas

SUSAN CLUBB, DVM
Diplomate, American Board of Veterinary Practitioners-Avian Practice Rainforest Clinic
for Birds and Exotics, Loxahatchee, Florida

ERIKA E. EVANS, DVM, MBA
Department of Small Animal Clinical Sciences, University of Tennessee College
of Veterinary Medicine, Knoxville, Tennessee

ADY Y. GANCZ, DVM, MSc, DVSc
Diplomate, American Board of Veterinary Practitioners-Avian Practice; The Exotic Clinic,
Herzliya, Israel

MICHAEL M. GARNER, DVM
Diplomate, American College of Veterinary Pathologists; Northwest ZooPath, Monroe,
Washington

PATRICIA L. GRAY, DVM, MS
Resident, Small Animal Clinical Sciences, Texas A&M University College of Veterinary
Medicine, College Station, Texas

VANESSA L. GRUNKEMEYER, DVM
Avian and Zoological Medicine Service, Department of Small Animal Clinical Sciences,
University of Tennessee College of Veterinary Medicine, Knoxville Tennessee

TARAH L. HADLEY, DVM
Diplomate, American Board of Veterinary Practitioners-Avian Practice; Atlanta Hospital
for Birds and Exotics, Inc, Conyers, Georgia

SHARMAN HOPPES, DVM
Diplomate, American Board of Veterinary Practitioners-Avian Practice; Assistant Clinical Professor, Small Animal Clinical Sciences, Texas A&M University College of Veterinary Medicine, College Station, Texas

MATTI KIUPEL, DrMedVet, MS, PhD
Diplomate, American College of Veterinary Pathologists; Fachtierarzt für Veterinär Pathologie, Associate Professor, Section Chief Anatomic Pathology, Department of Pathobiology and Diagnostic Investigation, Diagnostic Center for Population and Animal Health, Michigan State University, Lansing, Michigan

ERIC KLAPHAKE, DVM
Diplomate, American College of Zoological Medicine; Diplomate, American Board of Veterinary Practitioners-Avian Practice; Associate Veterinarian, Animal Medical Center, Bozeman; Head Veterinarian, ZooMontana, Billings, Montana

ANGELA LENNOX, DVM
Diplomate, American Board of Veterinary Practitioners-Avian Practice; Owner, Avian and Exotic Animal Clinic, Indianapolis, Indiana

MARLA LICHTENBERGER, DVM
Diplomate, American College of Veterinary Emergency and Critical Care; Owner, Milwaukee Emergency Clinic for Animals, Greenfield, Wisconsin

ROGER K. MAES, DVM, PhD
Professor, Section Head Virology, Department of Microbiology, Diagnostic Center for Population and Animal Health, Michigan State University, Lansing, Michigan

JÖRG MAYER, DMV, MSc
Diplomate, American Board of Veterinary Practitioners (ECM); Clinical Associate Professor, Head of Exotics Service, Department of Clinical Sciences, Tufts University Cummings School of Veterinary Medicine, North Grafton, Massachusetts

JERRY MURRAY, DVM
Animal Clinic of Farmers Branch, Dallas, Texas

SUSAN PAYNE, PhD
Associate Professor, Veterinary Pathobiology Department, Texas A&M University College of Veterinary Medicine, College Station, Texas

KATRINA D. RAMSELL, PhD, DVM
Northwest Exotic Pet Vet LLC, Beaverton, Oregon

NICHOLAS SAINT-ERNE, DVM
Technical Services Veterinarian, Aquatics Division, PetSmart, Inc, Phoenix, Arizona

H.L. SHIVAPRASAD, BVSc, MS, PhD
Diplomate, American College of Poultry Veterinarians; Diplomate, American College of Veterinary Pathologists; Professor, Avian Pathology, California Animal Health and Food Safety Laboratory System, Tulare, and University of California, Davis, California

MARCY J. SOUZA, DVM, MPH
Diplomate, American Board of Veterinary Practitioners-Avian Practice; Assistant Professor, Department of Comparative Medicine, University of Tennessee College of Veterinary Medicine, Knoxville, Tennessee

JOHN M. SYKES IV, DVM
Diplomate, American College of Zoological Medicine; Associate Veterinarian, Global Health Program, Wildlife Conservation Society, Bronx, New York

OLIVIER TAEYMANS, VMD, PhD
Diplomate, American Board of Veterinary Practitioners-Exotic Companion Mammal Practice; Assistant Professor of Radiology, Department of Clinical Sciences, Tufts University Cummings School of Veterinary Medicine, North Grafton, Massachusetts

IAN TIZARD, BVMS, PhD
Diplomate, American College of Veterinary Microbiologist; Professor and Director, The Schubot Exotic Bird Health Center, Veterinary Pathobiology Department, Texas A&M University, College Station, Texas

ROBERT WAGNER, DVM, PhD
Diplomate, European College of Veterinary Diagnostic Imaging; Associate Professor of Medicine, University of Pittsburgh, Division of Laboratory Animal Services, University of Pittsburgh, Pittsburgh, Pennsylvania

Contents

Preface: Advances and Updates in Internal Medicine   xiii

Kemba Marshall

**Diagnostic Techniques and Treatments for Internal Disorders of Koi
(*Cyprinus carpio*)**   333

Nicholas Saint-Erne

> The most common problems that occur in koi involve external pathogens
> and environmental conditions. Techniques for external fish examination
> and water quality analysis have been well described in the veterinary liter-
> ature. However, there are also some internal disorders of koi, such as gas
> bladder abnormalities affecting the fish's buoyancy, neoplasia, egg bind-
> ing (roe retention), and spinal disorders that can be diagnosed with com-
> mon veterinary medical procedures. Diagnostic techniques along with
> available treatments for these disorders are presented in this article.

Updates and Practical Approaches to Reproductive Disorders in Reptiles 349

John M. Sykes IV

> Reproductive biology and disorders are important facets of captive reptile
> management and are relatively common reasons for reptiles to present to
> the veterinarian. Although the factors and conditions for normal reproduc-
> tion differ between species depending on their natural histories, the gen-
> eral principles and common approaches to disorders are presented in
> this article. Frequently seen disorders addressed in this review include in-
> fertility or lack of conception, follicular stasis, dystocia, and reproductive
> organ prolapse. This article is divided into sections based on the taxo-
> nomic groups, although many of the predisposing factors for and the ap-
> proaches to these conditions are similar for all the groups.

A Fresh Look at Metabolic Bone Diseases in Reptiles and Amphibians   375

Eric Klaphake

> Metabolic bone diseases (MBDs) are a common presenting complaint in
> reptiles and amphibians to veterinarians; however, understanding of the
> causes and diagnostic and treatment options is often extrapolated from hu-
> man or other mammalian medicine models. Although the roles of UV-B,
> calcium, phosphorus, and cholecalciferol are better understood in some
> MBDs, there remain many X factors that are not. Likewise, quantitative di-
> agnosis of MBDs has been difficult not only in terms of staging a disease
> but also regarding whether or not a condition is present. Treatment options
> also present challenges in corrective husbandry and diet modifications,
> medication/modality selection, and dosing/regimen parameters.

Avian Renal System: Clinical Implications   393

Armando G. Burgos-Rodríguez

> The avian renal system differs anatomically and physiologically from the
> mammalian renal system. However, it is affected by similar disease

categories such as infectious, nutritional, degenerative, congenital, metabolic, and neoplastic conditions. The diagnosis of renal disease in birds can be challenging and, in many cases, diagnosis is made on postmortem examination. Successful treatment of avian renal disease requires early recognition of clinical signs and correct interpretation of diagnostic tools.

Advanced Diagnostic Approaches and Current Management of Avian Hepatic Disorders   413

Vanessa L. Grunkemeyer

Although the diagnosis of liver disease is common in avian patients, it is often based on subjective or inadequate evidence. Diagnosis of the inciting cause, determination of the severity of the tissue damage, and assessment of the remaining hepatobiliary function can be clinically challenging. A basic review of avian normal hepatic anatomy and function is included in this article as a foundation for further discussion of testing methods used to diagnose liver disease. Interpretation of abnormalities noted on the physical examination, clinical pathologic testing, and imaging studies in a patient with hepatic dysfunction are presented, and the methods of obtaining a hepatic biopsy are discussed. Therapies targeted at treating secondary complications of hepatic dysfunction and at supporting hepatocellular function and regeneration are also reviewed.

Management of Common Psittacine Reproductive Disorders in Clinical Practice   429

Tarah L. Hadley

The reproductive organs play a key role in the maintenance of normal homeostasis in psittacine birds. For this reason, sex determination should be part of the baseline data collected on every avian patient. Disorders of the psittacine reproductive tract can have a negative effect on the function of other organ systems in the body. Reproductive organs may be plagued by a multitude of problems ranging from infection and neoplasia to inflammation and idiopathic issues that affect fertility. Detection of reproductive problems may require the use of a variety of modalities. The ability to treat these problems often depends on the presenting complaint as well as the clinical condition of the avian patient. Different reproductive disorders of male and female psittacine birds, with their detection and treatment are discussed in this article.

Advanced Diagnostic Approaches and Current Medical Management of Insulinomas and Adrenocortical Disease in Ferrets (*Mustela putorius furo*)   439

Sue Chen

Endocrine neoplasia is the most common tumor type in domestic ferrets, especially in middle-aged to older ferrets. Islet cell tumors and adrenocortical tumors constitute the major types of endocrine neoplasms. Insulinoma is a tumor that produces and releases excessive amounts of insulin. Evaluation of fasted blood glucose levels provides a quick diagnostic assessment for the detection of insulinomas. Use of glucocorticoids, diazoxide, and diet modification are some of the medical treatment options for insulinomas. Adrenocortical neoplasia in ferrets usually overproduces one or more sex hormones. Sex hormones which can result in progressive alopecia, vulvar swelling in females, and prostagomegaly in males. Abdominal ultrasonography and sex hormone assays can be used to diagnose adrenocortical neoplasms. Drugs such as leuprolide acetate, deslorelin acetate, and the hormone melatonin can be used to treat adrenocortical neoplasms in ferrets when surgery is not an option.

Advanced Diagnostic Approaches and Current Management of Internal Disorders of Select Species (Rodents, Sugar Gliders, Hedgehogs) 453

Erika E. Evans and Marcy J. Souza

African pygmy and European hedgehogs, sugar gliders, and rodents such as rats, mice, gerbils, hamsters, guinea pigs, and chinchillas are becoming increasingly popular as pets in the United States, and more practitioners are being asked to examine, diagnose, and treat these animals for a bevy of disorders and diseases. Many procedures and techniques used in traditional small and large animal medicine are used for these species, with minor adaptations or considerations. This article examines available diagnostic tools and treatment methodologies for use in hedgehogs, sugar gliders, and selected rodents.

Advanced Diagnostic Approaches and Current Management of Proventricular Dilatation Disease 471

Ady Y. Gancz, Susan Clubb, and H.L. Shivaprasad

Proventricular dilatation disease (PDD) is a fatal inflammatory disease that affects mainly, but not exclusively, psittacine birds (Order: Psittaciformes). PDD has long been suspected to be a viral disease, but its causative agent, a novel Bornavirus, was only identified in 2008.

The Isolation, Pathogenesis, Diagnosis, Transmission, and Control of Avian Bornavirus and Proventricular Dilatation Disease 495

Sharman Hoppes, Patricia L. Gray, Susan Payne, H.L. Shivaprasad, and Ian Tizard

Proventricular dilatation disease (PDD) is a common infectious neurologic disease of birds comprising a dilatation of the proventriculus by ingested food as a result of defects in intestinal motility, which affects more than 50 species of psittacines, and is also known as Macaw wasting disease, neuropathic ganglioneuritis, or lymphoplasmacytic ganglioneuritis. Definitive diagnosis of PDD has been problematic due to the inconsistent distribution of lesions. Since its discovery, avian bornavirus (ABV) has been successfully cultured from the brains of psittacines diagnosed with PDD, providing a source of antigen for serologic assays and nucleic acid for molecular assays. This article provides evidence that ABV is the etiologic agent of PDD. Recent findings on the transmission, epidemiology, pathogenesis, diagnosis, and control of ABV infection and PDD are also reviewed.

Advanced Diagnostic Approaches and Current Management of Thyroid Pathologies in Guinea Pigs 509

Jörg Mayer, Robert Wagner, and Olivier Taeymans

The authors have encountered multiple clinical cases of clinical hyperthyroidism in the guinea pig, which responded positively to clinical treatment.

Hyperactive thyroids in the guinea pig appear to exist causing typical clinical signs. An early accurate diagnosis of this pathologic state is important in the clinical setting. One of the authors has encountered a few clinical cases of hypothyroidism in guinea pigs. Hypothyroidism appears to be a rare condition and has been described anecdotally in the German literature. Because of the rarity of hypothyroidism, the text focuses mainly on the guinea pig as a hyperthyroid case. A short description of the clinical presentation of the hypothyroid animal is included at the end of the text.

Updates and Advanced Therapies for Gastrointestinal Stasis in Rabbits   525

Marla Lichtenberger and Angela Lennox

Gastrointestinal stasis is currently a vaguely defined term for decreased gastrointestinal motility. The term gastric stasis syndrome was previously proposed, but falls short of an accurate description, as in many cases portions of the gastrointestinal tract other than the stomach are affected. The term rabbit gastrointestinal syndrome (RGIS) defines a complex of clinical signs, symptoms, and concurrent pathologic conditions affecting the digestive apparatus of the rabbit. When ill rabbits present for examination it is important to determine if RGIS is present and if so, begin treatment and a diagnostic workup to determine underlying contributing factors. Identification of underlying cause is often difficult; many rabbits present with evidence of RGIS whereby attempts to identify an underlying cause are unfruitful. In many cases, these rabbits respond positively to supportive therapy including fluids, hand feeding, and motility-enhancing drugs.

Ferret Coronavirus-Associated Diseases   543

Jerry Murray, Matti Kiupel, and Roger K. Maes

A novel coronavirus of ferrets was first described in 1993. This coronavirus caused an enteric disease called epizootic catarrhal enteritis (ECE). Recently, a ferret systemic coronavirus (FRSCV)-associated disease was discovered. This new systemic disease resembles the dry form of feline infectious peritonitis (FIP) and has been reported in the United States and Europe. This article addresses the clinical signs, pathology, pathogenesis, diagnosis, treatment, and prevention of this ferret FIP-like disease.

Disseminated Idiopathic Myofasciitis in Ferrets   561

Katrina D. Ramsell and Michael M. Garner

First described in 2003, disseminated idiopathic myofasciitis (DIM) has emerged as a new disease in young, domestic ferrets. DIM is a severe inflammatory condition that affects primarily muscles and surrounding connective tissues. The disease is characterized by rapid onset of clinical signs, high fever, neutrophilic leukocytosis, and general lack of response to therapeutic intervention. Until recently DIM was considered fatal, but a few surviving ferrets indicate there may be an effective treatment protocol. DIM is suspected to be an immune-mediated disease, but the etiopathogenesis is not known. This article reviews clinical and pathologic findings in DIM patients, covers recommended diagnostic procedures and clinical management of ferrets with DIM, and discusses potential etiologies for this newly recognized disease in ferrets.

Index   577

FORTHCOMING ISSUES

January 2011
Analgesia
Joanne Paul-Murphy, DVM, Dipl. ACZM,
Guest Editor

May 2011
The Exotic Animal Respiratory System
Cathy Johnson-Delaney, DVM,
DABVP-Avian, DABVP-Exotic Companion
Mammal, and Susan E. Orosz, PhD, DVM,
DABVP-Avian, DECAMS, *Guest Editors*

RECENT ISSUES

May 2010
Endoscopy and Endosurgery
Stephen J. Divers, BVetMed, DZooMed,
DACZM, DipECZM(herp), FRCVS,
Guest Editor

January 2010
Geriatrics
Sharman M. Hoppes, DVM,
Dipl. ABVP—Avian, and
Patricia Gray, DVM, MS, *Guest Editors*

September 2009
Bacterial and Parasitic Diseases
Laura Wade, DVM, Dipl. ABVP–Avian,
Guest Editor

RELATED INTEREST

Veterinary Clinics of North America: Small Animal Practice (Volume 38, Issue 3,
May 2008)
Advances in Fluid, Electrolyte, and Acid-Base Disorders
Helio Autran de Morais, DVM, PhD, and Stephen P. DiBartola, DVM, *Guest Editors*

THE CLINICS ARE NOW AVAILABLE ONLINE!

Access your subscription at:
www.theclinics.com

Preface
Advances and Updates
in Internal Medicine

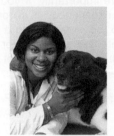

Kemba Marshall, DVM, DABVP-Avian
Guest Editor

Let the young know they will never find a more interesting, more instructive book than the patient himself.

—*Giorgio Baglivi*

Through our patients we, as veterinarians, learn and develop our anecdotes, our n = 1, and eventually our clinical impressions. It is through our patients that we experience the elation of being right and the cemented weight of being completely at a loss.

When I was in veterinary school, I asked one of my professors to give me advice on what I could do to become a better exotic animal practitioner. Poised with paper and pen, I was ready for whatever recommendations were to be given, or so I thought. My professor said to me, "Don't ever forget that medicine is medicine." I was initially somewhat offended; that seemed as informative to me as telling me that there are gravitational forces affecting the earth. Through the years, however, that simple statement has been its own gravitational, steadying force.

The contributions to this issue echo that same sentiment. Hyperthyroidism in guinea pigs still requires a minimum database and has a similar work-up as does hyperthyroidism in cats. Diagnostic imaging techniques are no different in koi than in canine patients. Prolonged anorexia has to be addressed in order for patients to receive daily nutritional requirements; stomach tubes work even when they are fed in through the nose.

With the help of contributing authors, the first portion of this issue attempts to provide updates on common diseases, such as reptile metabolic bone disease and avian renal disease syndromes. Where applicable, evidence-based research studies are cited to justify treatment modalities. When the research studies are lacking, the authors have cited their own opinions to explain therapies.

Vet Clin Exot Anim 13 (2010) xiii–xiv
doi:10.1016/j.cvex.2010.05.015
1094-9194/10/$ – see front matter © 2010 Elsevier Inc. All rights reserved.

vetexotic.theclinics.com

The second part of this issue focuses on advances; in general, this information is underreported, as in the case of guinea pig hyperthyroidism in the United States, or it is a new explanation of an old syndrome, like the exciting proventricular dilatation disease research presented. For all submissions, I am appreciative, and for the honor of being asked to guest edit this edition, I am humbled.

Use these articles for reference, information, and confirmation when seeing patients who look just like what an article describes. More importantly, if you have a question, contact the authors. We all learn when we share experiences. If, in communicating with authors, you see that n = 1 is really n = 5, consider writing a peer-reviewed article to advance the body of evidence based veterinary medicine for avian and exotic pets. If every patient is a book, just think of all the information yet to be discovered. So go palpate, go listen, and then go document.

Kemba Marshall, DVM, DABVP-Avian
PetSmart Store Support Group, 19601 North 27th Avenue
Phoenix, AZ 85027, USA

E-mail address:
petagrees@yahoo.com

Diagnostic Techniques and Treatments for Internal Disorders of Koi (*Cyprinus carpio*)

Nicholas Saint-Erne, DVM

KEYWORDS

- Fish • Carp • Koi • Diagnosis • Reproduction
- Internal medicine

Aquatic veterinary medicine is a fast-growing field in veterinary medicine, and aquatic veterinarians are involved in food fish production (aquaculture), natural fisheries management, research using fish as models, public aquarium maintenance, and ornamental fish keeping. The AquaVetMed.info Web site lists more than 700 veterinarians as practicing aquatic veterinary medicine. There are several worldwide organizations for veterinarians whose medical practice includes fish; including the World Aquatic Veterinary Medical Association (www.WAVMA.org) and the International Association for Aquatic Animal Medicine (www.IAAAM.org). The American Veterinary Medical Association (www.AVMA.org) survey of United States households' pet ownership, which is conducted every 5 years, indicates that in 2006 there were more than 9 million American households keeping a total of more than 75 million pet fish.[1] These numbers are 50% greater than in the previous 2001 AVMA survey!

Nishikigoi (Japanese for "brocaded carp"), or koi for short, are colorful variations of the common carp (*Cyprinus carpio*) that have been selectively bred in Japan for more than 200 years. In the last 50 years they have become very popular worldwide as ornamental fish. Koi can grow quite large (up to 100 cm) and live for many decades. Individual koi fish with perfect color patterns are valuable (**Fig. 1**). There are koi shows held all over the world, and a show-quality koi can be worth thousands, even tens of thousands of dollars. For this reason, along with their longevity and endearing personalities, koi are one of the fish species most often presented to the veterinarian for treatment of diseases.

Aquatics Division, PetSmart, Inc, 19601 North 27th Avenue, Phoenix, AZ 85027, USA
E-mail address: nsainterne@ssg.petsmart.com

Vet Clin Exot Anim 13 (2010) 333–347
doi:10.1016/j.cvex.2010.05.012
1094-9194/10/$ – see front matter © 2010 Elsevier Inc. All rights reserved.

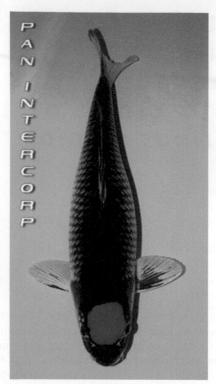

Fig. 1. A Tancho Goshiki (*red circle* on head of black patterned koi) that recently sold for well in excess of $10,000. (*Courtesy of* Pan Intercorp, Kenmore, Washington. www.Koi.com.)

DIAGNOSTIC TECHNIQUES

Disease diagnosis and treatment of koi or other ornamental fish in the veterinary hospital use techniques similar to those used for other animal species. Most of the needed equipment is already in the small animal veterinary hospital, except for water containers and filtration systems. One of the most important diagnostic tools is taking the history of the patient.[2] Discussing the patient's history with the owner is as necessary with fish as it is with other pets. History taking includes obtaining information on age, origin, length of ownership, previous diseases and treatments, feeding habits, aquatic habitat, water quality, and filtration systems. As with many exotic pets, knowing the environmental information is helpful in making an accurate diagnosis.

Many common clinical techniques can be used to diagnose diseases of koi, and these have been described in many other publications.[2–7] Diagnostic tests for external disorders are inexpensive, and can be performed using standard veterinary techniques.[6] Common diagnostic tests include skin, fin, and gill biopsies examined microscopically for diagnosing external parasites, culture and sensitivity testing for bacteria, polymerase chain reaction (PCR) tests for viruses, blood chemistry and serology, tissue and fluid aspiration cytology, radiology, and sonography. More advanced techniques available through specialty practices or veterinary colleges such as magnetic resonance imaging (MRI) and computed tomography (CT) are used for koi as well.

When handling fish for clinical procedures or diagnostic tests, the veterinarian and assistant should wear wet latex gloves to prevent damage to the fish's scales, skin, and glycocalyx (the mucus layer that protects the epidermis). Koi can be kept out of the water during examination, provided that the skin and gills are kept moist. Small fish (<20 cm in length) can be maintained out of the water for 5 to 15 minutes, larger fish for as long as 30 minutes or more, keeping in mind their health condition and monitoring their respiration. Use a wet towel or chamois cloth to lay the fish on and to wrap around it during handling.[7] Add dechlorinated water as needed to keep the koi wet. Cover the koi's eyes with a wet cloth to reduce light, and limit noise and vibrations around the area to help keep the fish calm while being examined.[8] The holding tank for the koi while in the clinic can also be opaque to reduce light and to prevent the fish from a sudden burst of motion if visually startled, resulting in injury from hitting the sides of the enclosure. The holding tank should be covered to prevent the fish from jumping out of the container. Use an aquarium water quality test kit to ensure that the holding tank water is ideal for keeping koi. The water should be kept aerated using an electric air pump or oxygen canister connected with plastic tubing to an air stone, producing fine bubbles in the water. **Table 1** lists the water quality tests and ranges appropriate for the holding tank water quality.[9]

Anesthesia techniques in fish are well described in a variety of publications.[7,10–12] Anesthetics can be useful with large koi to keep them still during examination and imaging, and to prevent injury during handling. Currently the US Food and Drug Administration has approved tricaine methanesulfonate powder, commonly called MS-222 (Finquel; Tricaine-S), as an anesthetic for fish. A buffered solution of MS-222 can be added to the water containing the fish at a dose of 30 to 40 mg/L to sedate koi for handling and examination, and a higher dose of 50 to 150 mg/L is used for anesthesia. Induction is fairly rapid, within 5 minutes, but recovery once the fish is placed into fresh water is dependent on how long the fish has been exposed to the anesthetic solution. Short-term anesthesia will have recovery times of 5 to 10 minutes, but long-term anesthesia, such as with surgical procedures, may result in prolonged anesthesia recovery times of 30 to 60 minutes. Isoeugenol (Aqui-S) is an investigational new animal drug, and works well as a fish tranquilizer to aid in handling koi. It is used at a dose of 30 to 60 mg/L and sedation occurs within 5 minutes, with a similar recovery time once the koi is placed in fresh water. The recovery water must be of appropriate temperature and be aerated with an air pump or with oxygen bubbled through the water. Use of an electrocardiogram or Doppler flow probe to measure the heart rate

Table 1		
Water quality parameters		
Water Test (Unit)	**Optimal**	**Acceptable Range**
Temperature (°F)	65	60–80 (will survive 39–95)
Dissolved Oxygen (mg/L)	9	6–12
Ammonia (mg/L)	0	0–0.02
Nitrite (mg/L)	0	0–0.02
Nitrate (mg/L)	0	0–40
pH (-Log[H+])	7.2	6.2–8.5
Hardness (mg/L)	100	75–250
Alkalinity (mg/L)	100	75–250
Salinity (%)	0.1	0–0.3
Chlorine (mg/L)	0	0–0.02

Data from Saint-Erne N. Water quality in the koi pond. In: Advanced koi care. Glendale (AZ): Erne Enterprises; 2002. p. 108.

and a pulse oximeter clipped onto the caudal fin to monitor blood oxygen saturation will help monitor patient status and depth of anesthesia.[7] Opercular motion (breaths) should also be observed and recorded during anesthesia and recovery. If opercular motion ceases during anesthesia, the depth of anesthesia may be excessive.

Radiographs can be taken successfully with standard veterinary radiology equipment.[3,6,7,13] In most cases, radiographs can be taken of koi without anesthesia by briefly restraining them in a sealed plastic bag with a small volume of water (**Fig. 2**A, B). The koi in the plastic bag can be placed directly onto the film plate or digital sensor, and the bag taped down if necessary to hold the fish in the correct position. Anesthetized koi can be briefly taken out of the water and positioned for radiographs (see **Fig. 2**C). Foam rubber supports are used if necessary to maintain the position of the koi. Radiographs are helpful in diagnosing gas bladder (swim bladder) abnormalities, spinal deformities, abdominal masses, and occasionally ingested foreign objects.[14] Normal radiographic anatomy can be seen in **Fig. 3**A, B. Abdominal viscera are not easily distinguishable in a radiograph. A flexible rubber tube can be inserted orally to place barium or iodinated contrast medium into the intestines (koi do not have stomachs) to perform contrast studies (**Fig. 4**) on the koi intestinal tract.[15] The dosage for barium is 5 to 10 mL/kg body weight and the iodinated medium is dosed at 1 to 2 mL/kg. Care must be taken not to leak barium into the oral cavity and onto the gills, which could impair oxygen diffusion through the gills.[16]

Ultrasound has been used on fish for sex determination for nearly 30 years.[17–19] Ultrasound imaging is easy with fish confined in a small container of water, as the

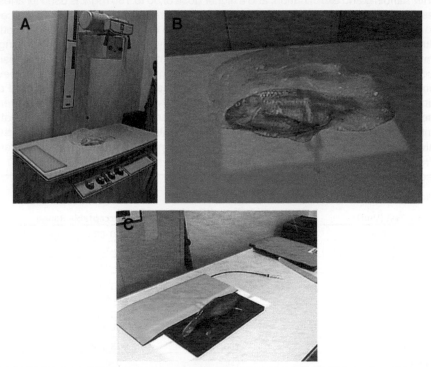

Fig. 2. (A) X-ray machine with koi restrained in plastic bag of water on tabletop for radiograph. (B) X-ray machine with koi in plastic bag with water on tabletop for radiograph. (C) Anesthetized koi positioned without restraint for radiographs. (*From* Saint-Erne N. Clinical procedures. In: Advanced koi care. Glendale, AZ: Erne Enterprises; 2002. p. 47–8; with permission.)

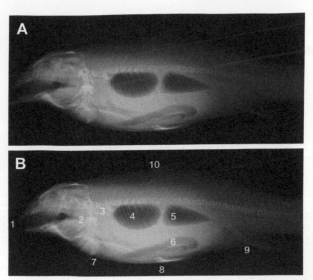

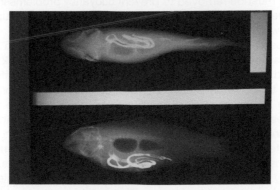

Fig. 3. (*A*) Normal koi radiograph. (*B*) Normal koi radiograph with anatomy labeled. 1, mouth opening; 2, pharyngeal teeth; 3, Weber's ossicles connecting the gas bladder to the inner ear; 4, cranial chamber of the gas bladder; 5, caudal chamber of the gas bladder; 6, gas in a loop of intestines; 7, pectoral fin; 8, pelvic fin; 9, anal fin; 10, dorsal fin. (*Modified from* Saint-Erne N. Clinical procedures. In: Advanced koi care. Glendale (AZ): Erne Enterprises; 2002. p. 36; with permission.)

water serves to couple the transducer to the fish's body, eliminating the need for ultrasound gel.[3] Transducers of 5 to 10 MHz work well for visualization of internal organs at depths up to 13 to 20 cm into the body, with lower frequency transducers producing images at greater depths of tissue penetration. If not waterproof, the transducer can be placed inside a plastic cover (eg, plastic bag, examination glove, condom) for protection. The transducer can be held several centimeters away from the koi if it is in the water, and the transducer repositioned until the desired image is obtained. Motion imaging can be used for guided tissue biopsy collection, abdominocentesis (**Fig. 5**), or to insert needles for aspiration of the gas bladder.[7] Anesthesia may be needed for biopsy sample collection. Echocardiography is helpful in assessing heart

Fig. 4. Koi radiograph with intestinal barium (3 hours post administration). (*Top*) Dorsal-ventral view. (*Bottom*) Lateral view. (*From* Saint-Erne N. Clinical procedures. In: Advanced koi care. Glendale (AZ): Erne Enterprises; 2002. p. 48; with permission.)

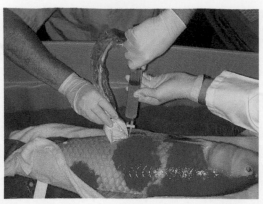

Fig. 5. Using ultrasonography to guide an abdominocentesis. (*Courtesy of* Gregory A. Lewbart, MS, VMD, Dipl ACZM, North Carolina State University College of Veterinary Medicine, Raleigh, NC, USA.)

rate during anesthesia.[16] The 2 chambers of a koi's gas bladder are highly visible using ultrasonography, as the contained air reflects back a white image. A deflated or fluid-filled chamber of the gas bladder can also be detected using ultrasonography. If the gas bladder contains water, it will transmit the sound waves and appear black.

Endoscopy can be used in tranquilized koi to examine the oral cavity, gill arches, and the pharynx. Flexible endoscopes can be passed through the esophagus into the intestines.[7] Koi have no stomach, but the proximal intestine is elastic and can distend to hold ingesta. The distal intestines are smaller in diameter. The koi's intestinal tract loops back and forth in the coelomic cavity, and is approximately 3 times the length of the body. Laparoscopy (coelioscopy) can be performed in year-old (~8 in [20 cm]) or larger koi to visualize internal organs or take biopsy samples. A small surgical incision can be made through an anesthetized koi's body wall to insert an endoscope. Coelomic cavity visualization is used to evaluate the liver (hepatopancreas), the gonads to determine gender or reproductive organ development,[20] the presence of adhesions or inflammation, the gas bladder position and status (inflamed, deflated, or fluid infused), or to conduct a tissue biopsy or collect an abdominal swab for bacterial culture. If the coelomic cavity has been insufflated with air during the procedure, the air must be removed to prevent buoyancy problems immediately after the procedure. The small incision can be closed with a simple interrupted absorbable suture, or sealed with methacrylate tissue adhesive.[21]

Surgery to expose the coelomic cavity in koi is performed through a ventral midline incision. The fish is positioned in dorsal recumbency on a foam block with a v-shaped notch, or on rolled wet towels.[21–23] Various surgical tables and platforms have been designed (**Fig. 6**) to aid in anesthetic administration during fish surgery.[22–27] Some surgeons remove scales in the operating area before cutting the skin; others cut through the scales (which can be more difficult in large koi) but then only remove the scales that are actually damaged during the surgery, reducing the number of scales that ultimately are removed. Scales will eventually regrow in most cases. Intracoelomic surgery is performed in the management of many disorders, including intestinal foreign body removal, tumor removal, elective gonadectomies, reproductive disorder treatments, gas bladder abnormalities and buoyancy problems, diagnostic exploration, and organ biopsy.[23] Gonadal neoplasms are encountered in mature koi, both male and female (**Fig. 7**). Such neoplasms can be surgically excised, with

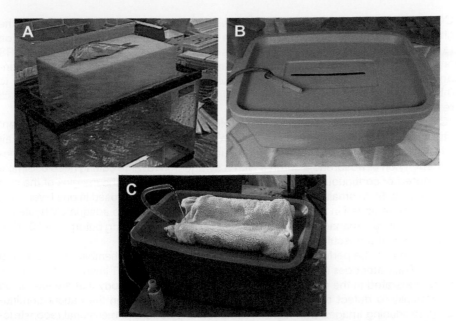

Fig. 6. (*A*) Anesthesia delivering surgical table for fish developed by Craig Harms and Greg Lewbart, North Carolina State University. (*B*) Portable surgical platform with anesthesia delivery. Water recirculates through slit in plastic lid down into container. Pump in container pushes water up through tube to koi. (*C*) Portable anesthesia delivering surgical platform showing water flowing from tube that can be inserted into the koi's mouth, and wet towels rolled to hold koi in position. (*From* Saint-Erne N. Clinical procedures. In: Advanced koi care. Glendale (AZ): Erne Enterprises; 2002. p. 51–2; with permission.)

great benefit if surgery is performed before significant damage has been done to the abdominal organs.[22,28]

Monitoring of the fish's condition while anesthetized during surgery can be accomplished by using electrocardiography (ECG). Hypodermic needles are inserted into the musculature of the koi at the base of the pectoral fins and near the anus (or vent) while the koi is out of the water in dorsal recumbency for surgery.[3,7] The metal clips of the

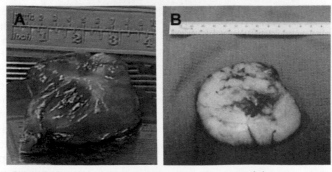

Fig. 7. (*A* and *B*) Surgically removed ovarian and testicular gonadal sarcomas. Note that tumor sizes range from 3 to 4 inches (7.5–10 cm) in diameter. (*From* Saint-Erne N. Neoplasia in koi. In: Advanced koi care. Glendale (AZ): Erne Enterprises; 2002. p. 136–7; with permission.)

ECG leads are attached to the metal needles (**Fig. 8**): the RA lead on the needle by the right pectoral fin, the LA lead on the needle by the left pectoral fin, and the LL lead on the needle by the vent. The P-QRS-T waves produced are of low amplitude (1 mV QRS complex), but similar to those of other animals. Heart rates are temperature dependant, as well as being affected by anesthesia. Normal heart rates for koi are 30 to 40 beats per minute (bpm), but can range from 15 to 100 bpm, and under anesthesia are 10 to 20 bpm.[7]

Closure of surgical incisions is accomplished by using absorbable monofilament suture material to close the muscle layer in a simple continuous pattern. Trapped air in the abdomen is removed by aspiration during closure. The skin is closed with monofilament nylon or absorbable sutures with a swaged-on reverse cutting needle. Simple interrupted or continuous suture patterns are used to oppose the margins of the skin incision (**Fig. 9**). In smaller fish, the muscles and skin may be closed in one layer. Skin sutures are removed in 2 to 3 weeks, or when the skin appears adequately healed.[22] Postsurgical pain management can be provided as needed using butorphanol 0.05 to 0.10 mg/kg intramuscularly.

CT scans can be performed on koi while they are in a small chamber of oxygenated water.[3] The water does not affect the image in a CT scan. The CT images are of narrow slices generated in the axial or transverse plane through the body that are examined sequentially to detect abnormalities. Helical CT methods scan the patient continuously, producing images with higher resolution and better 3-dimensional reconstruction (**Fig. 10**). Helical CT is also faster than standard CT scanning, so the koi is examined more quickly.[16]

MRI can produce very detailed images of the internal anatomy of koi.[3,16] Unfortunately, it is mostly available only at university and specialty veterinary hospitals; it is also still an expensive diagnostic technique. Because the patient must remain motionless during the imaging, anesthesia is necessary.

COMMON INTERNAL DISEASES AND THEIR TREATMENT

Abdominal (coelomic) enlargement in koi can result from bacterial infections producing ascites (dropsy), typically by bacteria in the genera *Aeromonas* or *Pseudomonas*. Granulomas of the liver or other organs can occur from bacterial infections caused by the zoonotic *Mycobacterium*. These infections require long-term injectable

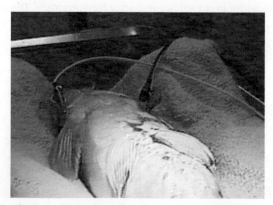

Fig. 8. Metal ECG leads clipped onto hypodermic needles inserted into pectoral musculature of a koi under anesthesia for surgery. (*From* Saint-Erne N. Clinical procedures. In: Advanced koi care. Glendale (AZ): Erne Enterprises; 2002. p. 55; with permission.)

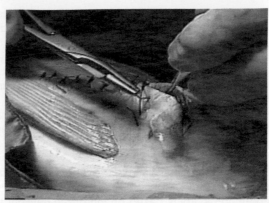

Fig. 9. Simple interrupted pattern of skin closure during surgery on a koi. (*From* Saint-Erne N. Clinical procedures. In: Advanced koi care. Glendale (AZ): Erne Enterprises; 2002. p. 56; with permission.)

and oral antibiotic administration. Percutaneous needle aspiration of ascitic fluid, especially guided by ultrasonography, and culture with sensitivity testing can help in determining appropriate antibiotic treatment. Noninfectious causes of coelomic enlargement include obesity, egg retention, neoplasia, gas bladder abnormalities, and intestinal obstructions, which can be differentiated using many of the diagnostic techniques described in the previous section.

Digestive system abnormalities can be caused by intestinal obstruction from an ingested foreign object such as a rock, plastic plant segment, coins, or debris in the water. Radiographs, especially with contrast media, help confirm the location of the obstruction. The obstruction sometimes can be retrieved orally using a flexible endoscope with biopsy forceps. Surgical removal via enterotomy can also be successful. One potential problem is that the condition may have been present for an extended time before the diagnosis is made, making prognosis less favorable.

Obesity is also not uncommon in well-cared for koi. The owners may have a tendency to overfeed the fish to get them to come up to the surface for viewing. Normal feed quantities should be 1% to 3% of the body weight daily, and a good rule of thumb is to feed only what the fish will consume in 3 to 5 minutes, once or twice

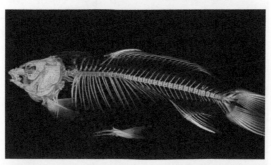

Fig. 10. CT image of a koi skeleton taken on a live koi. (*Courtesy of* Gregory A. Lewbart, MS, VMD, Dipl ACZM, North Carolina State University College of Veterinary Medicine, Raleigh, NC, USA.)

daily. Overfed koi may have a distended abdomen due to accumulated abdominal fat, and may have a hump at the nape of the neck where the skull ends and the scaled dorsum begins (**Fig. 11**). Hepatic lipidosis may accompany obesity from overfeeding and may occur due to feeding high-fat (>15%–18% fat) diets.[29] Fatty infiltration of the liver can also occur due to biotin or choline deficiency, or toxemias. Liver biopsies can be collected for histopathology examination through a small surgical incision or through endoscopic biopsy.[30] With hepatic lipidosis, the liver may appear yellowish and mottled, and be greasy when cut. Fatty infiltration results in intracellular oil droplets in the cytoplasm of the hepatocytes, not just fat between the liver cells. Treatment is to reduce feed quantity and fat content of the diet, and to feed a balanced, quality koi food.

Enlarged ovaries causing abdominal distension in female koi can be diagnosed with imaging techniques such as radiography, ultrasonography, or CT imaging (**Fig. 12**). Initiation of the reproduction in koi is based on increased daylight time in the spring and warming temperatures, which stimulate the release of gonadotropin hormones. When the water temperature reaches beyond 63° to 65°F (17.5°–18.5°C), the koi start to spawn. Koi that are kept indoors or in a heated pond during the winter that do not go through the normal cool to warm water cycle may not be stimulated to spawn. Over time, unspawned eggs are normally reabsorbed in a female as egg production is at the expense of stored mesenteric fat. But in an overfed female koi, this reabsorption of the eggs may not occur, resulting in a condition known as egg binding, or roe retention, whereby a large number of mature eggs are in the ovary and are unable to be released.[31] Eventually the distended ovaries can become necrotic, or impede normal hepatic or intestinal functions by causing a physical obstruction.

Egg binding tends to occur in overfed, fatty koi.[32] Reducing feeding after the normal spawning season so that females will reabsorb any remaining eggs may prevent egg binding. As a general guideline, reduce the feeding by half for a period of several weeks if the female koi still has abdominal enlargement after the spawning season in spring, depending on water temperature and body condition. See **Fig. 13** to determine normal body weight for koi length. Providing a cool-water period before spring can also help produce a normal spawning cycle in fish that are otherwise kept in a warm pond in the winter. Ovulation can also be induced by injections of carp pituitary extract (2–5 mg/kg intramuscularly, repeat in 9–12 hours), human chorionic gonadotropin (20–30 IU/kg intramuscularly, given twice, 6 hours apart), or Ovaprim (salmon

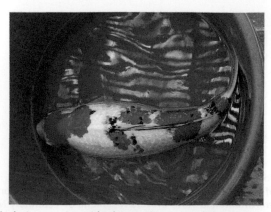

Fig. 11. Overweight koi; note the widening at the nape of the neck caudal to the skull.

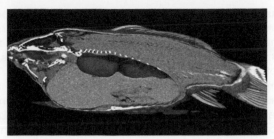

Fig. 12. CT image of a gravid female koi, sagittal section. The large egg mass (roe) is visible below the 2 chambers of the gas bladder. The white spots above the gas bladder are cross sections of the ribs. (*Courtesy of* Gregory A. Lewbart, MS, VMD, Dipl ACZM, North Carolina State University College of Veterinary Medicine, Raleigh, NC, USA.)

gonadotropin releasing hormone analog + domperidone). Ovaprim is dosed at 0.1–0.5 mL/kg of body weight, given intramuscularly or intracoelomically. Environment and temperature also play a significant role in the reproductive process, and may affect dose and timing. Ovaprim is effective in fish that are within or near their natural spawning season. Ovulation may occur in as little as 4 hours post treatment, so fish should be monitored accordingly.

Radiography, ultrasonography, CT imaging, and laparoscopy are useful in diagnosing abdominal (coelomic) neoplasia. These methods can also provide guidance

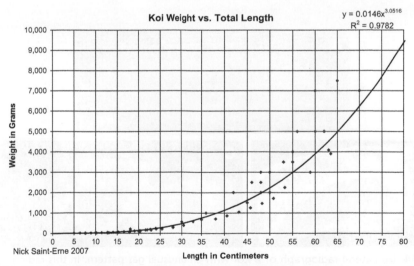

Fig. 13. Weight to length relationship in koi. This chart shows an approximation of the weight (in grams) to length (in centimeters) of koi fish. The black line is an extrapolated average value based on entered data points. Once koi begin to reach sexual maturity at 12 inches (30 cm), there begins to be a difference in weights between the sexes of the same length. Therefore, mature female koi will typically weigh more than the average depicted by the black line, and males will weigh less than the average value for each length. (*Modified from* data in Saint-Erne N. Advanced Koi Care. Glendale (AZ): Erne Enterprises; 2002. Used with permission.)

for excisional or aspiration biopsy. Excisional biopsy can be an important part of the treatment, as the neoplasm may be removed or debulked, which can provide a significant improvement in the quality of life for the fish.[33] Neoplasms in fish are generally less aggressive and more differentiated than neoplasia in mammals. In fish, a malignant neoplasm often results in local invasion, and metastasis is uncommon.[34] Neoplasms progress into space-occupying coelomic masses that can cause compression of the intestines, liver, or gas bladder and local tissue invasion. Necrosis will occur in the larger masses. Fish will survive for months with obvious abdominal distension. Surgical removal is often successful, but early intervention is important to prevent secondary complications (eg, tissue necrosis, intestinal compression, bacterial infection) that will lead to a poor prognosis. Internal neoplasia reported in koi include intestinal adenocarcinoma,[35] hepatoma,[36] and both male and female gonadal tumors.[22,37]

Gas (swim) bladder abnormalities occur in koi, which can make them negatively or positively buoyant, both of which require an increased expenditure of energy for the fish to move through the water. One or both of the koi's gas bladder chambers may become fluid filled (blood or water), overinflated with air, underinflated, ruptured, displaced by a coelomic mass, or have an abnormal structure (**Fig. 14**). Floating fish may become sunburned or have damage to the skin because of air exposure. Sinking koi may have a difficult time getting to the surface to eat, and may get abrasions on the ventral skin and pelvic fins from resting on the pond bottom (**Fig. 15**). Koi have physostomous gas bladders—a pneumatic duct connects the caudal chamber of the gas bladder to the pharyngeal esophagus. This location may be source of bacterial introduction into the gas bladder. Bacterial infections of the gas bladder result in

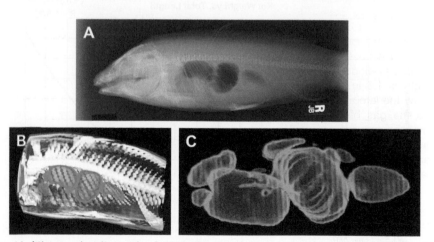

Fig. 14. (*A*) Lateral radiograph of a koi with an unusual gas pattern. In this radiographic image the cranial gas bladder appears shortened and the caudal gas bladder chamber appears rounded and displaced. There are several other abnormal gaseous objects that could be gas in loops of intestines. (*B*) CT image of mid body koi skeleton and gas bladder. Derived image, Technique 80 KVP, 100 mA, 2000 ms, slice thickness = 3.00 mm. (*C*) CT image of koi gas bladder; CT imaging on this same koi shows that the other abnormal gaseous images are superfluous extensions of the gas bladder. Derived image, Technique 80 KVP, 100 mA, 2000 ms, slice thickness = 3.00 mm. (*Courtesy of* Gregory A. Lewbart, MS, VMD, Dipl ACZM, North Carolina State University College of Veterinary Medicine, Raleigh, NC, USA.)

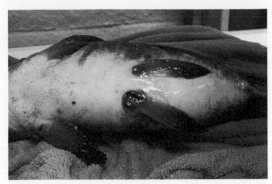

Fig. 15. Lesions on the ventral surface of a koi from scraping on the bottom of the pond due to a fluid filled gas bladder. (*From* Saint-Erne N. Infectious diseases. In: Advanced koi care. Glendale (AZ): Erne Enterprises; 2002. p. 68; with permission.)

granulomatous pneumocystitis with infiltration of macrophages, lymphocytes, and multinucleated giant cells.[38]

Radiographs are helpful in determining the size and position of gas bladders, and whether they are filled with air or fluid. When full of fluid the gas bladder has a homogeneous radiodensity with the viscera below it, and is difficult to delineate. Ultrasound is limited for detailed examination of the gas bladder due to echoes generated by the air in the gas bladder.[39] Ultrasonography can ascertain whether the gas bladder contains air or fluid. In some cases excess air causing positive buoyancy is not due to gas bladder disorder but to intestinal tympani (trapped gas in the intestines).

Pneumocystocentesis using a syringe and needle can be done to remove fluid from the gas bladder; some of the aspirated fluid should then be submitted for bacterial culture and sensitivity, and for cytology. To reach the caudal chamber of the gas bladder, use a syringe with a 22-gauge needle (for large koi a needle length of 1.5 in [3.8 cm] is necessary) and place it through the body wall slightly below the lateral line, angled cranially to obliquely pass through the body wall and into the gas bladder. Excess air can also be removed percutaneously through pneumocystocentesis, or the gas bladder can be surgically resected to drain the gas bladder and remove part of it to control overinflation.[40] Injections of antibiotics can be given directly into the gas bladder for treating internal infections of the gas bladder.

SUMMARY

Standard diagnostic techniques used in a small animal veterinary hospital can easily be applied for use with fish, especially koi. Koi owners are more than willing to have their pets treated by veterinarians interested in aquatic veterinary medicine. Although handling these wet pets takes a little getting used to compared with the other pets routinely seen in a veterinary practice, fish medicine can be very rewarding, challenging, and always interesting for a veterinarian willing to learn and wanting to try new things, especially since there is still much to be learned about the diagnosis and treatment of internal disorders of koi.

ACKNOWLEDGMENTS

The author would like to thank Joel Burkard of Pan Intercorp (www.Koi.com) and Dr Greg Lewbart (NCSU-CVM) for supplying some of the photographs and images for this article. All other photographs were taken by the author.

REFERENCES

1. American Veterinary Medical Association. U.S. pet ownership and demographics sourcebook. Schaumburg (IL): AVMA; 2007.
2. Stoskopf MK. Tropical fish medicine. Taking the history. Vet Clin North Am Small Anim Pract 1988;18(2):283–91.
3. Stoskopf MK. Clinical examination and procedures. In: Stoskopf MK, editor. Fish medicine. Philadelphia: WB Saunders; 1993. p. 62–78.
4. Noga EJ. Methods for diagnosing fish diseases. In: Fish disease diagnosis and treatment. St. Louis (MO): Mosby; 1996. p. 9–43.
5. Francis-Floyd R. Clinical examination of fish in private collections. Orcutt CJ, editor. Vet Clin North Am Exot Anim Pract 1999;2(2):247–64.
6. Smith SA. Nonlethal clinical techniques used in the diagnosis of diseases of fish. J Am Vet Med Assoc 2002;220(8):1203–6.
7. Saint-Erne N. Clinical procedures. In: Advanced koi care. Glendale (AZ): Erne Enterprises; 2002. p. 38–60.
8. Greenwell MG, Sherrill J, Clayton LA. Osmoregulation in fish: mechanisms and clinical implications. Hernandez-Divers SJ, Hernandez-Divers SM, editors. Vet Clin North Am Small Anim Pract 2003;6(1):177.
9. Saint-Erne N. Water quality in the koi pond. In: Advanced koi care. Glendale (AZ): Erne Enterprises; 2002. p. 94–109.
10. Brown LA. Tropical fish medicine. Anesthesia in fish. Stoskopf MK, editor. Vet Clin North Am Small Anim Pract 1988;18(2):317–30.
11. Brown LA. Anesthesia and restraint. In: Stoskopf MK, editor. Fish medicine. Philadelphia: WB Saunders; 1993. p. 79–90.
12. Roberts HE. Anesthesia, analgesia and euthanasia. In: Roberts HE, editor. Fundamentals of ornamental fish health. Ames (IA): Wiley-Blackwell; 2010. p. 166–71.
13. Love NE, Lewbart GA. Pet fish radiology: technique and case history reports. Vet Radiol Ultrasound 1990;38:24–9.
14. Lammens M. Radiography. In: The koi doctor. Belgium: A-Publishing; 2004. p. 57–9.
15. Saint-Erne N. Radiographic anatomy. In: Advanced koi care. Glendale (AZ): Erne Enterprises; 2002. p. 35–6.
16. Roberts HE, Weber ES, Smith SA. Imaging techniques. In: Roberts HE, editor. Fundamentals of ornamental fish health. Ames (IA): Wiley-Blackwell; 2010. p. 179–82.
17. Martin RW, Myers J, Sower SA, et al. Ultrasonic imaging, a potential tool for sex determination of live fish. N Am J Fish Manag 1983;3:258–64.
18. Bonar SA, Thomas GL, Pauley GB, et al. Use of ultrasonic imaging for rapid nonlethal determination of sex and maturity of Pacific herring. N Am J Fish Manag 1989;9:364–6.
19. Colombo RE, Wills PS, Garvey JE. Use of ultrasound imaging to determine sex of shovelnose sturgeon. N Am J Fish Manag 2004;24:322–6.

20. Swenson EA, Rosenberger AE, Howell PJ. Validation of endoscopy for determination of maturity in small salmonids and sex of mature individuals. Trans Am Fish Soc 2007;136:994–8.
21. Stoskopf MK. Surgery. In: Stoskopf MK, editor. Fish medicine. Philadelphia: WB Saunders; 1993. p. 91–7.
22. Saint-Erne N. Surgery. In: Advanced koi care. Glendale (AZ): Erne Enterprises; 2002. p. 52–6.
23. Roberts HE. Surgery and wound management in fish. In: Roberts HE, editor. Fundamentals of ornamental fish health. Ames (IA): Wiley-Blackwell; 2010. p. 185–95.
24. Reinecker RH, Ruddell MO. An easily fabricated operating table for fish surgery. Prog Fish Culturist 1974;36(2):111–2.
25. Courtois LA. Lightweight, adjustable and portable surgical table for fisheries work in the field. Prog Fish Culturist 1981;43(1):55–6.
26. Lewbart GA, Harms C. Building a fish anesthesia delivery system. Exotic DVM 1999;1(2):25–8.
27. LaVigne HR. An improved portable surgical table for the field and laboratory. N Am J Fish Manag 2002;22:571–2.
28. Lewbart GA, Spodnick G, Barlow N, et al. Surgical removal of an undifferentiated abdominal sarcoma from a koi carp (*Cyprinus carpio*). Vet Rec 1998;143:556–8.
29. Post GW. Nutrition and nutritional diseases of salmonids. In: Stoskopf MK, editor. Fish medicine. Philadelphia: WB Saunders; 1993. p. 354.
30. Boone SS, Hernandez-Divers SJ, Radlinsky MG, et al. Comparison between coelioscopy and coeliotomy for liver biopsy in channel catfish. J Am Vet Med Assoc 2008;233(6):960–7.
31. Wildgoose WH. Internal disorders. In: Wildgoose WH, editor. BSAVA manual of ornamental fish. 2nd edition. Gloucester (UK): BSVA; 2001. p. 132.
32. Strange R. Fish nutrition—egg binding. In: Roberts HE, editor. Fundamentals of ornamental fish health. Ames (IA): Wiley-Blackwell; 2010. p. 98.
33. Reavill D. Neoplasia in fish. In: Roberts HE, editor. Fundamentals of ornamental fish health. Ames (IA): Wiley-Blackwell; 2010. p. 204–12.
34. Groff JM. Neoplasia in fishes. Graham JE, editor. Vet Clin North Am Exot Anim Pract 2004;7(3):705–42.
35. Lewbart GA. Self-assessment color review of ornamental fish. Ames (IA): ISU Press; 1998. p. 111–2.
36. Garland MR, Lawler LP, Whitaker BR, et al. Modern CT applications in veterinary medicine. Radiographics 2002;22(1):55–62.
37. Ishikawa T, Takayama S. Ovarian neoplasia in ornamental hybrid carp (Nishikigoi) in Japan. Ann NY Acad Sci 1977;298:330–41.
38. Hobbie KR, Lewbart GA, Mohammadian LA, et al. Clinical and pathological investigation of "submarine syndrome" in a group of Japanese koi (*Cyprinus carpio*). In: Gulland FMD, editor. IAAAM Conference Proceedings. Algarve (Portugal), 2002. p. 31–2.
39. Wildgoose WH, Palmeiro B. Specific syndromes and diseases. In: Roberts HE, editor. Fundamentals of ornamental fish health. Ames (IA): Wiley-Blackwell; 2010. p. 214–22.
40. Britt T, Weisse C, Weber ES, et al. Use of pneumocystoplasty for over inflation of the swim bladder in a goldfish. J Am Vet Med Assoc 2002;221(5):690–2.

Updates and Practical Approaches to Reproductive Disorders in Reptiles

John M. Sykes IV, DVM, DACZM

KEYWORDS

- Reptile • Reproduction • Dystocia • Chelonian
- Lizard • Snake • Infertility

Reproductive biology and disorders are important facets of captive reptile management. When presented with any type of reptile patient, the clinician should investigate the specific biology of that species to help identify the potential environmental or husbandry-related causes of reproductive disorders. Although factors and conditions for normal reproduction differ between species depending on their natural histories, the general principles and commonalities are discussed in the following sections. Reproductive disorders are relatively common in captive reptiles.[1,2] Disorders addressed in this review include infertility or lack of conception, follicular stasis, dystocia, and reproductive organ prolapse. This article is divided into sections based on the taxonomic group, although many of the predisposing factors for and the approaches to these conditions are similar for all groups.

CHELONIANS
Normal Reproduction

In males, sperm is produced seasonally, depending on the natural history of the species. During breeding season, the testicles enlarge. The relaxed phallus is located within a groove in the ventral portion of the cloaca. Neither is the cloaca connected to the urinary system nor is it involved in excretion. During erection, the phallus becomes engorged and extends ventrally and cranially; it does not evaginate like the hemipenes of lizards and snakes (see discussion in the sections on lizards and snakes). The male mounts the female from behind. Sperm is delivered to the male's cloaca via the vas deferens and is then carried along the outer groove of the erect phallus to the female's cloaca. The phallus is then retracted but does not invaginate.[3–5]

Global Health Program, Wildlife Conservation Society, 2300 Southern Boulevard, Bronx, NY 10460, USA
E-mail address: jsykes@wcs.org

Vet Clin Exot Anim 13 (2010) 349–373
doi:10.1016/j.cvex.2010.05.013
1094-9194/10/$ – see front matter © 2010 Elsevier Inc. All rights reserved.

vetexotic.theclinics.com

Normal reproductive cycles and biology of female chelonians have been extensively reviewed elsewhere.[4,5] In brief, folliculogenesis generally begins with increased estrogen production, which stimulates the production of vitellogenin by the liver. Yolk is produced in the liver, transported by the blood, and deposited in the oocytes. Increased levels of testosterone, triglycerides, cholesterol, and calcium may be noted during this phase. The trigger for ovulation is poorly understood, and ovulation does not seem to require copulation in most species, even though the presence of a male may be required in some species (eg, loggerhead sea turtles [*Caretta caretta*][6] and some *Testudo* spp[4]). Ova then enter either oviduct and become fertilized. It is is to be noted that females may store sperm for an extended period and produce fertile eggs long after being separated from males. Albumen and shell are then added. The time for which eggs are retained in the oviduct ranges from 9 days to 6 months, although most species retain eggs for 1 to 2 months.[3] Females typically excavate a nest, deposit and cover the eggs, and then leave.[5] All chelonians are oviparous.[4]

Reproductive Disorders

Infertility

Individuals may exhibit a lack of desire or apparent inability to mate for many reasons. Medical causes may include reproductive pathology such as phallic infection or trauma. Underlying nonreproductive pathologic conditions may also result in lack of mating, so an evaluation of the entire animal is warranted. Husbandry-related causes can include lack of appropriate environmental conditions such as hibernation or rainy periods, incompatible size difference between male and female, or dominance by other individuals in the enclosure.[3] Long-term cohabitation may also suppress mating behavior; however, mating may occur if a pair is separated and then reunited. One should ensure that the individuals are of the same species and that the gender has been correctly determined.

Mature chelonians are often sexually dimorphic. Males typically have a longer tail with a more distal cloacal opening (**Fig. 1**) and a concave plastron (**Fig. 2**).[3-5] Freshwater (emydid) male turtles often have long nails on the front feet.[4,5] Some individual species have gender-specific traits such as red irises of male eastern box turtles (*Terrapene carolina carolina*) (**Fig. 3**) or long nails on the hindlimbs of female leopard tortoises (*Geochelone pardalis*). For species that have little dimorphism or for immature animals, other techniques are required to identify the gender. Males may be identified by elevated levels of plasma testosterone,[7,8] although females may have elevated testosterone levels during some stages of the reproductive cycle.[5] Karyotyping or genetic blood sexing of juveniles, as performed in many species of birds, is often not possible in chelonians because many species have temperature-dependent sex determination,[9] although some temperature-dependent species do have genetic differences between the sexes.[10] Ultrasonography may be used to identify gonads,[4,11] although this technique may be impractical with small individuals, and differentiation between quiescent ovaries and testicles may be challenging. Scanning with the animal immersed in a water bath can improve image quality, particularly in smaller individuals.[5] Laparoscopy has been used to reliably sex juvenile or hatchling turtles[7,12-14] and may become the preferred technique because it provides immediate results, can be performed quickly in small individuals without the need of a laboratory or blood collection, and offers the opportunity for biopsy in inconclusive cases. Techniques without the use of insufflation have been described,[7,15] although the use of lactated Ringer's solution for insufflation may provide better visualization and does not inhibit buoyancy in aquatic animals after the procedure.[14] Juvenile ovaries are located in the caudal coelom just cranial to the kidneys. They are thin and elongate, and the follicles

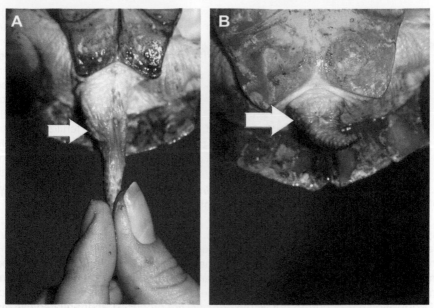

Fig. 1. Ventral views of the cloaca and tail of a male (*A*) and female (*B*) red short-neck turtle (*Emydura subglobosa*). Note the longer tail and more distal cloacal opening (*arrows*) of the male compared with the female.

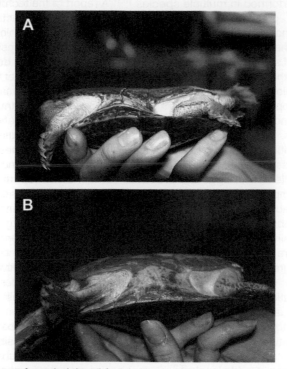

Fig. 2. Lateral views of a male (*A*) and female (*B*) red short-necked turtle (*E subglobosa*) held in dorsal recumbency. Note the concave plastron of the male and the convex plastron of the female.

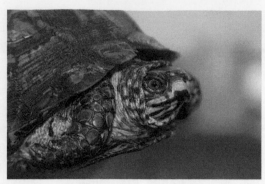

Fig. 3. Iris of a male eastern box turtle (*T carolina* subsp *carolina*). Males have red or bright orange iris, whereas females have brown or light-colored iris.

may be seen even in very young individuals.[14] Testicles are pink or yellow, oval, and located cranial to and extend ventral to the kidneys.[3] A study of endoscopic examinations found pain scores to be higher in animals receiving only local anesthetics when compared with those receiving general anesthesia; therefore, these procedures should be performed only under general anesthesia.[14]

If copulation has occurred but viable eggs are not produced, spermatogenesis may be investigated. Sperm may be collected by swabbing the cloaca of the male or female after copulation or found in reproductively active males' urine.[3] Electroejaculation has been performed in multiple species.[16,17] A report of the technique described anesthesia with propofol followed by successful semen collection in leopard tortoises.[18] Alternatively, specimens may be collected for testicular biopsy using laparoscopy. Males may produce sperm only seasonally, so multiple biopsies are required to confirm lack of spermatogenesis.[3] Although some work has been done,[13,17] semen characteristics other than the presence or absence of sperm have yet to be fully characterized in chelonians. As mentioned earlier, causes for aspermatogenesis may include lack of appropriate environment or underlying medical or nutritional disorders.

Females may not produce eggs after an apparent normal copulation with sperm-producing males. Lack of environmental triggers may be the cause. Alternatively, poor body condition or nutritional disease may inhibit folliculogenesis. Ultrasonography may be used to determine if folliculogenesis is occurring and to monitor the reproductive cycle.[3,6,19] If eggs are produced but fail to develop, uterine pathology is possible, but improper incubation parameters are more likely. It has been proposed that repeated radiography of free-ranging chelonians during sensitive stages of gamete and embryo development may cause damage to the germlines and/or embryos, increasing the risk of decreased fecundity or long-term genetic problems.[20] Although there are little data evaluating this risk, whenever possible it may be prudent to use ultrasonography rather than radiography for routine reproductive assessments. However, when evaluating individuals for reproductive disorders, radiography provides information critical to decision making (see later sections) and should be used in those situations.

Eggs that fail to develop may be fertile with inappropriate incubation or infertile. Differentiating between the 2 diagnoses can be difficult or impossible. Parameters that may influence incubation include temperature, humidity, substrate, ambient oxygen, and carbon dioxide levels.[3,21] Some species may require changes in incubation temperatures, such as a cooling period, before embryonic development.[22] Eggs that do not develop should receive a necropsy, including cultures.

Follicular stasis

Follicular stasis (also called preovulatory egg-binding or retained follicles) is commonly reported in lizards but can also occur in chelonians.[3,23] Possible causes include inappropriate nutrition or environmental conditions. Recent exposure to a male after prior isolation may lead to stasis.[24] Follicles that neither ovulate nor regress can become inspissated or necrotic and may progress to yolk coelomitis (**Fig. 4**). Clinical signs can include anorexia or lethargy,[24] and clinical pathologic findings may include elevated levels of calcium, albumin, total protein, and alkaline phosphatase, with anemia, leukopenia, and heteropenia.[23] Diagnosis can be made using ultrasonography to demonstrate the persistent presence of nonovulated follicles retained in the ovary. The recommended treatment at present is ovariectomy.[3] Recovery after ovariectomy in chelonians may be prolonged when compared with an iguana with the same condition.[24] A recent technique for celioscopy-assisted ovariectomy has been described.[25] Using this method, an endoscope is placed into the coelomic cavity of the anesthetized animal through an incision in the prefemoral fossa. The ovary is grasped and gently pulled out of the prefemoral incision; oocentesis or enlarging the prefemoral incision may need to be performed to exteriorize larger follicles. The ovarian vessels are then ligated, and the ovary is removed. Ovaries of immature animals may be too tightly attached to allow for exteriorization and would require intracorporeal surgery to remove, if a prophylactic ovariectomy was desired in a young animal.[25]

Dystocia

Dystocia has been defined as a failure to lay eggs within the period that is normal for a particular species and is often referred to as egg retention.[3,26] Because a normal

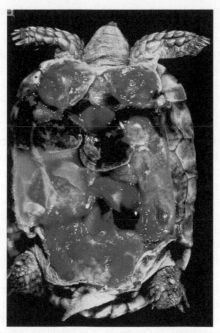

Fig. 4. Gross necropsy of a cape tortoise (*Homopus* sp) that died of yolk coelmoitis. Note the free yolk in the coelomic cavity and the associated adhesions. (*Courtesy of* Dr Ed Ramsay, DVM, Knoxville, TN, USA.)

gravid female can retain eggs in the uterus for an extended period, distinguishing between normally and pathologically retained eggs can be difficult.[26] Eggs may remain within the uterus well beyond the time they should normally be deposited, and cause no overt pathologic conditions. However, sequelae of chronically retained eggs can include debilitation, infectious salpingitis, rupture of the oviduct with resulting coelomitis (see **Fig. 4**), or urinary or colonic obstruction because of oversized eggs.

Husbandry parameters (such as failure to provide an appropriate nesting site, substrate, temperature, and humidity), in addition to social factors (such as competition for nest sites or interindividual aggression), may lead to egg retention.[27] Recommendations for the appropriate depth of substrate for nesting sites vary, but depths of at least 1 to 2 times the length of the carapace have been recommended.[3] Loosening the soil or the substrate may help the animal in digging the nest.[3] Medical causes for dystocia include mechanical obstruction, reproductive tract infections, nutritional deficiencies, or an underlying systemic illness.[3,27]

In the early stages of egg retention, often, no clinical signs other than being past the due date are noted. Some individuals may pass 1 or 2 eggs but not an entire clutch.[3] These cases can be treated conservatively or may not require treatment at all. As the eggs are retained for longer periods, other signs may develop either due to the retention of the eggs or due to a predisposing condition, including anorexia, lethargy, straining, cloacal discharge, constipation, urinary obstruction, cloacal prolapse, or hind-end paresis.[3,26]

Diagnosis of dystocia can be made based on the knowledge of a particular species' normal egg-retention time or an owner's previous experiences with a particular species. Eggs may be palpated in the inguinal area but should be distinguished from cystic calculi. Radiography is useful to identify the number, position, and apparent shell quality of eggs,[3] in addition to identifying possible predisposing factors such as metabolic bone disease or pelvic fractures/stenosis. Overly large or misshapen eggs may not be laid (**Fig. 5**), and very thick shells may indicate prolonged retention.[3] Ectopic eggs located in the coelom or bladder may be identified via radiography or ultrasonography,[28] although this may be a difficult distinction to make before surgery. Evaluation of underlying conditions should be conducted via routine blood evaluation. Hypocalcemia (ionized calcium <1 mmol/L) is often present and may be an indication of preexisting nutritional deficiencies or due to chronic calcium sequestration in the eggs. Aspiration of any coelomic effusion may be supportive of yolk coelomitis.

Chelonian dystocia is rarely an emergency and can often be resolved with husbandry changes or medical therapies. In apparently otherwise healthy individuals with a normal radiographic appearance of eggs, provision of an appropriate nest site and removal of social stressors can result in laying (oviposition). Oviposition can be medically induced using oxytocin, β-blockers, fluid therapy, and calcium supplementation. Any patient with dehydration or electrolyte imbalance should first be rehydrated and stabilized. Soaking may cure mild dehydration. For more severe dehydration, intracoelomic, intraosseous, or intravenous administration of fluids should be done before additional therapies. Medical induction of oviposition in a dehydrated or unstable animal is unlikely to be successful and may increase the risk of worsening the underlying metabolic disorders or rupturing a dehydrated friable oviduct. If the animal is hypocalcemic, parenteral calcium supplementation (intracoelomic, intramuscular, or subcutaneous administration of calcium gluconate, 50–100 mg/kg)[3,26] can aid in oviductal contractions.[26] Oxytocin, 1 to 20 IU/kg, can be administered intramuscularly[3,29–31] or, continuously, via an intraosseous catheter; the lower end of the dose range is often effective in chelonians. Oxytocin can be readministered if

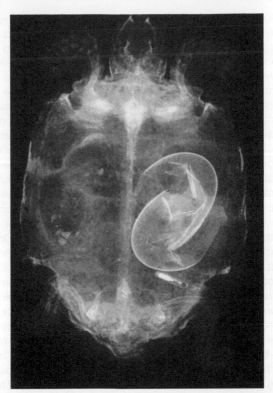

Fig. 5. Radiograph of a cape tortoise (*Homopus* sp) with a misshapen, collapsed egg within the oviduct. Eggs of this appearance should be surgically removed by either a prefemoral or a plastronotomy approach. (*Courtesy of* Dr Ed Ramsay, DVM, Knoxville, TN, USA.)

oviposition does not occur; various recommendations include administering thrice with an interval of 90 minutes with increasing doses[3] or 50% to 100% of the original dose 1 to 12 hours later.[26,32] McArthur[4] suggests the following protocol: rehydrate the patient; lubricate the cloaca; provide suitable nesting area, heat, and humidity; administer calcium, if needed, in the evening followed by atenolol (7 mg/kg by mouth) and oxytocin (1–3 IU/kg intramuscularly) the following morning; continue this protocol if eggs are being produced daily; and discontinue when oviposition stops. Arginine vasotocin is reported to be more effective in reptiles than oxytocin.[32] However, oxytocin works reasonably well in chelonians when compared with other groups of reptiles,[31] and arginine vasotocin is at present available only as a research drug.

Other adjunct medications may be beneficial, but their use has been studied little in chelonia. Prostaglandins may aid in oviposition and have been used in other reptiles.[33] A combination of oxytocin, 7.5 U/kg, and prostaglandin $F_{2\alpha}$, 1.5 mg/kg, given subcutaneously has been effective in inducing oviposition in red-eared sliders (*Trachemys scripta elegans*) (Mark Feldman, MD, personal communication, 2009), although it may be less effective in turtles that weigh more than 5 kg. Application of prostaglandin E gel on the cloaca has been recommended by Innis,[34] with no adverse or beneficial effects being noted. β-Blockers, such as atenolol (7 mg/kg) administered orally,[26] have been reported to potentiate the effects of oxytocin in chelonia. Propranolol, 1 mg/kg, intracoelomically has been used in lizards and may also be beneficial in chelonians.[33] Partial oviposition in 2 snapping turtles (*Chelydra serpentina*) sedated with medetomidine, 150 µg/kg, for repair of traumatic injuries has been reported.[34] Use of medetomidine may aid in relaxation of sympathetic tone in stressed individuals. Eggs that have progressed to the pelvic canal but have not been deposited may be expulsed via digital palpation of the patient within the prefemoral fossa under sedation.

More aggressive therapies are warranted, when conservative management is unsuccessful, abnormally shaped or sized eggs are present (see **Fig. 5**), and the animal shows signs of debilitation or is straining. Salpingotomy may be performed via a plastronotomy or a prefemoral approach. A plastronotomy is required if a large field of vision is required (eg, if yolk coelomitis is present), but the prefemoral approach is less invasive. Details of plastronotomy have been reported elsewhere.[35,36] A prefemoral celiotomy for ovariectomy or salpingotomy may be performed in species with a large prefemoral area and small plastron, such as sea turtles.[37] A celioscopy-assisted prefemoral approach for ovariectomy has been described for species with smaller prefemoral openings (see earlier discussion).[25] This technique may also provide adequate access for salpingotomy or salpingectomy. For eggs retained in the urinary bladder, a prefemoral celiotomy for cystotomy may be successful.[28]

Alternatively, ovocentesis may be performed via the cloaca.[3,26] A speculum (laryngoscope or rodent oral speculum) is helpful to visualize the egg, and a large-gauge needle is used to puncture the egg and aspirate its contents.[3,26] The egg usually fractures after aspiration, and the egg fragments may pass on their own or can be removed using forceps. For punctured eggs that do not pass, a novel technique has been described. The tip of a Foley catheter is cut such that the balloon is at the end of the catheter, the amount of air needed to inflate the balloon to the appropriate size for the egg to be removed is determined, and the infusion port is filled with water and placed in the freezer to improve the rigidity of the catheter. The catheter is then placed into the egg via the centesis hole, the balloon is inflated, and traction is applied to remove the egg. Care must be taken not to overinflate the balloon or tear the oviduct during this process.[34] McArthur[26] recommends irrigating the cloaca and oviduct after this procedure and continuing oxytocin and β-blocker administration. If the egg is adhered to the uterus, salpingotomy may be required. A similar technique of cystoscopy performed via the cloaca followed by implosion of the egg and removal of the fragments has been described to remove retained eggs within the bladder.[38]

Yolk coelomitis

Yolk coelomitis can be secondary to retained follicles, oophoritis, salpingitis, or dystocia. Clinical signs are often nonspecific and include anorexia, lethargy, diarrhea, or lack of fecal/urine production. Clinical pathologic changes may include hypercalcemia, hyperproteinemia, anemia, and/or azotemia. Ultrasonography and radiography may aid in identifying predisposing factors such as follicular stasis or dystocia (**Fig. 6**). In addition, ultrasonography may aid in guiding a needle for coelomic centesis. Laparoscopy can differentiate normal smooth, uniform, spherical follicles from degenerating hyperemic, brown or purple follicles and may help visualize free fluid or adhesions. In contrast to a chelonian with retained eggs in the oviduct, diagnosis needs to be made rapidly because these patients may decline very quickly once coelomitis has begun. Treatment consists of stabilizing the patient and then performing exploratory celiotomy (**Fig. 7**). The source of the egg material needs to be removed, so an ovariectomy, salpingotomy, and/or salpingectomy may need to be performed. Histopathologic and microbiologic examinations may help elucidate a cause for the condition. The coelom should then be thoroughly flushed to remove any remaining yolk material. Supportive care and appropriate analgesic and antimicrobial therapy should be continued postoperatively.

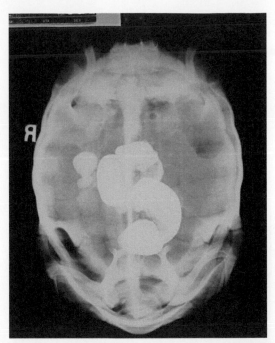

Fig. 6. Radiograph of a Burmese star tortoise (*Geochelone platynota*) with egg yolk coelomitis. The retained eggs were present unchanged within the uterus for 6 months before the sudden onset of profound lethargy and elevated uric acid level (170 mg/dL).

Phallus prolapse

Phallus prolapse may occur due to a variety of causes in chelonians (**Fig. 8**). General debilitation, neurologic dysfunction, excessive libido, trauma, lower urogenital or gastrointestinal tract infections, or causes of straining, such as constipation, parasites, gastrointestinal foreign bodies, or cystic calculi, may all predispose an animal to prolapse.[27] Nutritional metabolic bone disease may also lead to prolapse as the animal's soft tissue outgrows the shell and pushes the cloaca and phallus out.[3] A normal chelonian may erect the phallus during manipulation of the cloaca or handling of the caudal shell, but the penis should be retracted within a few hours.[3]

The prolapsed phallus should be cleaned and returned to the cloaca, if viable. Use of hypertonic solutions or cold compresses may aid in reducing swelling, and may require sedation or anesthesia. Trauma to the phallus from cagemates is common and may need to be treated before replacement of the phallus in the cloaca. Once replaced, a purse-string suture around the cloaca should be placed for 2 to 3 weeks, loose enough so that the animal can defecate but not reprolapse. If the tissue is nonviable or unable to be reduced, it may be amputated. Because the urinary system is separate from the phallus, amputation affects only the breeding potential. In small individuals, the base of the phallus can be ligated with encircling sutures or vertical mattress absorbable sutures, and the phallus is transected and removed. For larger individuals, the lateral vessels should be individually ligated and each corpus cavernosum should be separately ligated. The phallus can then be dissected free of the cloaca and transected. The cloacal tissue remaining after dissection can then be closed over the stump of the phallus in a simple continuous pattern.[3] Appropriate antibiotic and analgesic medications should be administered, and treatment of any underlying cause should be initiated.[39]

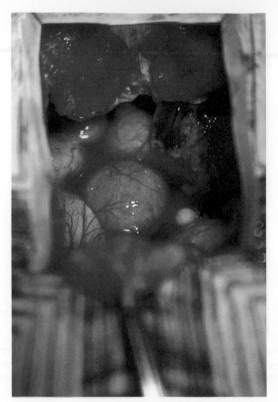

Fig. 7. Plastronotomy for egg removal, ovariosalpingectomy, and coelomic lavage for a Burmese star tortoise (*G platynota*) that was shown in **Fig. 6**. The animal made a complete recovery.

LIZARDS
Normal Reproduction in Lizards

Male lizards have paired hemipenes invaginated within the base of the tail. During copulation, only 1 of the 2 hemipenes is everted into the female's cloaca. Sperm is delivered to the male's cloaca via vas deferens and travels along a groove on the outside of the everted hemipenis to the female's cloaca. Similar to chelonians and snakes, the copulatory organ in lizards is not involved in excretion. Sperms within the female's reproductive tract may then fertilize ova or, in some species, may be stored for future use. Most male lizards have seasonal testicular enlargement and breeding behaviors.[40]

Female lizards can be oviparous (eg, monitors, most iguanids) or viviparous (eg, many skinks and chameleons).[40,41] The viviparous species provide varying degrees of nutrients to the developing embryo, directly via the placenta or indirectly via the preovulatory yolk.[41] Some species can be parthenogenic.[40]

Reproductive Disorders

Infertility
Causes of infertility may be similar to those for chelonians, although there is little published material addressing this concern in lizards. Correct identification of gender is important. Some species are dimorphic and gender can be readily identified but

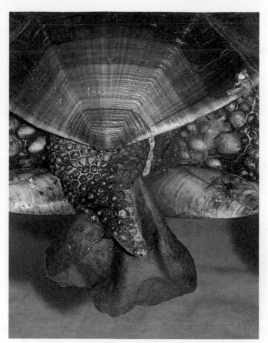

Fig. 8. Prolapsed phallus of an unknown species of tortoise. If unable to replace, the chelonian phallus can be surgically removed from its base without affecting urination. (*Courtesy of* Dr Jean Paré, DMV, DVSc, New York, NY, USA).

many are not. Some males can be identified by a hemipenal bulge at the base of the tail.[40,41] The vent can be probed in a similar manner as described in snakes in the following sections.[40] Femoral pores of male iguanids are generally larger than those of the females (**Fig. 9**).[41] Many species of monitor lizards (*Varanus* spp) have mineralization of the hemipenes, sometimes with an internal skeleton called hemibaculum, which can be identified radiographically (**Figs. 10 and 11**).[40,41] Follicles and possibly hemipenes may be identified using ultrasonography, and celioscopy can be used to confirm the gender.[15,42]

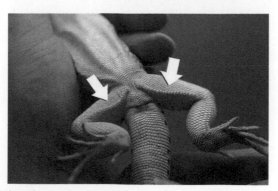

Fig. 9. Ventral thighs of a male desert iguana (*Dipsosaurus dorsalis*). Note the line of enlarged femoral pores that identify this individual as a male (*arrows*).

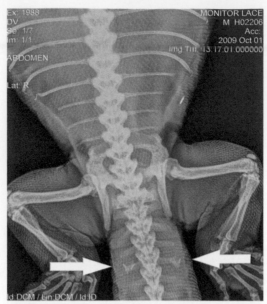

Fig. 10. Ventrodorsal radiograph of the tail and pelvic region of a quince monitor lizard (*Varanus melinus*). The mineralized hemibaccula in this individual (*arrows*) identifies it as a male.

Sperm evaluation and assisted reproductive techniques have not been extensively studied in lizards, although some work describing electroejaculation has been performed.[43] Hemipenal casts or plugs may interfere with normal copulation. These casts are formed from shed skin, sperm, and exudates (**Fig. 12**),[44] and can be gently removed before the onset of breeding season.

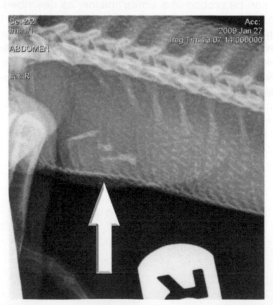

Fig. 11. Lateral radiograph of the tail and pelvic region of a quince monitor lizard (*V melinus*). The mineralized hemibaccula in this individual (*arrow*) identifies it as a male.

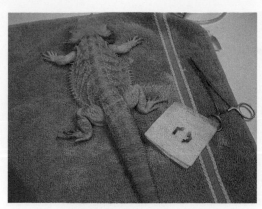

Fig. 12. Hemipenal casts of a bearded dragon (*Pogona vitticeps*). These casts are formed from glandular secretions and shed skin, and occur in lizards and snakes. The casts should be removed at the start of the breeding season to aid in successful copulation. (*Courtesy of* Dr Jean Paré, DMV, DVSc, New York, NY, USA.)

Follicular stasis (preovulatory egg binding)

Similar to chelonians, inappropriate husbandry conditions, including lack of appropriate environmental cues, lack of nesting substrate, and poor nutrition, can lead to follicular stasis or dystocia (postovulatory egg binding). In follicular stasis, follicles are produced by the ovary but fail to ovulate. Lack of an adequate nesting site seems to be a common cause of egg retention in iguanas (*Iguana iguana*),[32] in which this condition is particularly common.[1,45] Some lizards may normally have a long preovulatory follicular development,[46] which needs to be distinguished from stasis. Clinical signs of stasis include anorexia and lethargy; abdominal distention may also be observed.[32] Normal gravid iguanas may have decreased food consumption, particularly while nearing ovulation, and may lose some body condition during this period,[46] but persistently anorexic or emaciated animals are likely to be in stasis. Although follicles may be resorbed in some individuals, if left untreated, retained follicles may rupture, leading to yolk coelomitis, profound debilitation, and death. Gravid lizards that are depressed or unresponsive are likely to be in stasis or in dystocia, and should be rapidly evaluated and supported. In a captive collection of Fiji Island banded iguanas (*Brachylophus fasciatus*), coelomitis caused by yolk that leaked from preovulatory follicles undergoing atresia was a leading cause of death in sexually mature females.[47] In that collection, clinical signs ranged from none to skin discoloration and coelomic distention, although several animals had had previous reproductive disorders (eg, dystocia, lethargy associated with reproductive activity, and small or no clutches in the previous years).[47] Yolk coelomitis has also been identified as a major cause of death in captive Komodo dragons (*Varanus komodoensis*).[48] Specific causes for lack of ovulation or normal atresia without resulting in coelomitis have yet to be determined, but some type of behavioral or environmental cue is thought to be involved.

Diagnosis may be made using radiography or ultrasonography to confirm the presence of follicles. A space-occupying mass may be seen with radiographs in the mid-coelom to caudal coelom. A pneumocoelogram (created by injection of air into the coelom) may be used if follicles cannot be visualized on a plain radiograph,[40] although ultrasonography may be a faster and less-invasive methodology. Blood should be drawn to assess for underlying or concurrent conditions. Clinical pathologic

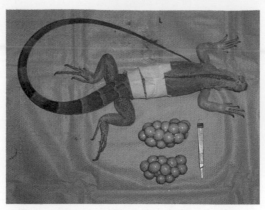

Fig. 13. Green iguana (*I iguana*) after ovariectomy for follicular stasis. Note that these retained follicles can occupy much of the available coelomic space. (*Courtesy of* Dr Ed Ramsay, DVM, Knoxville, TN, USA.)

abnormalities may include elevated levels of serum calcium and phosphorus[49] or indications of dehydration (hemoconcentration), although lizards with normal vitellogenesis may also have elevated levels of blood calcium and/or phosphorus[1] and some affected animals have normal clinical pathologic findings.[50] Heterophilia, particularly if there are toxic changes, may indicate marked inflammation and/or an infectious component.[1]

The treatment for follicular stasis is ovariectomy (**Fig. 13**). Induction of ovulation in a lizard (*Anolis carolinensis*) in a laboratory setting using follicle-stimulating hormone has been reported,[51] but to the author's knowledge, medical induction of ovulation in sick lizards with follicular stasis has not been described. The patient should be stabilized, which may require intravenous or intraosseous fluid administration. A ventral midline incision for celiotomy can be made, even though some investigators prefer a paramedian incision to avoid the ventral vein, which is suspended cranially just deep to the skin along the midline from the umbilicus (**Fig. 14**).[40,52] The ovary can

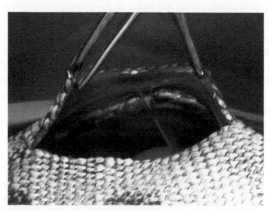

Fig. 14. Ventral abdominal vein of an unknown species of lizard. Note the close apposition of this vein with the ventral midline of the lizard. Many surgeons prefer to make a paramedian incision for celiotomies in lizards to avoid traumatizing this vein. (*Courtesy of* Dr Jean Paré, DMV, DVSc, New York, NY, USA.)

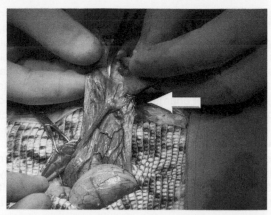

Fig. 15. Ovariectomy in a white-throated monitor lizard (*Varanus albigularis*) because of lethargy and oophritis. Note the use of sequentially placed hemoclips to ligate ovarian vessels and transect the pedicle (*arrow*).

be carefully retracted or exteriorized. Ovarian vessels are identified and ligated. The author prefers hemoclips to sutures for ligation because their use can significantly shorten the procedure time (**Fig. 15**). Often, both ovaries are affected and should be removed. Care should be taken to avoid damaging the vena cava when removing the right ovary and to leave the adrenal gland in place when removing the left ovary (**Fig. 16**). The oviduct can then be removed, if desired, although it may be preferable to leave the oviduct in place to shorten anesthetic time. Body wall and skin can be closed routinely. Postoperative supportive care, antimicrobials, and analgesia should be given as appropriate.

Dystocia

In this condition, follicles are ovulated into the oviduct but eggs fail to be laid. Predisposing factors can include environmental (eg, lack of appropriate nesting sites, inadequate temperature, humidity, or light cycle) or mechanical (eg, misshapen eggs,

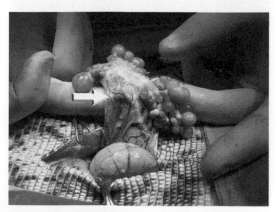

Fig. 16. Ovariectomy in a white-throated monitor lizard (*V albigularis*) because of lethargy and oophritis. Note the adrenal gland within the left ovarian pedicle (*arrow*). Care should be taken to leave this gland undisturbed.

maternal renomegaly or pelvic stenosis secondary to fractures, or metabolic bone disease) causes.[46] Affected lizards may be anorexic or lethargic, although some anorexia during gravidity is normal in many species during folliculogenesis.[46] Prolonged dystocia may result in signs consistent with hypocalcemia, such as weakness or tremors, because calcium is mobilized to the eggs (**Fig. 17**). Clinical pathologic findings may be nonspecific or may identify other predisposing factors (such as dehydration, renal disease). In a study of chameleons (*Chamaeleo chamaeleon*) with dystocia, elevation of the monocyte count and higher levels of aspartate aminotransferase (AST) were noted when compared with healthy gravid individuals.[53] The elevated level of AST was thought to be caused by tissue trauma.

Mechanical causes of dystocia can be diagnosed via cloacal examination and radiography. In animals without mechanical obstruction, medical therapy may be attempted. Oxytocin (5–30 IU/kg[32]) can be used, although it is less effective in lizards compared with chelonians. Arginine vasotocin, as the reptile equivalent of oxytocin,

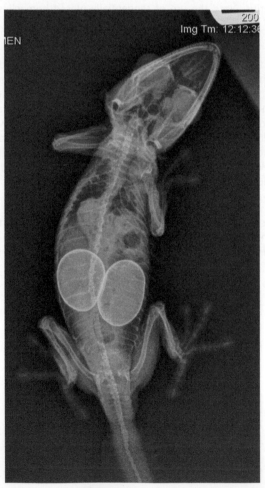

Fig. 17. Radiograph of a gravid leaf-tail gecko (*Uroplatus henkeli*). Note the thick shell on the eggs. This animal displayed signs of hypocalcemia (tremors, weakness), and a salpingotomy was performed to remove both eggs.

can be more effective but is available at present only as a research drug. In healthy, gravid, striped plateau lizards (*Sceloporus virgatus*), oviposition was induced using propranolol (1 µg/g) alone or followed by arginine vasotocin (500 ng/g) or prostaglandin $F_{2\alpha}$ (25 ng/g).[33] However, propranolol and prostaglandin $F_{2\alpha}$ were less successful in green iguanas.[54] Future investigation into the use of β-blockers and prostaglandins in lizards may be informative.

Similar to preovulatory follicles, eggs within the oviduct may rupture, leading to yolk peritonitis.[49] If medical therapies are unsuccessful in relieving the dystocia or if there are mechanical obstructions, salpingotomy is indicated. The approach to the oviduct is similar to that described for ovariectomy discussed earlier. The eggs may be removed from the oviduct or oviducts, and the oviduct is closed using absorbable suture in a simple continuous pattern.[52] If eggs are adhered to the oviducts or if they are damaged or ruptured, an ovariosalpingotomy should be performed. If the oviduct is removed, the ipsilateral ovary should also be removed to prevent ovulation into the coelomic cavity and subsequent coelomitis.

Hemipenal prolapse

Prolapse of the hemipenes may result from infection, trauma, or excessive or aggressive breeding (**Fig. 18**). It may be possible to clean and replace the hemipenes as described previously for penile prolapse in chelonia. Often however, if the tissue is traumatized or desiccated, it should be amputated. For amputation, the prolapsed hemipenes should be fully everted and clamped at its base. Horizontal mattress sutures of an absorbable material are placed at the base, and the hemipenes are transected and removed. The stump can then be replaced into the base of the tail. In case of infection, the caudal tail area should be carefully examined or explored to ensure that all affected tissues are recognized and treated. Amputation of one hemipenis preserves the animal's ability to breed.[39,40]

SNAKES
Normal Reproduction

Male snakes have hemipenes similar to lizards with each hemipenis invaginated caudal to the cloaca. One hemipenis is used at a time during copulation. Sperm is delivered in a manner similar to that described earlier for lizards. The epididymis is reportedly absent in snakes.[41]

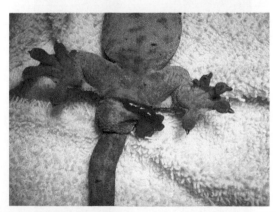

Fig. 18. Prolapsed hemipenes of an unknown species of gecko. If unable to replace, lizard hemipenes can be surgically removed from the base without affecting urination. (*Courtesy of* Dr Jean Paré, DMV, DVSc, New York, NY, USA.)

Female snakes can be oviparous (eg, pythons and most colubrids) or viviparous (eg, boas, all rattlesnakes, and most vipers).[41,44] Distinctions between viviparous and ovoviviparous species are no longer used, with all live-bearing snakes now being referred to as viviparous. Like lizards, some species may also be parthenogenic.[41]

Normal conditions to stimulate breeding behavior vary by the species. Similar to other groups of reptiles, temperature, humidity, light cycle, or social changes (ie, introduction of a male) may induce folliculogenesis and/or ovulation.[44] Many snakes may not reproduce if they do not have enough fat stores to produce follicles,[41] so a thorough examination before the onset of breeding season aids in successful reproduction.[44]

Reproductive Disorders

Infertility

Causes of infertility may be similar to those for chelonians and lizards, although there is little published material addressing this concern in snakes. As with other reptiles, accurate gender identification is critical for successful breeding and avoiding potential intraspecies aggression.[44] Snakes are rarely sexually dimorphic. Some exceptions include male boids, which often have larger cloacal spurs than females (**Fig. 19**), and some vipers, which may have color differences between the sexes (**Fig. 20**). In young snakes, it may be possible to evert the hemipenes by applying pressure and rolling the hemipenes out of the cloaca.[41,44] Alternatively, probing the hemipenes is a reliable method in most snakes. A round-ended sexing probe (snake sexing kits are commercially available) or a small, straight ball-tipped feeding tube can be lubricated, placed into 1 of the 2 openings at the lateral distal aspect of the cloaca, and directed caudally. Plastic-tipped straightened bobby pins have been recommended by Denardo,[41] because they can be discarded after a single use. The probe is easily

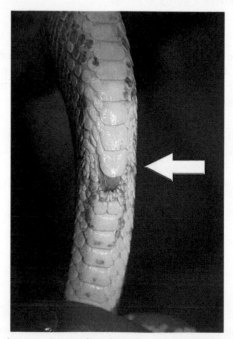

Fig. 19. Cloaca of a male emerald tree boa (*Corallus caninus*). Note the presence of cloacal spurs (*arrow*). These spurs are small or absent in females, and are a common trait in many boids.

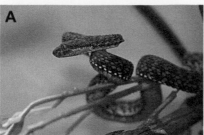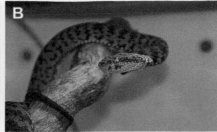

Fig. 20. Lateral views of the heads of a male (*A*) and female (*B*) Kanburian pit viper (*Trimeresurus kanburiensis*). Males have a white stripe on the lateral aspect of their head, which females lack. This stripe is present from birth.

advanced in males, much further than in females, which may have a short blind-ended sac in this area. A larger probe is preferred to a smaller one, because the larger probe is less likely to enter the female diverticula and gives an inaccurate result.[44] The number of scutes that the probe advances in males depends on the species, so it helps to have a pair of age-matched animals to compare with each other.

In animals for which manual eversion or probing is unsuccessful or indeterminate, hydrostatic eversion can be performed. A needle is inserted caudal to the end of the presumptive hemipenes, and sterile fluid is injected into the subcutaneous space. The fluid pressure causes the hemipenes and, potentially, portions of the cloaca to evert, and the hemipenes or oviductal papilla can be identified. Anesthesia may be required in larger individuals. Care should be taken to be as sterile as possible, to avoid the scent glands in this area, and to avoid injection or direct trauma to the hemipenes during this procedure.[41]

Hemipenal casts or plugs may interfere with normal copulation. These casts are formed from shed skin, sperm, and exudates (see **Fig. 12**).[44] They can be gently removed before the onset of breeding season.

Sperm assessment and assisted reproductive techniques have been studied in snakes and may become more widely used in the future.[55] Semen may be collected manually via massage[56,57] or through electroejaculation.[58]

Follicular stasis
Follicular stasis is rarely reported in snakes but may occur.[59] Treatment is ovariectomy, although multiple celiotomies may be required to remove the entire ovary (**Fig. 21**). Egg retention within the oviduct (dystocia) is much more common in snakes.

Dystocia
Causes for dystocia are similar to those described earlier for lizards. Inappropriate temperatures or humidity, lack of appropriate nest site, malnutrition, or social stressors may all contribute to dystocia. Many snakes oviposit within a covered box with damp moss or vermiculite inside.[44] For oviparous snakes, a common presentation is the recent oviposition of a clutch but retention of 1 to 2 eggs.[41,44] Retained eggs can often be palpated and possibly visualized. For viviparous species, lack of young after an expected due date may be observed. For both types of snakes, clinical signs may be absent, may be nonspecific, such as anorexia or lethargy, or may include straining or cloacal prolapse.

Retained eggs or young may be palpated or visible as swellings, but care should be taken during palpation as the oviduct can easily tear.[44] Radiographs may confirm the presence of young in viviparous species; uncurled young within the dam after the due

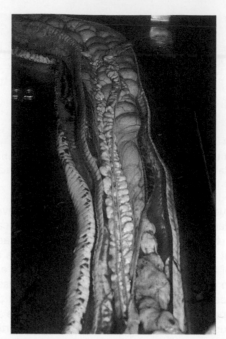

Fig. 21. Necropsy of an unknown species of python with retained follicles. Note the longitudinal extension of the ovaries. Often, multiple celiotomy incisions are required for ovariectomy in snakes because of this anatomy. (*Courtesy of* Department of Pathology, The University of Tennessee College of Veterinary Medicine, Knoxville, TN, USA; with permission.)

date or gas surrounding the young may indicate fetal death.[41,44] Plain radiographs are less useful for oviparous species as snake eggs are typically soft shelled and are poorly delineated with radiographs. However, the use of a contrast agent delivered orally or colonically may aid in identification of other structures in the caudal coelomic cavity that could be causing dystocia (**Fig. 22**). Ultrasonography may also be useful in identifying viviparous young or retained eggs, and it may be possible to detect fetal heartbeat or movement of the fetus.

Medical therapy can be attempted but is often unsuccessful. Possible obstructive causes for dystocia (eg, renomegaly or an overly large/malformed egg in the distal

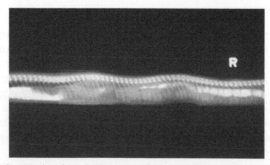

Fig. 22. Lateral radiograph of an unknown species of boa with egg masses within the oviduct. Note that the barium contrast within the intestinal tract identifies the masses as extraintestinal. (*Courtesy of* Dr Ed Ramsay, DVM, Knoxville, TN, USA.)

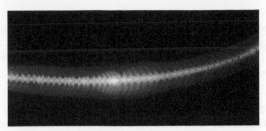

Fig. 23. Dorsoventral view of a rat snake (*Elaphe* sp) with a misshapen egg. Eggs of this shape should be surgically removed via celiotomy. (*Courtesy of* Dr Ed Ramsay, DVM, Knoxville, TN, USA.)

oviduct [**Fig. 23**]) should be first ruled out via physical examination, radiography, and possibly ultrasonography. If no obstruction is seen, oxytocin , 5 to 20 IU/kg, given intramuscularly may be effective, particularly if given within 2 to 3 days from the onset of dystocia;[44] however, in a reported case, live young were obtained after oxytocin administration 7 days after normal parturition had begun.[60] Arginine vasotocin may be more effective but is at present available only as a research drug. Use of additional medical therapies such as β-blockers or prostaglandins has received little attention in snakes.[61]

Eggs may be manually milked out of the cloaca, but this procedure carries a high risk of oviductal tearing and rupture of the follicles.[32] To be performed safely, the animal should be first anesthetized, and only gentle pressure should be applied to the eggs to move them toward the cloaca. Once near the cloaca, eggs may be visualized and aspirated/imploded via the cloaca as described earlier for chelonians. The remaining shell may be manually removed or left to pass on its own; however, care should be taken not to tear the oviduct because the shells may adhere to the oviductal mucosa if they have been in place for several days.[44] If the eggs cannot be removed medically or manually, surgery should be performed. A single paramedian celiotomy may be performed, but if there are many eggs or if they are adhered to the oviduct in multiple locations, multiple celiotomies may be necessary. Once eggs or fetuses are removed, an otherwise healthy oviduct can be closed in a simple continuous

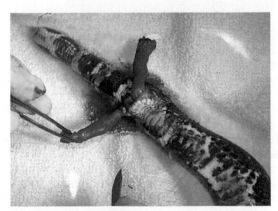

Fig. 24. Surgery to remove prolapsed hemipenes of a rat snake (*Elaphe* sp). Note that the hemipenes have been fully everted and are ligated with 2 encircling sutures before being transected. Removal of the hemipenes does not affect excretion in lizards or snakes. (*Courtesy of* Dr Jean Paré, DMV, DVSc, New York, NY, USA.)

pattern. If excessive inflammation or previous tearing has occurred, or if there is evidence of yolk coelomitis, the oviduct and ipsilateral ovary may need to be removed. Removal of the ovary often requires a long or multiple incisions to remove the entire organ (see **Fig. 21**).[62] The coelom can be closed in a simple pattern, and the skin can be closed using everting sutures.

Prolapse

The oviduct may prolapse secondary to straining from dystocia. If eggs are still present in the prolapsed tissue, it may be possible to remove the eggs, close the oviduct, and replace it within the cloaca. However, in most cases, the oviduct is too damaged to be replaced and should be surgically removed along with the ipsilateral oviduct as described previously.

The hemipenes may prolapse because of infection, trauma, or excessive use.[44] Therapy for hemipenal prolapse is as described earlier in lizards (**Fig. 24**).

ACKNOWLEDGMENTS

The author thanks Jean Paré and Ed Ramsay for contribution of their photographs and review of the manuscript. Special thanks to Jennifer Pramuk and Megan Baumer of the Department of Herpetology, Bronx Zoo for their assistance with the photography of sexually dimorphic traits.

REFERENCES

1. Campbell TW. Clinical laboratory evaluation of dystocia in lizards. Proceedings of the Association of Reptilian and Amphibian Veterinarians 1999;123–31.
2. Lloyd ML. Reptilian dystocias review: prevention, management, and comments on the synthetic hormone vasotocin. Proceedings of the American Association of Zoo Veterinarians 1990;329–36.
3. Innis C, Boyer TH. Chelonian reproductive disorders. Vet Clin North Am Exot Anim Pract 2002;5:555–78.
4. McArthur S. Reproductive system. In: McArthur S, Wilkinson R, Meyer J, editors. Medicine and surgery of tortoises and turtles. Oxford (UK): Blackwell Publishing; 2004. p. 57–63.
5. Kutchling G. The reproductive biology of the chelonia. Berlin: Spinger-Verlag; 1999.
6. Manire CA, Byrd L, Therrien CL, et al. Mating-induced ovulation in loggerhead sea turtles, *Caretta caretta*. Zoo Biol 2008;27:213–25.
7. Rostal D, Grumbles J, Lance V, et al. Non-lethal sexing techniques for hatchling and immature desert tortoises (*Gopherus agassizii*). Herpetological Monographs 1994;8:83–7.
8. Owens DW. Hormones in the life history of sea turtles. In: Lutz P, Musick JA, editors. Biology of the sea turtles. Boca Raton (FL): CRC Press; 1996. p. 315–41.
9. Madge D. Temperature and sex determination in reptiles with reference to chelonians. BCG Testudo 1994;2(3):9–14.
10. Demas S, Duronslet M, Wachtel S, et al. Sex-specific DNA in reptiles with temperature dependant sex determination. J Exp Zool 1990;253:319–24.
11. Stetter M. Ultrasonography. In: Mader D, editor. Reptile medicine and surgery. 2nd edition. St Louis (MO): Elsevier Inc; 2006. p. 665–74.
12. Kuchling G. 2006. Endoscopic sex determination in juvenile freshwater turtles, *Trachemys scripta*, a species with temperature dependent sex determination. Biol Reprod 1999;61:1275–80 – ordered.

13. Mitchell MA, Thompson D, Burgdorf A, et al. Coelioscopy as an antemortem method for confirming temperature dependant sex determination in Blanding's turtles (*Emydoidea blandingii*). In: Proceedings of the Association of Reptilian and Amphibian Veterinarians. Milwaukee (WI): 2009. p. 136.

14. Hernandez-Divers SJ, Stahl SJ. An endoscopic method for identifying sex of hatchling Chinese box turtles and comparison of general versus local anesthesia for coelioscopy. J Am Vet Med Assoc 2009;234(6):800–4.

15. Hernandez-Divers SJ, Hernandez-Divers SM, Wilson GH, et al. A review of reptile diagnostic coelioscopy. J Herp Med Surg 2005;3:16–31.

16. Platz CC, Mengden BS, Quinn H, et al. Semen collection, evaluation and freezing in the green sea turtle, Galapagos tortoise, and red-eared pond turtle. Proceedings of the American Association of Zoo Veterinarians 1980;47–54.

17. Wood F, Platz C, Critchley K, et al. Semen collection by electroejaculation of the green turtle, *Chelonia mydas*. Brit J Herpetol 1982;6:200–2.

18. Mitchell MA, Zimmerman D, Heggem B. Collection and characterization of semen from leopard tortoises. In: Proceedings of the Association of Reptilian and Amphibian Veterinarians. Milwaukee (WI): 2009. p. 166.

19. Cheng Y, Chen T, Yu P, et al. Observations on the female reproductive cycles of captive Asian yellow pond turtles (*Mauremys mutica*) with radiography and ultrasonography. Zoo Biol 2009;28:1–9.

20. Kutching G. How to minimize risk and optimize information gain in assessing reproductive condition and fecundity of live female chelonians. Chelonian Conserv Biol 1998;3(1):118–23.

21. Innis C. Infertility and embryonic death. In: McArthur S, Wilkinson R, Meyer J, editors. Medicine and surgery of tortoises and turtles. Oxford (UK): Blackwell Publishing; 2004. p. 63–8.

22. Ewert MA. Cold torpor, diapause, delayed hatching and aestivation in reptiles and birds. In: Deeming DC, Ferguson MWJ, editors. Egg incubation: its effects on embryonic development in birds and reptiles. Cambridge University Press, New York; 1991. p. 173–91.

23. McArthur S. Follicular stasis in captive chelonian, *Testudo* spp. In: Proceedings of the Association of Reptilian and Amphibian Veterinarians. Eighth Annual Conference, Orlando (FL): 2001. p 75–86.

24. McArthur S. Follicular stasis. In: McArthur S, Wilkinson R, Meyer J, editors. Medicine and surgery of tortoises and turtles. Oxford (UK): Blackwell Publishing; 2004. p. 325–9.

25. Innis CJ, Hernandez-Divers S, Martinez-Jimenez D. Coelioscopic-assisted prefemoral oophorectomy in chelonians. J Am Vet Med Assoc 2007;230(7):1049–52.

26. McArthur S. Dystocia. In: McArthur S, Wilkinson R, Meyer J, editors. Medicine and surgery of tortoises and turtles. Oxford (UK): Blackwell Publishing; 2004. p. 316–8.

27. McArthur S. Interpretation of presenting signs. In: McArthur S, Wilkinson R, Meyer J, editors. Medicine and surgery of tortoises and turtles. Oxford (UK): Blackwell Publishing; 2004. p. 273–80.

28. Thomas HL, Willer CJ, Wosat MA, et al. Egg-retention in the urinary bladder of a Florida cooter turtle, *Pseudemys floridana floridana*. J Herp Med Surg 2001; 11(4):4–6.

29. Johnson R. Dystocia in an injured common eastern long-necked turtle (*Chelodina longicollis*). Vet Clin North Am Exot Anim Pract 2006;9:575–81.

30. Tucker JK, Thomas DL, Rose J. Oxytocin dosage in turtles. Chelonian Conserv Biol 2007;6(2):321–4.

31. Feldman ML. Some options to induce oviposition in turtles. Chelonian Conserv Biol 2007;6(2):313–20.
32. DeNardo D. Dystocias. In: Mader D, editor. Reptile medicine and surgery. 2nd edition. St Louis (MO): Elsevier Inc; 2006. p. 787–92.
33. Gross T, Guillette LJ, Gross DA, et al. Control of oviposition in reptiles and amphibians. Proceedings of the American Association of Zoo Veterinarians 1992;143–50.
34. Innis CJ. Innovative approaches to chelonian obstetrics. In: Proceedings of the Association of Reptilian and Amphibian Veterinarians, Naples, Italy: 2004. p. 1–5.
35. McArthur S, Hernandez-Divers S. Surgery. In: McArthur S, Wilkinson R, Meyer J, editors. Medicine and surgery of tortoises and turtles. Oxford (UK): Blackwell Publishing; 2004. p. 403–59.
36. Mader DR, Bennett RA, Funk RS, et al. Surgery. In: Mader D, editor. Reptile medicine and surgery. 2nd edition. St Louis (MO): Elsevier Inc; 2006. p. 581–630.
37. Nutter FB, Lee DD, Stamper MA, et al. Hemiovariosalpingectomy in a loggerhead sea turtle (Caretta caretta). Vet Rec 2000;146:78–80.
38. Knotek Z, Jekl V, Knotkova Z, et al. Eggs in chelonian urinary bladder: is coeliotomy necessary? Proceedings of the Association of Reptilian and Amphibian Veterinarians 2009;118–21.
39. Barten SL. Penile prolapse. In: Mader D, editor. Reptile medicine and surgery. 2nd edition. St Louis (MO): Elsevier Inc; 2006. p. 862–4.
40. Funk RS. Lizard reproductive medicine and surgery. Vet Clin North Am Exot Anim Pract 2002;5:579–613.
41. Denardo D. Reproductive biology. In: Mader D, editor. Reptile medicine and surgery. 2nd edition. St Louis (MO): Elsevier Inc; 2006. p. 376–90.
42. Roberts J, Bechert U, Huber M, et al. Determination of gender in the bluetongued skink (Tiliqua scincoides) by ultrasonography and endoscopy with comparison of differentiating external morphologic parameters. Proceedings of the Association of Reptilian and Amphibian Veterinarians 2007;50.
43. Mitchell MA, Zimmerman D, Heggem B. Collection and characterization of semen from green iguanas. Proceedings of the Association of Reptilian and Amphibian Veterinarians 2009;165.
44. Stahl SJ. Veterinary management of snake reproduction. Vet Clin North Am Exot Anim Pract 2002;5:615–36.
45. Raiti P. Changing trends in diseases of the green iguana, Iguana iguana. Proceedings of the Association of Reptilian and Amphibian Veterinarians 1999;133–6.
46. Maxwell LK. Infectious and non-infectious diseases. In: Jacobson ER, editor. Biology, husbandry, and medicine of the green iguana. Malabar (FL): Krieger Publishing Co; 2003. p. 108–32.
47. Stacy BA, Howard L, Kinkaid J, et al. Yolk coelomitis in Fiji Island banded iguanas (Brachylophus fasciatus). J Zoo Wildl Med 2008;39(2):161–9.
48. Spellman LH. Medical management. In: Murphy C, Walsh T, editors. Komodo dragons: biology and conservation. Washington, DC: Smithsonian Press; 2002. p. 208–10 – ordered.
49. Backeus KA, Ramsay EC. Ovariectomy for treatment of follicular stasis in lizards. J Zoo Wildl Med 1994;25(1):111–6.
50. Scheelings TF. Pre-ovulatory follicular stasis in a yellow-spotted monitor, Varanus panoptes panoptes. J Herp Med Surg 2008;18(1):18–20.
51. Jones RE, Austin HB, Lopez KH, et al. Gonadotropin-induced ovulation in a reptile (Anolis carolinensis): histological observations. Gen Comp Endocrinol 1988;72: 312–22.

52. Lock B, Bennett RA. Anesthesia and surgery. In: Jacobson ER, editor. Biology, husbandry, and medicine of the green iguana. Malabar (FL): Krieger Publishing Co; 2003. p. 152–67.
53. Cuadrado M, Diaz-Paniagua C, Quevedo MA, et al. Hematology and clinical chemistry in dystocic and healthy post-reproductive female chameleons. J Wildl Dis 2002;38(2):395–401.
54. Innis C. Treatment with propranolol and PGF2a stimulates nesting behavior but not oviposition in a gravid green iguana. Bull Assoc Reptil Amph Vet 1996;6(2):1–4.
55. Mattson KJ, De Vries A, McGuire SM, et al. Successful artificial insemination in the corn snake, Elaphe gutatta, using fresh and cooled semen. Zoo Biol 2007; 26:363–9.
56. Zacariotti RL, Grego KF, Fernandes W, et al. Semen collection and evaluation in free-ranging Brazilian rattlesnakes (Crotalus durissus terrificus). Zoo Biol 2007; 26:155–60.
57. Fahrig BM, Mitchell MA, Eilts BE, et al. Characterization and cooled storage of semen from corn snakes (Elaphe guttata). J Zoo Wildl Med 2007;38:7–12.
58. Quinn H, Blasedel T, Platz CC. Successful artificial insemination in the checkered garter snake. Int Zoo Yearbook 1989;28:177–83.
59. Denardo D, Barten SL, Rosenthal KL, et al. Dystocia. J Herp Med Surg 2000; 10(2):8–17.
60. Lock BA. Treatment of interrupted parturition with delivery of viable young in a Brazilian rainbow boa, Epicrates cenchria cenchria. Bull Assoc Reptil Amph Vet 1998;8(2):11–3.
61. Nathan R. Treatment with ovicentesis, PGE2, and PGF2a to aid oviposition in a spotted python. Bull Assoc Reptil Amph Vet 1996;6(4):4.
62. Lock BA. Reproductive surgery in reptiles. Vet Clin North Am Exot Anim Pract 2000;3(3):733–52.

A Fresh Look at Metabolic Bone Diseases in Reptiles and Amphibians

Eric Klaphake, DVM, DACZM, DABVP (Avian)

KEYWORDS

- Nutritional secondary hyperparathyroidism
- Renal secondary hyperparathyroidism • Calcium • Phosphorus
- Metabolic bone disease • Reptiles • Amphibians

Metabolic bone diseases (MBDs) are a group of conditions that continue to plague and perplex veterinarians and pet owners. Although the reptile and amphibian (herptile) veterinary knowledge base has grown understanding of the causes and diagnostic and treatment options are often extrapolated from human or other mammalian medicine models. Although the roles of UV-B radiation (280–315 nm wavelength), calcium, phosphorus, and cholecalciferol (vitamin D_3) are better understood in some MBDs, there remain many "X" factors that are not. Likewise, quantitative diagnosis of MBDs has been difficult not only in terms of staging a disease but also regarding whether or not a condition is present. Treatment options also present challenges in corrective husbandry and diet modifications, medication/modality selection, and dosing/regimen parameters.

Green iguanas (*Iguana iguana*) have provided the classic presentations of the most commonly seen MBDs, nutritional secondary hyperparathyroidism (NSHPT) and renal secondary hyperparathyroidism (RSHPT), for many years. Although the popularity of the green iguana as a pet has waned, other herptiles have now filled the void, with MBDs still a common primary presentation to veterinarians for those animals. Lizards and chelonians are the most common groups represented, but snakes, anurans, and urodeles/caudates may also develop and present with MBDs.

With a switch in the common species presenting with MBDs comes new challenges in how to identify and how to correct these diseases. I have seen MBDs in bearded dragons (*Pogona vitticeps*), Asian water dragons (*Physignathus cocincinus*), various chameleon species, leopard geckos (*Eublepharis macularius*), uromastyx (*Uromastyx* spp), *Testudo* spp, and *Geochelone* spp. Instead of the typical diurnal basking, herbivorous green iguana habitat, the entire spectrum of potential environments and dietary

Animal Medical Center, 216 North 8th Avenue, Bozeman, MT 59715, USA
E-mail address: dreklaphake@msn.com

Vet Clin Exot Anim 13 (2010) 375–392
doi:10.1016/j.cvex.2010.05.007
1094-9194/10/$ – see front matter © 2010 Elsevier Inc. All rights reserved.

vetexotic.theclinics.com

options now needs to be addressed for MBDs. Although the classic presentation of rubber jaw and popeye arms and legs is noticeable in some species, in other species there are myriad clinical signs to be aware of.

Radiographs and initial blood work are the standards to start better quantifying the diagnosis, but it is critical to try to apply evidence-based medicine techniques to initially assess, diagnose, treat, and prevent these conditions if veterinary medicine is to advance in addressing them. Anecdotal reports are often helpful as starting points, but peer-reviewed scientific studies will continue to be necessary to support and validate theories, test results, and treatment regimens or to debunk those that are ineffective or even potentially harmful. Where possible, this article references such studies, few though they are at this time. In other cases, well-respected anecdotal herptile veterinary articles or review articles are referenced, with extrapolations directly from human/mammalian studies and personal anecdotal observations referred to at times as necessary.

CALCIUM HOMEOSTASIS

Although each MBD is different, there are some basic concepts that address the physiology behind why these diseases occur. It is critical for this to be understood by veterinarians, veterinary staff, and owners, particularly in terms of future prevention. **Fig. 1** shows these basics facts of calcium/phosphorus/cholecalciferol homeostasis and how when one part goes wrong, the ramifications affect the other parts and even parts outside the standard system. **Fig. 2** is a handout provided by me to all herptile-owning clients, whether or not their pet has an MBD. Readers are welcome to contact me for a copy of this to use with their own clients, as long as appropriate credit is provided and it is not modified.

As a review, calcium is a mineral that needs to be consumed in a herptile's diet (perhaps as part of the environmental water). Calcium is critical for bone development

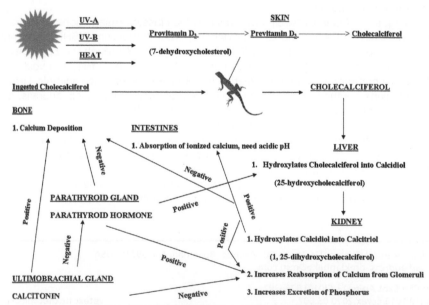

Fig. 1. Calcium and cholecalciferol homeostasis and disease pathlophysiology.

NUTRITIONAL SECONDARY HYPERPARATHYROIDISM Better Known As "METABOLIC BONE DISEASE"

Eric Klaphake, DVM, DACZM, DABVP (Avian)

Nutritional secondary hyperparathyroidism (NSHP) is the most common presentation of metabolic bone disease (MBD) in reptiles & amphibians. MBD encompasses a number of syndromes including NSHP, osteoporosis (bone mass loss), osteomalacia (failure of adult bone to calcify), rickets (juvenile form of osteomalacia), fibrous osteodystrophy (excessive bone resorption and replacement with fibrous tissue), or hypocalcemia (low blood calcium levels).

1. Assume all reptiles & amphibians are either clinical for MBD (showing outward signs) or sub-clinical (it's waiting to happen).

2. We all know that calcium is extremely important to strong bones. But it is probably more important at the cellular level for muscle contractions (especially the heart). It even plays a role in allowing blood to clot. Too much can cause heart attacks and seizures, so there can be too much of a good thing.

3. The third concept is how calcium is taken in, monitored, and maintained. The following diagram may help.

Natural sunlight or an indoor bulb with 2-12% UVB hits the skin, converting the inactive form of vitamin D3 into the active form. This is what determines how much calcium is absorbed from the intestine. Oral forms of vitamin D3 (cholecalciferol) in inappropriate species can cause excessive uptake of calcium and cause blood vessels and internal organs to be calcified. This is how many rat poisons work. The sunlight or UVB will not work through glass, plastic, fine screening or if the UVB is more than 2 feet from the reptile and amphibians.

The kidneys ideally reabsorb calcium as urine is filtered, and selectively excrete phosphorus. However, when the kidneys are dehydrated or damaged, needed calcium is lost and undesired phosphorus is retained, skewing the ratio.

Calcium is ingested in the diet. It must be in an absorbable form and its ratio with phosphorus in the diet should be 2:1 or more.

Blood carries the calcium to the muscles, along with all the hormones that regulate the calcium. When blood calcium is low, things are bad.

***Bone is the calcium warehouse, too much loss leads to rubbery bones that easily break.

MORE ON THE BACK!

Fig. 2. Handout provided to clients to explain MBDs (especially NSHPT). (*Courtesy of* the Animal Medical Center, Bozeman, MT; with permission.)

Anything affecting a part of this diagram can mess everything up. In some cases, this is easy to fix, but in most, recovery is long and drawn out at best. As the old saying goes, "prevention is the best cure." It is important to realize that we do not know the perfect set-up for any species or individuals. Reptile/ amphibian medicine is changing rapidly, thus it is important to keep in touch with your reptile/amphibian veterinarians for the latest information.

How can you prevent this or help correct an already existing problem?
By doing the following:

1. **FEEDING THE RECOMMENDED DIET, IN THE CORRECT PROPORTIONS, AT THE CORRECT TEMPERATURE.** See species specific handouts/get diet instructions directly from veterinarian.

2. **USE THE CORRECT BULBS, WITH CORRECT LEVELS OF UVB, SET UP IN THE RECOMMENDED MANNER, WHEN NATURAL SUNLIGHT CAN NOT BE USED.** UVB levels should be 0-12%, dependent on species (ask vet if uncertain) within 2 feet of the animal, with no barriers between, & should be changed every 6 months. Use ZooMed®'s T-Rex®'s fluorescent bulbs or their mercury vapor lamps.

3. **SOAK YOUR REPTILE ONCE DAILY FOR 15 MINUTES IN A SHALLOW, WARM WATER BATH.** Certain species may not have this recommended for them. Keep the temperature at what a small child should be bathed at, and the water should be only one half the height of the reptile, less if they are sick or weak. This helps keep them hydrated, and their kidneys at their peak level of function.

4. **DO NOT USE ORAL VITAMINS CONTAINING VITAMIN D3 OR PHOSPHORUS. DO NOT USE THE SUN SPRAYS OR MOON SPRAYS.** Pet stores often sell products in ignorance, if there is a new product you are interested in, ask your veterinarian. I like to use Tums ® ground up into a powder as a calcium source.

5. **DO NOT FEED ANY ANIMAL-BASED PROTEINS SUCH AS MONKEY CHOW/ BISCUITS, DOG FOOD, CAT FOOD, OR OTHER MEATS TO VEGETARIAN REPTILES. FEED HIGH QUALITY PROTEIN TO THE CARNIVORES.**

**These make our reptiles/amphibians real big, real fast, but it damages their kidneys, and severely shortens their lifespans. Remember this when purchasing an older animal, it might have occurred in its past. They like the taste of these products, "but just cuz it tastes good don't mean it's good for 'em!"

What are the signs to look for in your reptile or amphibian?
1. fractured legs
2. inability to stand upright
3. paralysis
4. swollen "Popeye" arms and legs
5. rubber jaw, upper jaw longer than swollen lower jaw
6. finger, toe, tongue, and pupil tremors
7. stunted growth
8. unable to eat, though hungry
9. abnormal shell growth in turtles and tortoises
10. scoliosis of the back (S-curved)
11. inability to urinate and defecate
12. weakness and collapse
13. DEATH

All of these are signs which indicate your reptile/amphibian needs to be seen by your veterinarian. There are some diagnostic tests that can determine severity of the MBD, secondary complications (dehydration, infection, liver disease), and the best course of action. Likewise there are treatment regimes that can buy more time or even correct the situation. MBD TAKES A LONG TIME TO DEVELOP & A LONG TIME TO CORRECT IN THOSE SITUATIONS WHERE CORRECTION IS POSSIBLE!

Fig. 2. (*continued*)

and maintenance, egg production, and cellular/muscle activity, with the last including the heart, the gastrointestinal tract (GIT), and the brain. Calcium comes in several forms and, as discussed later, the form plays a significant role in how much calcium is absorbed and how it is used. Calcium absorption is regulated by the type of calcium, levels of phosphorus in the diet, the health of the GIT, cholecalciferol (vitamin D_3) levels, calcitonin levels, and PTH levels. Calcium and phosphorus form a conglomeration, called hydroxyapatite, which is the main component of bone and teeth. As in mammals, magnesium, among other factors, may also play roles in calcium regulation; however, supportive evidence is lacking for roles or lack thereof at this time.

The next factor to consider is cholecalciferol. How this works depends on the type of herptile. For most snakes,[1] crocodilians, some chelonians, and some amphibians, life-style (nocturnal) and ingestion of whole prey seem to have led to an evolution whereby cholecalciferol is completely (or nearly completely) collected orally from the diet (see later discussion on UV-B). For many commonly kept lizards that are diurnal and insectivorous or herbivorous, some chelonians, and some amphibians, UV-B (280–315 nm wavelength) and UV-A (315–400 nm wavelength) are necessary to activate the cholecalciferol pathway (see **Fig. 1**). Provitamin D_3 (7-dehydrocholesterol) in the skin is converted by UV-B and UV-A to previtamin D_3. Previtamin D_3 is thermochemically isomerized into cholecalciferol in the skin, with higher temperature increasing the rate of isomerization; however, if excessive levels of cholecalciferol develop, the same process can break it down into inert tachysterol or lumisterol or back into provitamin D_3.[2] It is undetermined whether or not this reversal mechanism works in herptiles relying completely on dietary cholecalciferol, particularly in the case of ingestion of toxic levels; however, it can be surmised that the system is built to reduce mild or slowly increasing excesses, not a sudden rush.

Once cholecalciferol is inside the body, whether or not from diet or from UV-B/UV-A conversion, the next steps are the same. Cholecalciferol travels to the liver, where it is hydroxylated into calcidiol (25-hydroxycholecalciferol), then travels to the kidney for a final hydroxylation to become calcitriol (1,25-dihydroxycholecalciferol)—the biologically active form of vitamin D_3.

Calcitriol is what increases calcium and phosphorus absorption from the GIT, increases bone release of calcium (demineralization), induces immune system stimulation (in mammals at least), and creates a relatively inhospitable microenvironment for neoplastic cells (in mammals at least).[2] In certain situations, calcitriol is regulated by estrogen, prolactin, and growth hormone in mammals; although regulation is likely similar in herptiles, further research needs to be done to confirm and perhaps elucidate the presence of other factors influencing calcitriol levels and effects.[2] Current levels of calcium and phosphorus, among other parameters, can affect renal hydroxylation of calcidiol. Parathyroid hormone (PTH) release promotes increased renal hydroxylation, so that more calcitriol is produced. In opposition, increased levels of calcitonin from the ultimobrachial glands inhibit demineralization of bone (and thus enhance remineralization) and have a negative feedback directly on PTH release. Although calcitonin evolved back at least as far as fish, PTH likely evolved in amphibians and was retained further up the evolutionary tree.[2] Although PTH has several redundant effects duplicated by other organs or hormones, from an evolutionary perspective, there developed a need for that redundancy.

Bone serves as a repository, releasing or storing calcium and phosphorus as directed by calcitriol, calcitonin, or PTH, thus filling a passive role. The kidneys are the final piece of the puzzle. They play a hydroxylation role in the final steps of converting calcidiol. They also respond to calcitriol to increase calcium reabsorption in the glomerulus and increase phosphorus secretion. Effects of PTH and calcitonin can affect hydroxylation activity in the kidney and, therefore, indirectly affect calcium homeostasis (discussed previously).

TYPES OF METABOLIC BONE DISEASES

There are many types of MBDs and, although a layperson may use the singular term, MBD, veterinarians must first identify which type of MBD exists in terms of: diagnostics, treatment, ramifications, prevention, and prognosis. There is an excellent summary of MBDs by Mader in *Reptile Medicine and Surgery*.[3] Many pictures and diagrams in the chapter demonstrate the clinical presentations of the disease, and the author strongly encourage readers to take advantage of the information provided in Dr Mader's chapter.

The two most commonly presented and identified types of MBDs are NSHPT and RSHPT. Most MBDs present to a veterinarian late in the disease process due to a combination of owner ignorance, animal stoicism, and slow progression. This is an important concept to remember when presenting initial findings and recommendations to a client for the first time. This is also relevant when discussing prognosis, diagnostics, treatment, and prevention; the latter three are particularly concerning in terms of financial and emotional costs.

NSHPT presents in most cases as a juvenile or immature herptile. Owners are usually new to owning herptiles in general or, although owning that particular species, or they have lost several herptiles over a period of time and have self-diagnosed MBD or just want to stop losing these animals. Most are quite progressed by the time an owner realizes a problem (or decides to address a problem) or even when a veterinarian recognizes a problem. In these cases, inadequate oral calcium, a poor calcium/phosphorus ratio, inadequate oral cholecalciferol/UV light, inappropriate heating/humidity, or often a combination of several of these factors leads to a physiologic response to depleted calcium levels by increasing PTH production. Because needs are not met, calcium depletion from bone becomes clinical and the overall shortages start affecting muscle calcium needs.

In most lizards, there may be a history of several individuals housed in the same cage or in close proximity. This stress seems to predispose to a variety of secondary diseases, including NSHPT. Bearded dragons tend to develop better individually when housed in confined spaces. Additionally, bearded dragons not allowed to bask in ideal areas for heat and UV light and forced to eat undesired leftovers in food bowl have compounded stressors. They often lay down flat most of the time and may have a rubber jaw with lip deformations and secondary chelitis/gingivitis/stomatitis and intention tremors in the extremities and tongue. These pets want to eat but select soft foods if they eat at all. Prehension may be slowed or may not occur, thus drawing out the eating process. Constipation affects many species in all types of MBDs. With calcium's effect on GIT motility, cloacal prolapse or diarrhea may also be presenting complaints.[3,4] Pathologic fractures of the long bones or mandible are common. Temporary paralysis of the caudal limbs acutely or severe spondylosis due to vertebral fracture and callus can be seen. Pelvic fractures and malunions can lead to dystocia or constipation. In chameleons and anurans, an inability to retract their tongues after attempted prey capture has been noted. Chelonians often have very soft, squishy shells, malformed rhamphothecas (beaks), and caudal paresis. In advanced stages, seizures, respiratory/cardiac compromise, and death occur. In my opinion, it is likely that described UV-B deficiency seen in some snake species (discussed later) is a variation of NSHPT, although again that is purely conjecture on at this point.

RSHPT tends to be a condition of older animals, where a slow decline in kidney function eventually leads to an inability to respond to signals for the kidneys to selectively retain calcium and secrete extra phosphorus. Often gastrointestinal absorption can compensate for this declining function, but eventually the combination of this issue and the inability to hydroxylate calcidiol to calcitriol leads to a nonresponsiveness of the system to PTH and the hypertrophy of the parathyroid glands. Of greater concern seems to be the resultant hyperphosphatemia due to loss of selective secretion of excess phosphorus. Unlike with NSHPT, many of these herptiles have not even begun to tap far into their bone calcium reserves. These animals often present with seizures and collapse or intention tremors occasionally due to acute loss of calcium but more commonly due to hyperphosphatemia. More often than not, RSHPT herptiles present as anorexic or lethargic. Initial blood work results often indicate the diagnosis. When palpable, kidneys may be swollen, normal, or nonpalpable—potentially indicating chronic renal failure at various stages.

Hypertrophic osteodystrophy has been reported only in lizards. Clinical signs include lameness, painful limbs, and reluctance to move. As with mammals, pulmonary pathology is reported, although with no mention of clinical manifestations; in lizards this condition has an idiopathic etiology.[3] In reptiles, osteopetrosis usually manifests as lameness due to bone brittleness and fracturing.[3] Osteitis deformans has been described in herptiles; more recent literature suggests that it may actually be a progression of osteomyelitis to a chronic osteoarthrosis and spondylosis, particularly in snakes.[3,5]

Although not reported in herptiles, in theory a parathyroid gland neoplasm (primary hyperparathyroidism) could lead to a calcium imbalance. Likewise, some birds can so deplete their bone reserves from chronic egg production and laying that pathologic fractures as seen in herptiles with NSHPT can occur but again, to my knowledge, this phenomenon has not been reported in herptiles. Reptiles have much less calcium in the shells of their leathery eggs and amphibians have even less.

RAMIFICATIONS

Addressing the presenting symptoms and underlying cause needs to be considered. As in all clinical presentations, make sure to rule in or out other conditions and particularly watch for concurrent issues or secondary opportunistic conditions. These animals often need special nutritional support, potentially for many months. Secondary, opportunistic infections from otherwise benign parasites, bacteria, or fungi can occur. In mammals, most MBDs are considered extremely painful. Unfortunately, pain models in reptiles are only beginning to be developed and, although they exist in anurans at least, in all herptiles there is a challenge to evaluate analgesic options, dosages, and regimens for these stoic animals. Veterinarians need to discuss the ethics, the frustrations, the emotional exhaustion, the quality of life, and often guarded prognoses with clients early in the process and make sure that progression in managing a case is in the patient's best interest, not the client's or veterinarian's. Long-term and short-term prognoses in MBD herptiles are often guarded to poor, owning to the chronicity of disease before diagnosis and treatment plan are made. Likewise, an owner who is told that an initial estimate for diagnostics and treatment will run into the hundreds of dollars for a 25% chance of long-term success, added to hundreds of dollars more for often complete revamping of the herptile's environment, often pushes the only feasible options to a choice of euthanasia and hopefully client education to minimize recurrence in future animals.

DIAGNOSTICS

Begin with an extremely thorough history, particularly regarding environment and diet. Physical examination and signalment likewise can fuel suspicions of an MBD. A complete blood cell count may not directly enhance this diagnosis, but concurrent issues often set the table for overall therapy and prognosis. A plasma chemistry panel can be a first step to indications of an MBD. Look particularly at total calcium and phosphorus, their individual values and their relationship. Hypocalcemia, hyperphosphatemia, a less than 1:1 total calcium/phosphorous ratio, and occasionally hypercalcemia (can be high, however, in females and even normal in some species, such as indigo snakes) are initial indicators of potential MBDs. With many animals, lymphatic vessels and sinuses are often in close proximity to blood collection sites, and contamination with significant amounts of lymphatic fluid or pericardial fluid of cardiac phlebotomy may skew those results.

Ionized calcium has been closely studied for its value in diagnosing MBDs in green iguanas.[6] It is important not to draw conclusions from one herptile to all others. With few literature reports, however, veterinarians are often forced to do that in practice. Many blood parameters seem to be well conserved across orders and even classes and, if results are interpreted in light of the clinical presentation, decisions and interpretations can be made. In a study evaluating healthy green iguanas, the mean ionized calcium concentration measured in blood was 1.47 ($\pm$0.105 mmol/L), with no significant variation by gender or age.[6] I have seen otherwise healthy immature green iguanas have measured values approaching 2.0 mmol/L on repeated assessments with no apparent clinical manifestations. Challenges with this test include the correct collection/storage of sample and delivery to an outside laboratory. Contacting the primary diagnostic laboratory before sample collection is recommended to confirm correct technique. In mammalian and bird species, portable instant blood evaluation units have been used for faster results.

Several studies have looked at vitamin D_3 levels in the blood or, more specifically, calcidiol (25-hydroxycholecalciferol).[7–11] Commercially, this test is available through the Michigan State University Diagnostic Center for Population and Animal Health (DCPAH Endocrine Diagnostic Section, PO Box 30076, Lansing, MI 48909-7576; [517] 353-0621; www.animalhealth.msu.edu). It is highly recommended to contact the laboratory before sample collection to determine sample type, shipping requirements, and necessary quantities required. They have panels that also include ionized calcium, PTH, and an option for veterinary endocrinologist interpretation. In red-eared sliders (Trachemys scripta elegans), calcidiol concentrations differed significantly between turtles provided supplemental UV radiation (71.7 $\pm$ 46.9 nmol/L) and those not provided UV radiation (31.4 $\pm$ 13.2 nmol/L).[7] A study of 22 healthy, adult tortoises (Testudo hermanni, T graeca, and T marginata) of mixed gender kept in captivity under natural unfiltered sunlight in southern England with no dietary sources of cholecalciferol found that the concentration of calcidiol did not vary significantly with the seasons. The concentrations in the female tortoises, however, were significantly lower than in the males.[8] Calcidiol values for 22 wild Ricord's iguanas (Cyclura ricordii), 7 wild rhinoceros iguanas (C cornuta cornuta), and 13 captive rhinoceros iguanas held outdoors were sampled. In a separate study, mean concentrations of calcidiol were 554 nmol/L for wild Ricord's iguanas, 332 nmol/L for wild rhinoceros iguanas, and 317 nmol/L for captive rhinoceros iguanas. On the basis of these results, serum concentrations of at least 325 nmol/L for calcidiol were considered normal for healthy Ricord's and rhinoceros iguanas.[11] A group of captive adult Fijian iguanas (Brachylophus fasciatus) and (B vitiensis) had their calcidiol status compared with that of agamid and iguanid lizards housed in indoor enclosures under artificial UV light or exposed to natural sunlight (wild-caught or captive animals housed outdoors). Those under artificial lighting had a significantly lower calcidiol status than those housed exclusively outdoors, whereas the calcidiol status of Fijian iguanas that had received intermittent exposure to natural sunlight was intermediate and not significantly different from that of animals housed exclusively outdoors. Captive Fijian iguana eggs, however, had substantially lower calcidiol content compared with eggs from outdoor iguanid and agamid animals. Artificial UV light, therefore, might not be an adequate substitute for natural sunlight to maintain vitamin D status of lizards.[10] Voluntary exposure to higher UV-B irradiance (70 vs 1 μW/cm^2) resulted in greater circulating calcidiol levels in female panther chameleons (Furcifer pardalis) (1510 to 230 nmol/L 604 vs 92 ng/mL).[9]

Radiographs have been used in many cases as a primary diagnostic tool for MBD. Radiographs only detect 30% or greater change in bone density, however, and if total bone density is poor, then evaluation is often subjective for nonradiology specialists, particularly in immature, small, or reproductively active animals. The advent of digital radiology does seem to have removed a great amount of technique error, although current machine limits (particularly with small specimens), poor positioning, and over-interpretation of findings can affect diagnosis. Again, the author refer readers to Dr Mader's chapter for photographic examples of these conditions.[3]

A diagnostic tool used in humans to better quantify bone density, particularly in women with osteoporosis, is the dual energy x-ray absorptiometry (DXA) scan, some-times referred to as a bone density scan. I have used this modality in a RSHPT green iguana to quantify current bone density and monitor therapeutic response. In humans, child values cannot be compared with adult values due to overall bone mass differ-ences. Likewise, as with routine radiographs, most DXA scans are 2-D so cannot account as well for individuals with dense bones. These two limitations may also apply to herptiles. Challenges with this diagnostic tool include the need to position as rec-ommended for humans; it is challenging to account for the tail. This positioning usually requires anesthesia because lack of movement beyond breathing is critical and the scan can take some time depending on an animal's size (scan for a mature male took 30 minutes). A DXA scan generally reads to estimated calcium levels in individual bones, although they can be summed to estimate whole body calcium levels. In the published study using DXA scan, reference bone density values in relation to body weight, gender, and MBC were collected in 28 green iguanas. The regions of interest were the head, lumbar spine, right, and left femur. Body weight had the strongest rela-tionship with bone density. Within regions of interest, for iguanas of average weight (710 g), statistically significant differences between healthy and sick animals were found: head (0.140 vs 0.090 g/cm^2), lumbar spine (0.164 vs 0.107 g/cm^2), right femur (0.103 vs 0.076 g/cm^2), and left femur (0.103 vs 0.078 g/cm^2).[12]

Ultrasound as a modality can be used to visualize the kidneys and as a guide for fine-needle aspirates. Use of this modality requires an understanding of kidney loca-tion; the kidneys may be more in the pelvic canal versus the abdomen. Kidneys in the pelvic canal will require a more unique approach for visualization.

Glomerular filtration rate was evaluated in 2-year-old healthy green iguanas by IV administration of iohexol (75 mg/kg) into the ventral coccygeal (tail) vein. The mean (SD) glomerular filtration rate was 16.56 mL/kg/h ($\pm$3.90).[13] This is a helpful value to use for determination of RSHPT.

Another, more advanced diagnostic modality to better evaluate reptilian kidneys is nuclear medicine. A limitation is having the necessary facility and, again, it general requires sedation without movement. Radiopharmaceuticals need to be injected into the bloodstream, as described for two different herptiles (discussed later). Ten healthy green iguanas were evaluated for the determination of kidney morphology and function by the use of scintigraphy involving technetium Tc 99m diethylenetri-amine pentaacetic acid (99mTc-DTPA) or technetium Tc 99m dimercaptosuccinic acid (99mTc-DMSA). The researchers found that the use of 99mTc-DTPA for renal scintigraphy was nondiagnostic because of serum protein binding and poor renal uptake of the isotope. Renal uptake of 99mTc-DMSA produced distinct visualization of both kidneys. Renal uptake and soft tissue clearance of 99mTc-DMSA increased over the 20-hour imaging period with a mean renal uptake of 11.31% ($\pm$3.06%) at 20 hours. Results indicated that the kidneys of iguanas can be evaluated scintigraph-ically by use of 99mTc-DMSA.[14] The efficacy of three radiopharmaceuticals, 99mTc-DTPA, 99mTc-DMSA, and 99mTc-mercaptoacetyltriglycine (99mTc-MAG3), for renal imaging was examined in 16 corn snakes (*Elaphe guttata guttata*). All snakes received the radiopharmaceutical via an intracardiac injection. The kidneys could not be visualized in the three snakes that received 99mTc-DTPA or in the three snakes that received 99mTc-DMSA but were well delineated in all 10 snakes receiving 99mTc-MAG3. These snakes were anesthetized and a dynamic frame mode acquisition was obtained for 30 minutes immediately after injection. A 60-second single static frame mode image was then obtained with the snake in a curled position. Pericardial injections could be a potential contributor to erroneously interpreted results. The mean renal uptake was 25% (±9.8%). Correction for remaining radioactivity in the heart did not seem to be necessary if it is was than 10% of the total dose. 99mTc-MAG3 provided consistently high-quality images of the kidneys and further studies are warranted to evaluate its sensitivity for detecting decreased function in snakes with renal disease.[15]

Biopsies are another component of MBDs. The results depend, however, on the quality and location of the bone sample and the experience of pathologists in evaluating herptile samples versus more common mammalian samples. Also, the results need to be considered in conjunction with other findings. Herptile bones seem to be less dense than mammalian bones, so collection technique needs to be appropriate; also, many suspect cases are in animals with pathologic weakening of the bone, so avoiding iatrogenic fractures is critical. With RSHPT, bilateral endoscopic renal evaluation and biopsy can provide tissue samples of excellent diagnostic quality, although proper equipment and training, especially geared toward unique anatomic features of green iguanas, are necessary.[13] It is assumed that endoscopic renal visualization and biopsy can also be useful in other herptile species.

HUSBANDRY AND DIET FACTORS

Husbandry and diet are two critical areas of management for MBDs and often require point-by-point, in-depth recommendations for clients. These expectations and how nothing will change if they are not addressed must be reiterated with clients, in-person and in discharge handouts. Veterinarians must continue to keep current on those recommendations because they constantly change, often requiring World Wide Web research or discussion with successful herpetologists of a particular species in zoos or the general public. Further research into their natural history and environments also provides insight into specific species' care. Finally, everyone must realize that the requirements to keeping a particular herptile in an ideal captive situation varies significantly by geographic location.

Temperature is an often overlooked factor for ideal reptile health and in particular for the prevention of MBDs. Uptake and action of UV radiation (UV-A and UV-B) needs to occur in a microenvironment that is of the appropriate temperature. Many times, herptiles can self-regulate temperature appropriateness if given a temperature gradient to select from. Many herptiles seem to shun warm areas because of bright light in their eyes or that they feel exposed in the heat and light because of a lack of hiding opportunities. Each species has species-specific temperature ranges. Clients also need to recognize that changes in indoor house temperature due to seasonal variation require the modification of heating set-ups dependent on strategic placement of digital thermometers. For me, in summer, some of my reptiles require supplemental only at night whereas in winter in colder climates, three separate ceramic heat emitters may be needed 24 hours per day to maintain the same temperature. Owners often do not notice this. One option in colder climes is to encourage owners to have summer and winter enclosures, with the latter smaller but easier and more economical to heat.

UV-B radiation exposure, dietary cholecalciferol, and skin-generated vitamin D_3 synthesis were compared between adult males of two species of Jamaican anoles (*Anolis* spp). The more shade-tolerant and thermal-conforming *A lineotopus merope*, rarely exposed to full sun, experienced less UV-B irradiation in its shady environment than the more heliophilic and thermophilic *A sagrei*, which frequently basked in full sun during morning. Both species obtained detectable levels of cholecalciferol in their diet, but the heliophilic *A sagrei* obtained more. To compensate for less availability of UV-B and cholecalciferol, the skin of *A lineotopus merope* seems to have acquired a greater sensitivity than that of *A sagrei* regarding UV-B–induced vitamin D_3 photobiosynthesis, which was assessed by observing a greater conversion of provitamin D_3 to photoproducts in skin exposed to UV-B from a sunlamp. The reduced skin sensitivity of *A sagrei* regarding vitamin D_3 photobiosynthesis may reflect a correlated response associated with less need for vitamin D_3 photobiosynthesis and a greater need for UV-B screening capacity as an adaptation to a more damaging UV-B environment. The possibility, however, that adaptations for photobiosynthesis of vitamin D and for protection from skin damage could involve independent mechanisms needs investigation.[16]

There is no substitute for unfiltered, natural sunlight. For several reasons, however, many pet reptiles cannot get adequate exposure to this. And what constitutes adequate exposure? Latitude, time of year, temperature, species, and elevation need to be considered. The right answer is neither obvious nor easy to determine. If clients can take their herptiles outside, they need to watch for overheating, UV burns (usually on the dorsum or eyes—hard to differentiate from thermal burns), and the fact that many herptiles become extremely active and fast moving in natural warm sunlight, leading to a herptile potentially engaging in aggressive or evasive action.

In the laboratory, panther chameleons exhibited a positive phototaxis to greater visible UV-A and UV-B light. With equivalent high irradiances of UV-A or UV-B, however, their response to UV-B was significantly greater than to UV-A. Exposure of in vitro skin patches of panther chameleons to high UV-B (90 $\mu W/cm^2$) for 1 hour significantly enhanced cholecalciferol concentration.[9] Voluntary exposure to higher UV-B irradiance (70 vs 1 $\mu W/cm^2$) resulted in greater circulating calcidiol in female panther chameleons (604 vs 92 ng/mL). Depending on dietary intake of cholecalciferol, chameleons adjusted their exposure time to UV-B irradiation as if regulating their endogenous production of the hormone. When dietary intake was low (1–3 IU/g), they exposed themselves to significantly more UV-producing light; when intake was high (9–129 IU/g), they exposed themselves to less. Vitamin D_3 photoregulation seemed to be an additional component of the function of basking.[9] Panther chameleons with low dietary cholecalciferol intake significantly increased exposure to UV in natural sunlight compared with those with high dietary cholecalciferol intake. All lizards fed low dietary cholecalciferol regulated within optimal UV levels with extreme effectiveness (ability to regulate within optimal UV levels relative to available UV). Chameleons of both dietary treatments regulated UV exposure with great precision, exhibiting little variation among individuals within treatments. This demonstrated the importance of basking for nonthermoregulatory purposes and as an integral mechanism for the regulation of vitamin D_3. Panther chameleons behaviorally regulate exposure to UV in natural sunlight with high precision, accuracy, and effectiveness.[17] A study of red-eared slider turtles post estivation found that the mean calcidiol levels differed significantly between turtles provided supplemental UV radiation (71.7 nmol/L) and those not provided UV radiation (31.4 nmol/L).[7] As discussed previously, anoles showed selective exposure behavior when exposed themselves to natural UV as needed,[16] and varying UV levels opportunities should be provided in captivity for herptiles also, as recommended for heat. Places to hide from UV radiation and to partial expose only certain parts of body to UV can allow for better opportunities. Likewise, UV exposure with varying thermal opportunities is important. As with red-eared sliders, juvenile Blanding's turtles (Emydoidea blandingii), had significantly higher circulating calcidiol levels when supplemented with UV-B radiation. This leads to the recommendation for UV supplementation for a second basking site, if several semiaquatic chelonians are housed in the same enclosure.[18]

What follows is a simplification of how I have interpreted scientific studies and natural history observational reports on species; however, each species is unique and research should be performed on unfamiliar species to see whether or not these rules of thumb are applicable. Opportunities to get out of this intense level of UV-B, as in the wild, are critical to avoid UV radiation and thermal burns.

- For desert-dwelling diurnal lizards or chelonians, high UV-B levels (10% or full unfiltered sun, 12 hours) are recommended.
- For diurnal arboreal lizards or semiaquatic basking chelonians, moderate levels of UV-B (5%, 12 hours) are recommended.
- For diurnal terrestrial lizards or chelonians from a forested environment, low levels of UV-B (5%, 6 hours) are recommended.
- For nocturnal lizards or amphibians, low levels of UV-B (2%, 6 hours) are recommended.
- Snakes they seem to get adequate levels of calcium and cholecalciferol from the ingestion of whole vertebrate prey (or earthworms—usually Lumbricus terrestris in the case of many minute snake species or juveniles). An exception to this, anecdotally, may be diamond pythons (Morelia spilota spilota), indigo snakes (Drymarchon corais), some aquatic species, the insectivorous rough and smooth green snakes (Opheodrys aestivus and O vernalis), and other arboreal, diurnal snakes.[2] I have had cases of pathologic rib fractures in green tree pythons (M viridis) with minimal handling that anecdotally resolved with the addition of low level UV-B. There are no known studies, however, that have more thoroughly evaluated this urban legend in these snake species.
- There are differences of opinion on the need for UV-B for crocodilians and many chelonians, although it may be best to default to at least minimal to moderate levels of UV-B until studies better determine their needs.
- Albino (amelanistic), hypomelanistic, snow, blizzard, pastel, tangerine, lavender, yellow, pied, anerythristic, leucistic, xanthochromistic, or any other genetic mutant with less than normal levels of melanin are more susceptible to UV light burns of the eyes and dorsal skin, so lower levels of UV supplementation (if any) should be provided with plenty of hiding spots and close monitoring of the skin.

For most captive herptiles, it has been recommended to supplement the diet with calcium of some sort, except for those eating whole prey. Unfortunately, there are few scientific studies evaluating calcium types in herptiles, so medical research is extrapolated from humans with osteoporosis or children with MBDs. In mammals, an acidic intestinal pH is required for calcium absorption. Calcium is also absorbed in the ionized form. How herptiles actually eat their food seems important in how they process or digest the nutrients. Do they swallow the prey whole, or do they chew it? The answer to the question may determine whether or not prey should be gut loaded or dusted and why there are conflicting studies on the benefits of these two techniques. In juvenile leopard tortoises, one group was fed a basic low-calcium feed for 6 months, and the other 3 groups were fed the same basic diet supplemented with 1, 3, and 9 times the amount of calcium recommended as a supplement to the diet of reptiles. The animals' bone mineral content and bone mineral density were estimated by DXA scan. Those receiving no calcium supplement had bone calcium depletion, and the shell of the tortoises receiving the recommended level of calcium did not calcify to the extent expected. Tortoises receiving 3 times the recommended level of calcium supplementation had the highest growth rate and were thriving. Metastatic calcifications were observed post mortem, however, in the 2 groups that were given the highest doses of calcium.[19]

Calcium comes in many forms. Although there is a lot of debate on which form is best, it is important to understand the strengths and weaknesses of each type, at least as they are understood in humans. Calcium carbonate (Tums, coral calcium, or cuttlebones) is the least expensive and should be taken with food. It requires low pH levels for proper absorption in the intestine. In humans, calcium absorption from calcium carbonate is similar to the absorption of milk calcium from milk. Calcium carbonate is 40% elemental calcium (1000 mg = 400 mg of calcium). Calcium citrate does not need to be taken with food, is less likely to cause constipation and gas, and has a lower risk of contributing to kidney stone formation. Calcium citrate is 21% elemental calcium (1000 mg = 210 mg calcium). It is more expensive and more of it must be taken to get the same amount of calcium. Calcium phosphate splits the difference in cost, is easily absorbed, and is the least likely to cause constipation and gas. Calcium lactate has similar absorption as calcium carbonate but is more expensive. Calcium lactate, calcium gluconate, and calcium glubionate are less concentrated forms of calcium and are not practical oral supplements in humans often due to volume.[20] Calcium glubionate is still commonly used, however, especially for treatment of MBDs in reptiles, particularly because of safety. I select and prefer using human products with calcium carbonate. Unfortunately, nutraceutical products for animals, such as vitamin and mineral supplements, are not heavily regulated and there are significant concerns based on published studies as to what certain animal products report to contain and what they actually contain, whether or not there is batch variation or even if every sample is tested for quality control. My opinion is that there is no purpose in supplementing any human or pet product for a herptile containing phosphorus without evidence of a phosphorus deficiency. High percentages of calcium in the diet can affect palatability to certain herptiles. Calcium sand as substrate has been found to cause impactions in herptiles and is not recommended to use as a substrate or as a calcium supplement.

As discussed previously, oral cholecalciferol supplementation is necessary in herptiles not entirely reliant on UV radiation for vitamin D_3 creation. Yet, how to do this and deciding which products to use present a conundrum. Does dusting provide much nutrient benefit or is it a wasted effort altogether? Use a product with added calcium? What is benefit to having phosphorus in the mixture? Should human products be used instead of pet products because of the higher standards they must meet (albeit fewer standards than for medications)? For some species, an ideal situation seems to be using a combination of UV radiation and oral cholecalciferol. How much is needed and how much is too much? Should it be gut loaded into the invertebrates' gastrointestinal system or applied topically? These are all questions that need scientific, evidence-based answers and until then, we are often left guessing or extrapolating. Hemolymph collected from six wild-caught, subadult goliath birdeater spiders (*Theraphosa blondi*) was analyzed for calcidiol and was detected in all of the spiders with a mean of 5.7 nmol/L (±1.5 nmol/L). How they got calcidiol was unknown; UV radiation was thought unlikely and dietary from prey invertebrates was thought possible.[21]

Gut loading and dusting of invertebrates has been recommended for many years to compensate for their naturally poor calcium content (exceptions are snails and earthworms [*Lumbricus terrestris*] fed calcium-rich soil). Gut loading refers to feeding the invertebrate a calcium-rich diet, then feeding the invertebrate to provide calcium to the herptile. Diets too high in calcium, however, are considered unpalatable in many crickets (*Acheta domesticus*). Dusting (or shake and baking) invertebrates may provide some extra calcium; however, toxicity reports in certain anurans and the rapid loss of the calcium dust from the invertebrate, should it not be eaten immediately, need to be considered.[22] Some invertebrates, such as wax worms (*Galleria Mellonella*) and Phoenix worms (*Hermetia illucens*) are not able to be gut loaded, so any supplemental calcium or cholecalciferol could be at best dusted on them. Phoenix worms, the larval form of the soldier fly, may have a moderately good calcium/phosphorous ratio, but there have been anecdotal reports by my colleagues of unpalatability, undigestibility, and even potential gastrointestinal rupture. This can vary by species of herptile fed to, but caution and further research are recommended. A recent study found that feeding of Mazuri Hi-Ca Cricket diet (http://www.mazuri.com/PDF/5m38. pdf) to mealworms (*Tenebrio molitor*) and superworms (*Zophobas morio*) enabled the nutrient composition of the larvae to reach a calcium/phosphorus ratio of 1.31:1 in mealworms (or 2.42 g/kcal) and 1.47:1 in superworms after 48 hours of feeding on the diet. These ratios are reported to be slightly lower than those recommended for rats (1.66:1); however, there are no nutritional evaluations for the needs of any herptile.[23] Two studies looked at various diets fed to crickets and found that certain calcium-fortified diets increased the crickets' calcium levels compared with controls but found several of the diets advertised as calcium fortified did no better than an unfortified control diet.[24,25] Donoghue[22] has an excellent chart in her chapter in *Reptile Medicine and Surgery* that shows the natural, unsupplemented calcium and phosphorus levels of many commonly fed invertebrates. Earthworms were the only ones with a better than a 1:1 calcium/phosphorus ratio, with most other ratios approaching an inverted 1:6 versus the recommended 2:1 or greater. Most vertebrates have an adequate ratio of calcium to phosphorus, although immature specimens, such as 1-day-old chickens (*Gallus domesticus*) or pinkie mice (*Mus musculus*), are considered inadequate for long-term calcium sources.

For herbivores, the key portion of the diet from a calcium perspective is lots of leafy greens. These are often best purchased in a prepackaged salad mix, with the spring mix best in my opinion. Many older references recommend other greens, such as kale or chard, but these greens have strong flavors and can be rejected by herbivorous reptiles. Noniceberg lettuces have great calcium/phosphorous ratios, sprouts tend to have inverted ratios, and most other vegetables have at best a 1:1 ratio, but many are inverted. With fruits, most are inverted ratios; however, berries often are 1:1. Prickly pear cactus and alfalfa hay have excellent ratios, with timothy hay less so and orchard grass having an inverted one. Oxalates are a compound found in some plants that bind calcium. Spinach, rhubarb, cabbage, peas, potatoes, and beet greens contain these and should be avoided in MBD reptiles.[22]

A concern with aquatic species, such as semiaquatic chelonians, semiaquatic lizards and snakes, and amphibians, is the effect of calcium in the environmental water. Distilled and demineralized water have all minerals, including calcium salts, removed. These should particularly be avoided with amphibians. Softened water has sodium replacing calcium and magnesium. Calcium-enhanced water leads to significantly greater absorption of calcium in humans when compared with dairy products; however, this has not been studied in herptiles.[22] With RSHPT, ideal species hydration is obvious. Many herptiles not only drink water but also engage in cloacal drinking, passive absorption of the water into the cloaca for storage in urinary bladders, the cloaca itself, or even ureters in those species lacking a urinary bladder. I recommend mandatory soaks 1 to 7 times weekly for many herptiles, depending on their hematocrit and plasma protein levels, owner's geographic location, and environmental conditions of the immediate enclosure. Many arboreal species are ill suited for soaking, and many desert species may not handle evenly slightly deep water well. I recommend reptiles be soaked in a separate container, at a depth of one-quarter the height of the animal's body at approximately 43°C (110°F). Amphibians differ by a recommended temperature of no greater than 27°C (82°F). Usually amphibians' environments are very humid, so this recommendation generally pertains more to terrestrial salamanders and anurans, in particular toads. In most cases, the water cools significantly within 10 to 15 minutes, so the water should be refreshed or the process completed. If there is concern with a specific individual animal, put the container at a slight tilt so the deep end meets the one-quarter height requirement and the shallow end allows the head to be free of water. Many substrates used in cages (chips, barks, and recycled newspaper pellets) are by their nature dehydrating and can contribute to an animal's subclinical chronic dehydration, particularly in nondesert species.

A side note is a condition in chelonians known as pyramiding. The carapaces of captive-raised tortoises often develop a pyramid-shaped osseous growth centrally within the horny plates. With few exceptions (Indian star tortoises [*Geochelone elegans*]), this conical growth pattern is considered pathologic. Fifty recently hatched African spurred tortoises (*G sulcata*) were raised for 5 months under artificial conditions of varying environmental humidity and dietary protein content (14% vs 19% vs 30% crude protein in dry matter). Dry environmental conditions (24.3%–57.8% and 30.6%–74.8% relative humidity) produced taller humps than humid conditions (45%–99% relative humidity). Hump formation differed significantly between these three groups kept under different humidity conditions. Variable dietary protein had a minor, positive impact on this pathologic formation of humps. Levels of calcium and phosphorus in the blood led to no further explanation as to the development of the humps.[26,27] More studies needed to further elucidate complete etiology behind this condition and perhaps calcium metabolism may play a role.

A final environment-related note for herptiles with MBDs is consideration of limiting opportunities for animals with potentially extremely brittle bones to fall or otherwise injure themselves. Removal of climbable items is recommended for many herptiles that can adapt well to a single level environment; however, species, such as chameleons, may require instead cushioning below needed branches, using uncompacted and hydrated sphagnum moss or even old pillows.

TREATMENT

Once an MBD is diagnosed, treatment options can be selected but should be based in many cases on total calcium, ionized calcium, and other diagnostic test results. Previous sections of this article have focused on recommendations for developing a normal environment and diet, and often implementing these recommendations is where efforts are best directed, from an energy and financial perspective. There are some medical therapeutics, however, that may enhance the recovery of these patients; however, there are few, if any, studies in herptiles documenting their effectiveness, so most recommendations are based on anecdotal evidence or extrapolation from human or mammalian medicine. Intravenous (or intramuscular [IM] or subcutaneous) calcium is often considered for MBDs; however, its use is controversial and can be fatal. Very low total calcium in certain mature herptiles has been responsive to IV calcium in a handful of my cases but is usually only given to seizuring animals or those that are comatose and with requisite low calcium values as a last resort. I have had only 5 cases in 13 years respond out of approximately 25 attempts. Giving calcium IM or subcutaneously seems to have little benefit and is painful, so extremely aggressive intervention (IV) should be performed or, due to the chronicity of these cases, oral supplementation is generally the best approach. Other practitioners have had some success, however, in treating hypocalcemic tetany with IM or intracoelomic calcium.[3]

Salmon calcitonin has been used by many practitioners, including me, to manage certain cases of MBDs. It is critical to not administer this if an animal has low blood calcium so is often provided once a patient is stabilized. In humans, salmon calcitonin provides an analgesic effect for the pain usually found with MBDs. In monitoring salmon calcitonin's benefits for patients by monitoring calcium levels, it must be remembered that it only has an effect on ionized calcium levels.[3] Calcitriol supplementation has been discussed previously and is often necessary; however, parenteral administration of a vitamin D product should be carefully considered and is generally not recommended. Bisphosphonates are a class of drugs used in humans to prevent the loss of bone mass and to treat osteoporosis, osteitis deformans, bone metastasis (with or without hypercalcaemia), multiple myeloma, primary hyperparathyroidism, osteogenesis imperfecta, and other conditions that feature bone fragility. Bisphosphonates inhibit the digestion of bone by osteoclasts by encouraging osteoclasts to undergo apoptosis. These may be a future area of research for potential treatment in herptiles with MBDs.

Never underemphasize the necessity of fluids for the MBD-afflicted patients. Fluids can be administered in many different ways, from IV/interosseously to oral to cloacal drinking, but whether or not the diagnosis is RSHPT or some other type, rehydration must be addressed. Nutritional support of a balanced diet in the critical phases is addressed by me by using the carnivore or herbivore critical care diets from Oxbow Animal Health (Murdock, Nebraska; http://www.oxbowhay.com).

In some cases, these herptiles may have suffered fractured bones. Often these fractures healed quickly, albeit via malunion. With spinal fractures, prognoses are often guarded, although some regain hind limb function once swelling and remodeling have resolved. In the short term, an honest discussion of quality of life needs to occur with owners, and regular enemas to help express feces and urine are required, if an animal is unable to urinate or defecate on its own. With limb fractures, surgical repair (internal and external) should be avoided whenever possible, because the likelihood of anesthetic recovery is lower in MBD animals and the likelihood of iatrogenic additional fractures is higher. Splinting limbs to the body or tail or using smoothed syringe cases as splints has worked for me in the past. Pain in these patients with MBDs, whether or not fracture, is described as considerable in some humans and mammals and should be assumed to be so in herptiles until proved otherwise. Management of pain is in its infancy in terms of understanding in herptiles, so guidance on ways to manage this are best left for future articles on pain management.

REFERENCES

1. Available at: http://www.uvguide.co.uk/whatreptilesneed.htm. Accessed January 16, 2010.
2. Antwis RE, Browne RK. Ultraviolet radiation and vitamin D-3 in amphibian health, behaviour, diet and conservation. Comp Biochem Physiol A Mol Integr Physiol 2009;154(2):184–90.

3. Mader D. Metabolic bone disorders. In: Mader D, editor. Reptile medicine and surgery. 2nd edition. St. Louis (MO): Saunders/Elsevier; 2006. p. 841–51.
4. Wright K. Two common disorders of captive bearded dragons (*Pogona vitticeps*): nutritional secondary hyperparathyroidism and constipation. Journal of Exotic Pet Medicine 2008;17(4):267–72. Available at: http://www.exoticpetmedicine.com/issues/contents?issue_key=S1557-5063%2808%29X0005-9. Accessed May 4, 2010.
5. Isaza R, Garner M, Jacobson E. Proliferative osteoarthritis and osteoarthrosis in 15 snakes. J Zoo Wildl Med 2000;31(1):20–7.
6. Dennis PM, Bennett RA, Harr KE, et al. Plasma concentration of ionized calcium in healthy iguanas. J Am Vet Med Assoc 2001;219(3):326–8.
7. Acierno MJ, Mitchell MA, Roundtree MK, et al. Effects of ultraviolet radiation on 25-hydroxyvitamin D3 synthesis in red-eared slider turtles (*Trachemys scripta elegans*). Am J Vet Res 2006;67(12):2046–9.
8. Eatwell K. Plasma concentrations of 25-hydroxycholecalciferol in 22 captive tortoises (*Testudo* species). Vet Rec 2008;162(11):342–5.
9. Ferguson GW, Gehrmann WH, Karsten KB, et al. Do panther chameleons bask to regulate endogenous vitamin D3 production? Physiol Biochem Zool 2003;76(1):52–9.
10. Laing CJ, Trube A, Shea GM, et al. The requirement for natural sunlight to prevent vitamin D deficiency in iguanian lizards. J Zoo Wildl Med 2001;32(3):342–8.
11. Ramer JC, Maria R, Reichard T, et al. Vitamin D status of wild Ricord's iguanas (*Cyclura ricordii*) and captive and wild rhinoceros iguanas (*Cyclura cornuta cornuta*) in the Dominican Republic. J Zoo Wildl Med 2005;36(2):188–91.
12. Zotti A, Selleri P, Carnier P, et al. Relationship between metabolic bone disease and bone mineral density measured by dual-energy X-ray absorptiometry in the green iguana (*Iguana iguana*). Vet Radiol Ultrasound 2004;45(1):10–6.
13. Hernandez-Divers SJ, Stahl SJ, Stedman NL, et al. Renal evaluation in the healthy green iguana (*Iguana iguana*): assessment of plasma biochemistry, glomerular filtration rate, and endoscopic biopsy. J Zoo Wildl Med 2005;36(2):155–68.
14. Greer LL, Daniel GB, Shearn-Bochsler VI, et al. Evaluation of the use of technetium Tc 99m diethylenetriamine pentaacetic acid and technetium Tc 99m dimercaptosuccinic acid for scintigraphic imaging of the kidneys in green iguanas (*Iguana iguana*). Am J Vet Res 2005;66:87–92.
15. Sykes JM 4th, Schumacher J, Avenell J, et al. Preliminary evaluation of 99mTechnetium diethylenetriamine pentaacetic acid, 99mTechnetium dimercaptosuccinic acid, and 99mTechnetium mercaptoacetyltriglycine for renal scintigraphy in corn snakes (*Elaphe guttata guttata*). Vet Radiol Ultrasound 2006;47(2):222–7.
16. Ferguson GW, Gehrmann WH, Karsten KB, et al. Ultraviolet exposure and vitamin D synthesis in a sun-dwelling and a shade-dwelling species of *Anolis*: are there adaptations for lower ultraviolet B and dietary vitamin D3 availability in the shade? Physiol Biochem Zool 2005;78(2):193–200.
17. Karsten KB, Ferguson GW, Chen TC, et al. Panther chameleons, *Furcifer pardalis*, behaviorally regulate optimal exposure to UV depending on dietary vitamin D3 status. Physiol Biochem Zool 2009;82(3):218–25.
18. Mitchell M, Thompson D, Augustine R, et al. Effects of ultraviolet radiation on 25-hydroxyvitmain D3 synthesis in juvenile Blanding's turtles (*Emydoidea blandingii*). Proceedings of the Annual Conference of the Association of Reptilian and Amphibian Veterinarians. Milwaukee (WI): Omnipress; 2009. p. 137.
19. Fledelius B, Jørgensen GW, Jensen HE, et al. Influence of the calcium content of the diet offered to leopard tortoises (*Geochelone pardalis*). Vet Rec 2005;156(26): 831–5.

20. Available at: http://en.wikipedia.org/wiki/Calcium. Accessed January 19, 2010.
21. Zachariah TT, Mitchell MA. Vitamin D_3 in the hemolymph of goliath birdeater spiders (*Theraphosa blondi*). J Zoo Wildl Med 2009;40(2):344–6.
22. Donoghue S. Nutrition. In: Mader D, editor. Reptile medicine and surgery. 2nd edition. St. Louis (MO): Saunders/Elsevier; 2006. p. 251–98.
23. Latney L, Toddes B, Wyre N, et al. Evaluation of the nutrient composition of *Tenebrio molitor* and *Zophobas morio* fed supplemental diets utilized to improve the nutrition of insectivorous animals. Proceedings of the Annual Conference of the Association of Reptilian and Amphibian Veterinarians. Milwaukee (WI): Omnipress; 2009. p. 173.
24. Finke M, Dunham S, Kwabi C. Evaluation of four dry commercial gut loading products for improving the calcium content of crickets, *Acheta domesticus*. J Herp Med Surg 2005;15(1):7–12.
25. Finke M, Dunham S, Cole J. Evaluation of various calcium-fortified high moisture commercial products for improving the calcium content of crickets, *Acheta domesticus*. J Herp Med Surg 2004;14(2):17–20.
26. Wiesner CS, Iben C. Influence of environmental humidity and dietary protein on pyramidal growth of carapaces in African spurred tortoises (*Geochelone sulcata*). J Anim Physiol Anim Nutr (Berl) 2003;87:66–74.
27. Available at: http://en.wikipedia.org/wiki/Bisphosphonate. Accessed January 22, 2010.

Avian Renal System: Clinical Implications

Armando G. Burgos-Rodríguez, DVM, ABVP-Avian

KEYWORDS

• Avian • Renal • Diagnostics • Diseases • Treatments

Avian renal disease is common in veterinary practice.[1] However, it is often diagnosed during an advanced stage of disease. In the last few years, avian medicine has advanced in the recognition of kidney disease, but there is still a dearth of knowledge that needs to be rectified to better understand these diseases. This article serves as a guide to the current literature as well as some review topics pertinent to clinical avian renal disease.

ANATOMY AND PHYSIOLOGY

The avian renal system has anatomic and physiologic specificities that influence disease processes, diagnostics and treatment modalities. The kidneys are deeply imbedded within the renal fossae, the ventral depression of the synsacrum.[2] This is clinically relevant in cases of trauma and in the interpretation of imaging techniques. Nerves from the sacral and lumbar plexus pass through the kidneys.[2,3] Because of the close association with the kidney, any case of renal enlargement can cause nerve impingement, leading to paresis or paralysis. The kidneys account for approximately 1% of the bird's body weight.[2,3] They are symmetric and contain 3 lobes: cranial, middle, and caudal.[2] There are some species variations; for example, in passerines the middle and caudal lobes are fused.[2] In several species, such as herons, puffins, and penguins, the caudal lobe of the kidneys are fused at the midline.[2] Three main arteries supply each lobe of the kidney: the cranial, middle, and caudal renal artery, each supplying blood to its respective lobe.[2] The external iliac artery runs between the cranial and middle lobes, and the ischiadic artery runs between the middle and caudal lobes.

In birds, the most clinically significant renal anatomic feature is the renal portal system. The renal portal system is a ring of vasculature composed of cranial and caudal renal portal veins that branch off the left and right external iliac veins and left and right common iliac veins.[4,5] The renal portal system receives blood from the caudal mesenteric vein, the ischiatic vein, the internal vertebral venous sinus, and the internal iliac vein.[3] The renal portal system has a valve in the common iliac vein

The author has nothing to disclose.

Clínica Veterinaria San Agustín, #26 Marginal 65 de Infantería, Río Piedras, Puerto Rico 00923

E-mail address: burgosag@hotmail.com

Vet Clin Exot Anim 13 (2010) 393–411

doi:10.1016/j.cvex.2010.05.001

vetexotic.theclinics.com

that is responsible for diverting blood away from or to the kidneys[4,5] The renal portal system is under adrenergic and cholinergic stimulation.[3] When the valve is closed as a result of stimulation by acetylcholine, blood is diverted straight to the kidneys and, when it is open as a result of stimulation by epinephrine, blood goes directly into the vena cava. This arrangement has clinical implications because blood from the caudal part of the body can travel directly to the kidneys. Although intramuscular injections in the legs are not routinely given in avian species, it is important to understand the function of the renal portal system, particularly when using potentially nephrotoxic drugs or drugs that may be cleared by the kidneys.

Avian kidneys differ from mammalian kidneys in that there is no defined cortex, medulla, or renal pelvis.[3] The avian kidney has 2 types of nephrons; the reptilian type and the mammalian type.[2] The mammalian type has cortical proximal and convoluted tubules and a loop with thin and thick segments descending into the medullary cones. The reptilian-type nephrons are smaller and more numerous, with only a short, poorly defined intermediate segment between the proximal and distal convoluted tubules with no loop of Henle.[3,5] The avian glomerulus has a similar structure and function to its mammalian counterpart.[6]

In the normal bird, most protein is excluded from the glomerular filtrate. The concentrations of glucose, amino acids, and electrolyte in the filtrate are the same as in plasma.[6] Glucose, most sodium, chloride, and amino acids are reabsorbed with water in the proximal convoluted tubule. The loop of Henle of the mammalian-type nephrons creates an osmotic gradient, resulting in an isotonic filtrate. In the distal convoluted tubules the filtrate becomes hypotonic as additional sodium is removed. This filtrate passes through the collecting ducts, which are impermeable to water, to produce hypotonic urine.[6]

The ureter starts at the cranial division of the kidney and courses caudally then branches to the middle and caudal renal lobes ending in the urodeum.[2] The ureter is lined by mucus-secreting pseudostratified epithelium that facilitates the excretion of urates in colloidal suspension.[2,4] The ureteral walls contain fibrous connective tissue and smooth muscle.[2]

Avian urine is stored in the urodeum where it can reflux back into the hindgut for water and electrolyte homeostasis.[4] In addition, in some species there is a supraorbital gland that contributes to water and electrolyte homeostasis.[4,7] This paired gland opens in the nasal cavity and responds to an increased plasma osmolality by secreting a watery fluid that is hyperosmotic to plasma.[4]

In mammals, the end product of protein metabolism is urea. Birds only produce small amounts of urea because they lack a functional urea cycle because of the absence of at least 2 of the essential enzymes.[3] In addition, most of the urea is completely excreted and is affected by hydration status.[8]

Uric acid is the predominant nitrogenous waste in birds and is produced mostly by the liver, with a small portion synthesized by the kidney.[3,9] Most of the uric acid is actively secreted by the proximal tubules.[2,4,10] Approximately 65% of the uric acid is protein bound.[5] In comparison with urea, which requires large quantities of water, uric acid can be excreted as a semisolid suspension with small amounts of water.[11]

Uric acid secretion is independent of water reabsorbtion, so it is minimally influenced by hydration status.[10] This is clinically significant because, as uric acid continues to be secreted, it cannot be flushed away from the ureter; this causes accumulation of uric acid within the tubules and possible ureteral obstruction (**Fig. 1**).

The avian kidney is also involved in regulation of water and electrolytes, production of vitamin D metabolites, excretion of metabolic wastes, and detoxification and secretion of endogenous and exogenous toxins.[3]

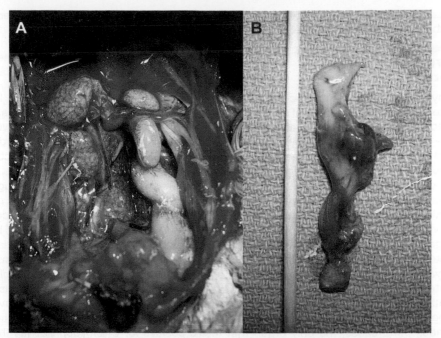

Fig. 1. (*A*) Severe dilation of the left ureter; note the atrophic left kidney and the enlarged right kidney, likely caused by a compensatory mechanism. (*B*) The ureter next to a cotton-tipped applicator to appreciate dilation.

CLINICAL SIGNS

In birds, clinical signs of renal disease are nonspecific. Possible signs include lethargy, weakness, crop stasis, vomiting, polyuria, polydipsia, lameness, muscle atrophy, deposition of urates in joints, feather-damaging behavior or self-mutilation over the synsacrum, and changes in urate character.[12–15] These signs can be present in a plethora of disease processes. For example, polyuria may not be of primary renal origin, and may be associated with diabetes, neoplasia, systemic infections, or other disease syndromes.[6]

RENAL INJURY

Renal injury in any species is a complex process and it is influenced by many factors. In mammals, an inflammatory cascade occurs during renal disease.[9] Although these same processes may not occur in the same manner in avian species, they may provide valuable insight into treatment modalities. During renal ischemia and vasoconstriction, prostaglandin and thromboxane production is increased.[9] This in turn causes changes in vascular resistance, blood flow, and recruitment of inflammatory cells. As a result of vasoconstriction and mesangial cell contraction and the effects of thromboxane A, a decreased glomerular filtration rate (GFR) can occur, leading to renal tubular damage from decreased oxygen and nutrient delivery.

DISEASES

There are several diseases that affect the avian renal system. These diseases can be of infectious origin (bacterial, viral, fungal, and parasitic) as well as noninfectious origin (metabolic, nutritional, toxic, congenital). In a study in which 605 renal samples were submitted, 223 (37%) had renal lesions.[3]

INFECTIOUS CAUSES
Bacteria

Any bacterial organism associated with sepsis may be found in avian renal tissue.[1] In a retrospective study, 50% of nephritis cases were associated with bacterial disease.[4] Bacteria can gain access by an ascending infection from the cloaca to the ureter or via the hematogenous route.[2] Ascending infections have been reported in some birds with ulcerative cloacitis caused by a *Salmonella* infection.[3] In cases of colitis, infectious agents, toxins, and inflammatory products can gain access to the kidneys if blood draining from the colon is diverted into the renal vasculature.[9] It has been suggested that the renal portal system creates the potential for exposure of microbial or toxic agents from the alimentary tract to the kidneys.[4] *Staphylococci* and *Streptococci* have been reported as causative agents for renal disease in finches and canaries.[2] In pigeons, *Salmonella* infections have caused interstitial nephritis.[16,17] Enterobacteriaceae (*Escherichia coli*, *Klebsiella*, *Listeria*, *Yersenia*, and possibly *Proteus*) in chickens, *Erysipelothrix rhusiopathiae* in Coturnic quail and *Pasteurella* have also been implicated in renal disease.[2,3,9] *Mycobacterium* and *Chlamydophila* infections can cause pathology of the kidneys, but they usually cause systemic diseases.[2] There have been reports of *Chlamydophila* infection, but only affecting the kidneys in psittacines.[18] In 2 cases, the only organ that tested positive for *Chlamydophila* was the kidney, despite other organs being affected.

Viruses

Two of the viruses affecting the renal system are adenoviruses and polyomavirus, both causing renal enlargement.[2,3] Adenoviral infections are usually not clinically relevant and tend to be an incidental finding during histopathology.[3] In contrast, polyomavirus infection has been associated with clinical disease in passerines and psittacines.[2,3,6,15] In Gouldian finches, chronic renal disease with glomerular sclerosis is seen in those that survived acute polyomavirus infection.[2] Lesions such as interstitial nonsuppurative inflammation and mesangial cell necrosis may be seen in psittacine birds with avian polyomavirus disease.[2] As many of 70% of these birds will develop secondary glomerulopathy. This lesion is caused by the deposition of dense aggregates of immune complexes within the capillary lumen and the mesangium.[2] Ascites and anasarca have been reported in several species of parrots that are polymerase chain reaction (PCR)-positive for polyomavirus.[2] The ascites and anasarca are attributed to a protein-losing nephropathy or decreased hepatic production of albumin as a result of polyomavirus-induced hepatic necrosis.[2] Other viruses that can cause a nonsuppurative inflammation of the renal interstitium include reovirus, paramyxovirus, and West Nile virus.[2]

Fungi

Fungal infection affecting the kidneys is associated with extension of a fungal air sacculitis or systemic infection (fungal thrombosis).[2,6] The kidney is rarely involved in either case.[3] In 11 cases of systemic mycotic disease, 2 had renal involvement.[3] Both cases had renal infarction associated with thrombi containing fungal hyphae, suspected to be *Aspergillus* species. Large fungal granulomas can affect renal function as a result of a mass effect, but they can also locally invade the kidneys.[6] Unless the kidney is severely affected, renal function is not typically affected in fungal infections.[6] If renal function is affected with a mycotic infection, the bird usually has other signs of severe fungal disease.[6] These signs can include weight loss, labored or open-mouth breathing, voice change, or decreased vocalizations.

Parasites

Parasitic infections affecting the kidneys are not usually found in pet birds. They are often found in waterfowl and marine species.[2,9] Renal coccidiosis is the most common avian renal parasite and has been associated with clinical disease in several species of waterfowl, such as ducks, graylag geese, and a loon.[2,9,19,20] The renal tubules are affected, and severe tubular destruction can occur as well as interstitial nephritis.[9] Systemic protozoan disease in zebra finches has also been reported.[21] *Cryptosporidium* is not a common parasite affecting the kidney in avian medicine, but sporadic cases have been reported.[22,23] *Encephalitozoon hellem* has been associated with nephritis in lovebirds and budgies.[2] *E hellem* has been involved in severe disease in immunocompromised patients. In a study of healthy lovebirds, 25% of birds sampled had spores for *E hellem*.[24] Lovebirds that were PCR-positive for psittacine beak and feather disease were 3 times more likely to shed microsporidian spores.[24]

Renal trematodes have been reported in species such as waterfowl, passerines, poultry, pigeons, barbets, and psittacines.[2,25,26] In 2 barbets, these parasites were not associated with clinical signs and were considered an incidental finding.[25] In 3 psittacine birds, (2 macaws and a white-eared parakeet), clinical signs were associated with *Paratanasia robusta* infection.[26] All 3 birds had enlarged kidneys with yellowish-brown discoloration and irregular cortical surface. Histology showed a granulomatous nephritis with adult worms present within the dilated tubules. Paratanasia infection requires the ingestion of a terrestrial snail, and the authors of the article believed that the *Paratanasia* infection of these birds was accidental, as snails are not normally part of the psittacine diet.[26]

NONINFECTIOUS CAUSES
Nutrition

Renal disease such as nephritis, renal calcification (**Fig. 2**), and gout resulting from nutritional problems in avian species have been associated with high calcium and vitamin D, low vitamin A, or high protein levels in the diet.[2,9,11,27,28]

In nestling and adult budgies, diets containing 0.7% or more of calcium caused metastatic mineralization of the kidney.[2] In 1 case of a salmon crested cockatoo in which the diet contained 20 times the recommended amount of vitamin D_3, metastatic calcification of the kidneys, lungs, and proventriculus was present.[12] Recommendation of 1000 IU per kilogram of food has been made for psittacine birds.[12] Nephrosis and nephritis were present in poultry fed diets high in protein and calcium, containing urea, or deficient in vitamin A.[27,28] Hypovitaminosis A may also lead to renal disease.[9] Vitamin A deficiency causes metaplastic changes of the ureters and collecting ducts as well as decreased secretions of mucus within the ureter.[2,10] These metaplastic changes and decreased mucus secretion can lead to ureteral obstruction.[2,10] In poultry, diets low in vitamin A can lead to renal disease. Renal lesions include dilation and impaction of the collecting ducts with cellular debris, inflammatory cells and urates, tubular degeneration, and necrosis.[29] In psittacine birds, some diets are mostly seed based. Because of the likely low vitamin A level present in seeds, a similar association between renal disease and hypovitaminosis A can be made in pet birds.

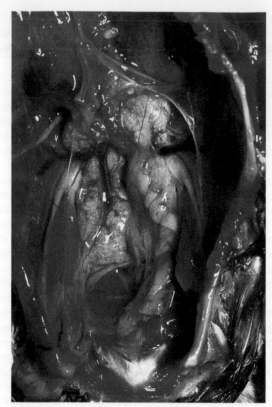

Fig. 2. Severe renal calcification in a cockatiel. (*Courtesy of* Drury Reavill, DVM, ABVP-Avian, ACVP).

Amyloidosis

Renal disease in avian species has been associated with amyloidosis.[9] Amyloidosis is not commonly seen in pet birds but is reported mostly in waterfowl, gulls, shorebirds, and small passerines.[2] Amyloidosis typically affects multiple organs and has been associated with end-stage renal disease.[2,9] It is usually associated with prolonged periods of stress and chronic inflammatory diseases.[30] In a flamingo that died with necrogranulomatous and septic air sacculitis hepatic capsulitis, and atherosclerosis, severe systemic amyloidosis was present. The amyloid deposit in the kidneys was severe and was considered to be the cause of death.[9] It has also been reported that pet geese have been presented with end-stage renal failure with renal amyloidosis.[9]

Lipidosis

Renal tubular lipid deposition has been reported in several avian species such as poultry, psittacines, and captive merlins.[2,15] It has been associated with high-fat or low-protein diets, starvation, biotin deficiency, and chronic liver disease.[2,15] Of clinical relevance in psittacine birds is the presence of chronic active hepatitis in Amazon parrots and cockatiels, which in turn can cause lipid deposition in the kidneys.[2] In pigeons fed diets supplemented with cholesterol, a high incidence of end-stage renal disease was seen compared with pigeons fed a control diet.[16] In psittacine birds this is clinically relevant, because high-fat diets are commonly present and may affect the kidneys.

Myoglobinuric Nephrosis

Myoglobinuric nephrosis has been associated with exertional rhabomyolysis or severe crushing injury.[2] A similar presentation with anuric renal failure and increased uric acid levels has been reported in an ostrich.[3] Myoglobinuria has also been reported in a flamingo with capture myopathy.[15]

Gout

During dehydration there is decreased urine flow, leading to sludging of urate crystals within the tubules. If dehydration is transient, the lesion is reversible; persistent dehydration will result in renal failure.[2] In addition, dehydration can lead to decreased uric acid elimination. As uric acid levels increase in the blood and exceed the solubility of plasma, uric acid precipitation can occur, leading to gout.[2,9]

Two forms of gout occur in the avian species: visceral and articular gout.

Visceral gout occurs as a result of increased plasma uric acid levels, resulting in deposition of urates on various organs, particularly the pericardium, liver, spleen, and kidney (**Fig. 3**).[9,30]

Articular gout occurs when uric acid crystals accumulate within the synovial capsules and tendon sheaths of the joints.[9] In cases of articular gout, deposition of urates in the viscera typically does not occur.[29] Clinical signs include lameness, inability to ambulate, and swellings along the metatarsophalangeal and interphalangeal joints (**Fig. 4**).

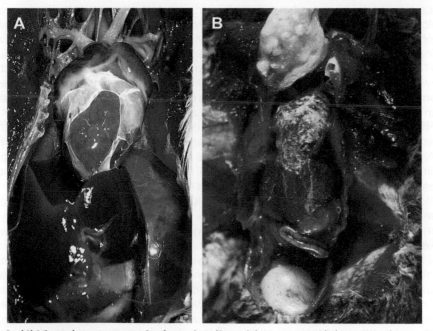

Fig. 3. (*A*) Visceral gout present in the pericardium. (*B*) Urate crystal deposit in the pericardium and hepatic surface. (*Courtesy of* Connie Orcutt, DVM, ABVP-Avian).

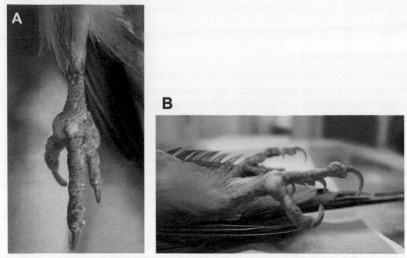

Fig. 4. (*A, B*) Articular gout present on metatarsus and interphalangeal joints.

Toxicity

In many cases, renal toxins cause similar gross and histologic lesions.[2] During the examination, a thorough history is needed to establish a list of potential toxins. The toxic substances affecting birds include rodenticides (vitamin D3 analog), aminoglycosides (gentamicin), lead, and zinc.[2] Renal nephrosis and acute tubular necrosis have been reported in avian species with lead and zinc toxicity.[31] This is clinically significant; this damage to the tubules can lead to further compromise of the patient because uric acid cannot be excreted appropriately, leading to potential uricemia. Calcium EDTA, one of the treatments for metal toxicity, has been associated with nephrotoxicosis in mammals. Calcium EDTA produces acute but reversible necrotizing nephrosis of the proximal convoluted tubules.[32] In birds of prey, calcium EDTA has been used in prolonged therapy (up to 23 days) with no deleterious effect.[33] However, no mention of histopatholgy to evaluate the kidneys of the birds of prey was mentioned. The author has also used calcium EDTA for prolonged treatment (3 weeks) with no clinical side effects in waterfowl and an African gray parrot.

Nephrotoxicity has been seen with the use of aminoglycosides in avian species.[34] In scarlet macaws and galahs, gentamicin administration for 7 days was associated with polyuria and polydipsia.[34] Renal tubule cells have an intrinsic ability to accumulate aminoglycosides via lumenal and basolateral transport in mammalian species.[35] It is presumed that this also occurs in birds but it has not been defined.

Nonsteroidal antiinflammatory drugs (NSAIDs) have the potential for nephrotoxicity in avian species.[36,37] Flunixin meglumine has been associated with nephrotoxicity in flamingos, cranes, and northern bobwhite quail.[38] Diclofenac, a new NSAID, was linked to a decrease in a population of vultures that ingested animals treated with this medication.[36] Acute renal necrosis and visceral gout was present in these birds. Similar histopathologic findings were present in pigeons, broiler chicks, Japanese quail, and mynah experimentally treated with diclofenac.[36] Mycotoxins such as ochratoxin and oosporein have also been associated with renal disease in avian species.[9] Oosporein toxicity has been associated with dehydration, stunted growth, nephromegaly, and death in chickens and turkeys.[9] Ochratoxin is produced by *Aspergillus* and *Penicillium* species that grow on moldy food, usually stored in high-moisture conditions.[39] Oosporein is produced by *Chaetomium* sp and has been found in animal feeds, corn, and food products.[9,40] Although most of the reports have been in poultry, there is the potential for mycotoxins in pet birds because similar feeds, grains, and seeds are used in their diets, and these may be contaminated.

Neoplasia

Renal carcinoma and nephroblastoma are the most common tumors of the avian kidney (**Fig. 5**).[2,41] Other renal neoplasms include adenoma, cystadenoma, fibrosarcoma, and lymphosarcoma.[2]

Most commonly, clinical signs associated with renal tumors are abdominal distension and unilateral or bilateral lameness.[13,41] In a survey of 74 abdominal tumors in budgies, 63.5% were of renal origin.[41] An association with avian leukosis virus was investigated but the presence of antigen did not correlate with the presence or absence of tumors.[41] In 1 case of a cockatiel with a renal adenocarcinoma, osteopenia and muscle atrophy was noted in 1 of the limbs.[13] Prognosis for renal neoplasia is often poor because of the anatomic location of the kidneys, renal vasculature, and lack of response from chemotherapeutic agents.

Congenital Diseases

Congenital diseases occur in avian species but are often considered incidental findings. In a survey of poultry, one of the major defects involved the renal system.[42] Reported abnormalities were renal hypoplasia, dilated ureter, and remnant ureters.

Compensatory hypertrophy of the opposite kidney is generally present.[2]

Renal cysts can be solitary or multiple. This condition usually occurs as a result of incomplete fusion of the cortical portion of the tubule with ureteral tubules. In severe cases, this can lead to renal failure.[2] Glomerular hypervasculatiry, which has also been reported in a canary, leads glomerular deformation but does not result in immediate renal failure.[2]

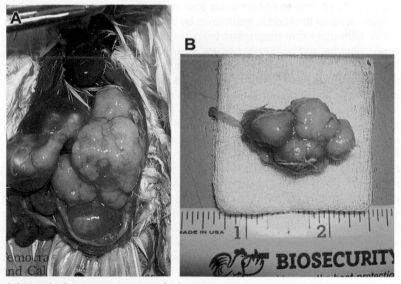

Fig. 5. (*A*) Renal adenocarcinoma on a budgerigar (*Melopsittacus undulatus*). (*B*) Mass after removal from the coelomic cavity.

Urolithiasis

Urolithiasis is a condition seen primarily in caged layer hens.[29] Lesions present within the kidney include tubular degeneration, renal atrophy, and enlargement and thickening of the ureter. The ureter contains accumulated mucus and ureteral stones. The cause of ureterolithiasis is unknown.[29] Possible causes may include water deprivation, excess calcium in the diet, viral infection, dietary/electrolyte imbalances, and hypovitaminosis A.[29,43]

Although not commonly seen in avian species, urolithiasis has been reported in a parrot and a penguin.[44,45] An ureterotomy was performed in an Amazon parrot with chronic ureteral stones.[44] Extracorporeal lithotripsy was performed in a Magellanic penguin (Spheniscus magellanicus) to remove renal stones.[45] In the case of the parrot, 2 ureteroliths were present and required multiple surgeries to remove them. This is partly a result of the complex anatomy of the avian renal system; because the kidneys are imbedded in the synsacrum, the ureter is closely adhered to the kidneys and the caudal aspect of the ureter is located in the dorsal aspect of the cloaca. The lithotripsy used in the penguin is a viable, noninvasive option to remove uroliths, because it uses shock waves to break up calculi, allowing the body to excrete them. One disadvantage is the need for specialized equipment to perform the procedure. As in any animal with urolithiasis, in addition to relieving any obstruction, treatment should include fluids, pain medications, and possibly antibiotics.

DIAGNOSTICS
Bloodwork

Renal function is determined in mammalian species by measuring glomerular filtration. GFR decreases in response to shock, blood loss, dehydration, glomerular or tubular disease, and postrenal obstruction.[6] Accurate determination of GFR requires measurement of clearance of exogenous (inulin) or endogenous compounds that are filtered through the kidneys within a 24-hour period.[6] In avian species, this is not a viable option because of the need for extensive anesthesia and cannulization of the ureter for extended periods of time to obtain urine that has not been contaminated with feces. For that reason, renal function is estimated by the measurement blood analytes such as uric acid, although other diagnostic tests may become available in the future.

Increased plasma uric acid only occurs when renal function is less than 30%, and can occur as a result of severe dehydration, damaged proximal tubules, obstruction, or congenital abnormality.[2,6,10] It only reflects the functional capacity of the renal tubules and is minimally affected by hydration status.[3] In 1 study with pigeons, high levels of plasma uric acid did not correlate with histopathologic changes in the kidneys.[46] The author has seen cases in which the uric acid has been within normal limits and, during postmortem examination and histopathology, the kidneys were severely affected.

Plasma uric acid levels have been shown to be increased after a meal in penguins, birds of prey, and broiler chickens.[47–49] It is therefore important to fast these species approximately 24 hours before blood sampling to get a more accurate value. In psittacines, studies conducted to evaluate changes in uric acid secondary to high-protein diets did not show a positive correlation.[50–52] Only cockatiels fed 70% protein in their diet had an increase in uric acid levels: no renal pathology was found in these birds.[52]

Urea has been used as an indicator for dehydration in birds.[10] Urea is produced in small amounts and is almost entirely excreted in the hydrated animal. In dehydrated pigeons, it has been shown that a large amount of urea is reabsorbed, thus suggesting urea as a potential indicator of dehydration in birds.[8]

Creatinine is excreted as creatine in the urine before its conversion, hence its clinical value is questionable.[5,10,46] Other parameters, such as protein, potassium, calcium, and phosphorus, have been used to aid in the diagnosis of renal disease in mammalian species. These values have not been consistent in the diagnosis of renal disease in birds, although changes in these values should be further investigated.

Urinalysis/Urate Character

Urinalysis is a valuable tool in general veterinary medicine. Urine dipsticks to assess renal disease are routinely used in mammals. In avian practice, urinalysis is not routinely performed.[10] One of its complications is the mixture of urine with fecal contents.[53] This makes the value of urine as a diagnostic tool debatable. A technique has been described to collect urine for urinalysis in pigeons, but this procedure can be time consuming.[54] In this procedure, the pigeon was fastened to a board and a cannula (cutoff 1-mL syringe without the plunger) was placed in the cloaca. Fecal matter from the cloaca was manually removed and periodic checks were performed to remove any feces. Four milliliters of urine were collected from the pigeons. In falcons, urine values for urinalysis were determined by aspirating and then centrifuging the urine portion from the droppings and then using the supernatant for analysis.[55] Birds may have polyuria as a stress response during examination; this may not represent the bird's eliminations at home (**Fig. 6**).[30]

Avian urine specific gravity is typically between 1.005 and 1.020 g/mL because of birds' decreased capacity for concentrating urine; only 10% to 30% of avian nephrons have loops of Henle.[6,7] The presence of abnormal specific gravity, cellular casts, proteinuria, glucosuria, ketonuria, or hematuria can have significant value.[10] Cellular casts in the urine may occur in diseased renal tubules.[30]

Urate color can indicate kidney disease, although other organ such as the liver may be involved. Normally, urates are white but, in presence of hepatic disease, biliverdinuria may occur, causing the urates to turn green or yellow.[6,30] This occurs because of the

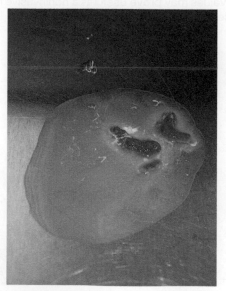

Fig. 6. Polyuria in an African gray parrot; likely stress related, because no evidence of renal disease was found in this bird. Note the excessive urine portion of the dropping.

accumulation of biliverdin, which is normally removed by the liver.[30] Unlike mammals, birds produce small amounts of bilirubin because of the decreased production of an enzyme (biliverdin reductase) that coverts biliverdin into bilirubin.[66] Hence, in a urinalysis, bilirubin should not be present.[6] Bile pigment nephrosis is a common finding in birds with liver disease.[6] Heavy metal toxicity in Amazon parrots causes hemoglobinuria, leading to a red or brown urate color.[6] Hematuria can be present from kidney disease or from cloacal, reproductive, or gastrointestinal origins (**Fig. 7**).[5,30]

Some clinicians have proposed using measurements of urine enzymes to help diagnose renal damage.[4,55] During renal damage, intracellular enzymes are not released into systemic circulation, but are present in the urine. The renal tissue in budgerigars and houbara bustards has high levels of lactate dehydrogenase, aspartate aminotransferase, creatine kinase, alkaline phosphatase, glutamate dehydrogenase, and alanine aminotransferase.[55] Determination of these enzymes may prove useful in the diagnosis of avian renal disease.

N-Acetyl-β-D-Glucosaminidase

N-Acetyl-β-D-glucosaminidase (NAG) is an exoglycolytic enzyme located in renal tubule lysosomes that has been used in mammals as a marker for renal damage.[57] This enzyme also exists in the avian kidney.[57] In pigeons, the kidney has the greatest NAG activity, although NAG is also present in the liver and intestines.[58] NAG is excreted during damage to the renal tubules (gentamicin, destruction of tubular epithelium, and increase in intracellular calcium concentrations in tubular cells). In hens, levels of NAG in the urine were increased after a 40-day supplementation of vitamin D 3.[57] In another study, pigeons that were given gentamicin had significantly increased urine NAG values compared with baseline.[58] In the hen study, timing of NAG measurement was suggested as a critical point in sample collection to provide a valid marker for kidney damage.[57] NAG values in the urine are normally higher in children and men, which may be of importance as normal avian values are developed.[58] Although further studies are needed regarding species variation, gender, and age, measuring urine NAG values may prove useful as a noninvasive measurement of renal disease in avian species.

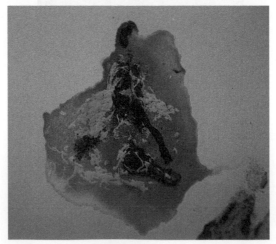

Fig. 7. Hematuria present in an Eclectus parrot with lead toxicity. (*Courtesy of* Lauren Powers, DVM, ABVP-Avian).

Radiographs

The kidneys are located within the synsacral fossae, making it difficult to visualize them. Diverticula from the abdominal air sacs extend between the kidneys and the pelvis.[3] This is visible on a lateral view, and loss of this rim of air is interpreted as a sign of pathologic swelling of the kidney.[3] Increased renal opacity has been associated with dehydration or renal mineralization.[10] Renal tumors in the caudal division will displace coelomic organs in a cranial and ventral direction.[30] Tumors in the cranial and middle division will tend to displace the intestines caudally and ventrally and the ventriculus and liver cranially and ventrally. In some cases, urinary calculi are seen in the ureter (**Fig. 8**). Contrast studies of the gastrointestinal tract may help isolate the location of the kidneys.[5]

Ultrasound

Ultrasound studies to evaluate the kidneys are limited because of the presence of air sacs.[5,30] It does have applications in cases of suspected renomegaly, renal cysts, and ascites in which the kidney may be evaluated.[5] To perform an ultrasound in birds, a small head probe, 7.5-Mhz, 60-degree sector transducer should be used.[5] In some cases, a gel pad standoff may be needed, because the distance from the scanner to the target organ is short. Avian patients should be fasted for at least 3 hours to decrease food material within the gastrointestinal tract.

Advanced Imaging

Other imaging techniques such as magnetic resonance imaging (MRI), computed tomography (CT) scan, and nuclear scintigraphy have been used in avian species to evaluate the renal system, but these may not be readily available. Nuclear scintigraphy has been used to evaluate renal function in pigeons.[46] In this study, it was determined that technetium-99 dimercaptosuccinic acid (DMSA) can be better used to determine renal morphology, and that Tc 99m diethylenetriaminepentacetic acid (DTPA) should be used to evaluate renal function. Although valuable information can be obtained with this type of study, it does require a facility that routinely performs nuclear medicine procedures.

Renal Biopsy

To confirm renal disease antemortem, a renal biopsy is needed. Endoscopic-guided biopsy has been widely used in avian medicine. One of the main advantages of

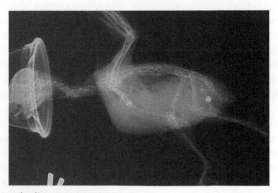

Fig. 8. Two urinary calculi in a psittacine.

endoscopic examination is the direct visualization of both kidneys as well as other coelomic organs.[4] Endoscopic examination of the kidneys is often recommended in cases in which there is persistent uric acid increase, polyuria, anuria, oliguria, and renomegaly on radiographic examination.

The endoscopic approach is usually into the left caudal thoracic air sac.[5] The limb can be retracted caudally or cranially.[59] The landmarks for the caudal technique are the last rib, the iliotibialis muscle, and the synsacrum.[5,59] In the cranial technique, the entry point is caudal to the pelvic limb and behind the last rib.[59] In birds of prey, an approach directly into the abdominal air sacs is not recommended because a large mass of tail muscles has to be penetrated, increasing the risk of bleeding.[4] The middle and caudal renal lobe are preferred kidney biopsy sites because the renal artery near the cranial lobe is more superficially located.[4,10]

A surgical biopsy technique to obtain kidney samples via a dorsal pelvic approach has been described.[60] An advantage of this procedure is that it requires minimal equipment. Also, iatrogenic trauma to the ureter, vas deferens, and caudal renal vein may be avoided.[60] Disadvantages include lack of visualization of other organs and the entire kidney, as with endoscopy. In addition, this procedure is more invasive than endoscopy.

Murexide Test

In cases in which articular gout is suspected, a small amount of aspirate from the suspected lesion is placed on a microscope slide and mixed with nitric acid. After allowing the mixture to dry over a flame, a drop of ammonia is added. If a mauve color develops, uric acid crystals are present.[4]

TREATMENT

Treatment of avian renal disease follows, for the most part, the treatment principles for mammalian renal disease. Because of anatomic and physiologic differences, it is difficult to achieve similar drug concentrations and durations between the 2 classes.[7] Allometric scaling has been used to help calculate drug dosages, taking into consideration the differences in anatomy, physiology, biochemistry, and pharmacokinetics in animals.[7] However, this equation has not been proven to be consistent, so it should be used with caution.[7,35] An overview of this topic has been published.[7]

Fluid Support

Different factors should be taken into consideration before fluid therapy administration, such as dehydration status, anorexia, and urine output. Once- to twice-daily weight measurements in critical patients may aid in determining fluid requirements.

In cases in which weight gain is not being achieved despite supportive care, hydration status must be assessed. Total fluid body requirement is about 4% of body weight in birds.[4] Maintenance fluid dosing for birds is typically 40–50 mL/kg/d.[9,15] Depending on hydration status and stability of the patient, several fluid routes are available. In cases in which the animal is stable and minimally dehydrated, subcutaneous fluids may be given. In more severe cases, intraosseous or intravenous fluids may be needed. Subcutaneous fluid administration is less invasive and does not require placement of catheters that the bird may remove. One major disadvantage is that the rate of absorption is much slower than intravenous or intraosseus fluid administration. Intravenous and intraosseus fluid administration has the advantage of more rapid fluid delivery to the patient, but thus requires the use of catheters that the bird may not tolerate. Caution should be taken to avoid fluid overload during fluid administration.

Antibiotics

As previously mentioned, 50% of avian nephritis cases have been associated with bacterial disease. For this reason, the use of antibiotics in renal disease should be strongly considered. It has been recommended that antibiotic administration should extend for 4 to 6 weeks in cases of bacterial renal disease.[9] Dosages for several antibiotics and other medications used in renal disease have been published.[61] Certain antibiotics should be used with caution, particularly aminoglycosides, in cases in which renal disease is suspected, because these are nephrotoxic.[2]

Nutrition

In cases of renal disease, the bird can also be malnourished or on a seed-based diet. In anorexic animals, hand-feeding formulae can be used to aid with nutrition, by providing essential nutrients needed for recovery. In cases in which hypovitaminosis A is suspected, supplementation of vitamin A should be implemented at a recommended dose of 2000 to 5000 IU/kg intramuscularly once a day for 2 weeks, followed by a lower dose of 1000 IU orally daily.[15] ω-3 fatty acids have been used as an adjunct therapy for renal disease because of their antiinflammatory, lipid-stabilizing, and renal-protective properties, among others.[9] Although no controlled studies in avian species exist regarding the use of ω-3 fatty acids, ω-3 fatty acids have been shown to reduce thromboxane A synthesis and increase production of vasodilatory prostaglandins in dogs.[62] In addition, fatty acid–supplemented dogs had a decreased tubular necrosis secondary to gentamicin administration, compared with control groups. Clinically, ω-3 fatty acids, alone or in combination with low-dose aspirin, have been used successfully in avian cases with confirmed glomerulopathy.[9]

The author has observed that a significant number of psittacine birds are on seed-based diets. These birds need to be gradually switched to a pellet-based diet supplemented with fresh fruits and vegetables. The author recommends that 50% of the diet be pellets, with 25% for fruits and vegetables, 15% for nuts, and 10% for seeds.

TREATMENT OF GOUT/HYPERURICEMIA

Overall, prognosis for gout tends to be poor, as treatment is usually not rewarding and clinical signs tend to interfere with quality of life. Several medications have been used in an attempt to reduce plasma uric acid levels. Surgery has been proposed to help remove the uric acid crystals in articular gout lesions.[9] This procedure is painful, so pain medications should be used. Medical treatments of hyperuricemia have included allopurinol, colchicines, and urate oxidase.[15]

Allopurinol

Allopurinol is a competitive xanthine oxidase inhibitor that blocks the metabolic pathways from hypoxanthine via xanthine to uric acid, thus decreasing uric acid production.[9,63] Allopurinol must be used with caution in birds of prey, because it has been shown that allopurinol increases uric acid levels and may lead to gout.[63] In a study with red-tailed hawks given allopurinol at doses of 50 mg/kg once a day, there was an increase of oxypurinol, a nephrotoxic metabolite of allopurinol, and xanthine, which is believed to reduce renal function.[63]

Urate Oxidase

Urate oxidase catalyzes the conversion of urate and oxygen into allantoin and hydrogen peroxide; allantoin might be further degraded to, and excreted as, allantoic acid.[4] It has been studied in pigeons and red-tailed hawks and may be useful for the treatment of hyperuricemia.[8]

Colchicine

Colchicine has been used in humans to treat gout and has been used clinically in avian species.[9] Colchicine reduces uric acid levels by reversibly inhibiting xanthine dehydrogenase. A recommended dose of 0.0 to 0.04 mg/kg by mouth once or twice a day has been published.[15]

SUMMARY

Although renal disease is frequently diagnosed in avian species, it is often not recognized clinically until its advanced stage. In addition, because the clinical picture in many cases is often similar to other diseases, accurate diagnoses are further complicated. For these reasons, it is imperative to recognize early clinical signs of renal disease and use diagnostic tests to aid in the treatment regimen. Fluid therapy, nutritional support, vitamin A supplementation, ω-3 fatty acids, and broad-spectrum antibiotics are a good initial treatment plan while further diagnostics are performed. It is of utmost importance to address any nutritional deficit that the diet may have, particularly in psittacine birds.

REFERENCES

1. Schmidt RE. Types of renal disease in avian species. Vet Clin North Am Exot Anim Pract 2006;9:97–106.
2. Schmidt RE, Reavill DR, Phalen DN. Urinary system. In: Pathology of pet and aviary birds. Ames (IA): Iowa State Press; 2003. p. 95–107.
3. Phalen DN, Ambrus S, Graham DL. The avian urinary system: form, function, diseases. In: Association of Avian Veterinarians Annual Conference Proceedings. Boca Raton (FL): Association of Avian Veterinarians; 1990. p. 44–57.
4. Lumeij JT. Pathophysiology, diagnosis and treatment of renal disorders in birds of prey. In: Lumeij JT, Remple D, Redig P, et al, editors. Raptor biomedicine III. Lake Worth (FL): Zoological Education Network, Inc; 2000. p. 169–78.
5. Lierz M. Avian renal disease: pathogenesis, diagnosis, and therapy. Vet Clin North Am Exot Anim Pract 2003;6:29–55.
6. Phalen D. Avian renal disorders. In: Fudge AM, editor. Laboratory medicine: avian and exotic pets. Philadelphia: WB Saunders; 2000. p. 61–8.
7. Frazier DL, Jones MP, Orosz SE. Pharmacokinetic considerations of the renal system in birds: part I. Anatomic and physiologic principles of allometric scaling. J Avian Med Surg 1995;9(2):92–103.
8. Lumeij JT. Plasma urea, creatinine and uric acid concentrations in response to dehydration in racing pigeons. Avian Pathol 1987;16:377–82.
9. Echols MS. Evaluating and treating the kidneys. In: Harrison GH, Lightfoot TL, editors. Clinical avian medicine. Palm Beach (FL): Spix Publishing; 2006. p. 451–91.
10. Speer BL. Diseases of the urogenital system. In: Altman RB, Clubb SL, Dorrestein GM, et al, editors. Avian medicine and surgery. Philadelphia: WB Saunders; 1997. p. 625–44.
11. Dorrestein GM. Physiology of the urogenital system. In: Altman RB, Clubb SL, Dorrestein GM, et al, editors. Avian medicine and surgery. Philadelphia: WB Saunders; 1997. p. 622–5.

12. Schoemaker NJ, Lumeij JT, Beynen AC. Polyuria and polydipsia due to vitamin and mineral over supplementation of the diet of a salmon crested cockatoo (*Cacatua moluccensis*) and a blue and gold macaw (*Ara ararauna*). Avian Pathol 1997;26:201–9.
13. Freeman KP, Hahn KA, Jones MP, et al. Right leg muscle atrophy and osteopenia caused by renal adenocarcinoma in a cockatiel (*Melopsittacus undulates*). Vet Radiol Ultrasound 1999;40(2):144–7.
14. Müller K, Göbel T, Müller S, et al. Use of endoscopy and renal biopsy for the diagnosis of kidney disease in free-living birds of prey and owls. Vet Rec 2004; 155(11):326–9.
15. Pollock C. Diagnosis and treatment of avian renal disease. Vet Clin North Am Exot Anim Pract 2006;9(1):107–28.
16. Klumpp SA, Wagner WD. Survey of the pathologic findings in a large production of pigeons, with special reference in pseudomembranous stomatitis and nephritis. Avian Dis 1986;30:740–50.
17. Gevaert D, Nelis J, Verhaeghe B. Plasma chemistry and urine analysis in *Salmonella*-induced polyuria in racing pigeons. Avian Pathol 1991;20: 379–86.
18. Shivaprasad HL, Crespo R, Woolcock PR, et al. Unusual cases of chlamydiosis in psittacines. In: Association of Avian Veterinarians Annual Conference Proceedings. Monterey (CA); 2002. p. 205–7.
19. Montgomery RD, Novilla NM, Shillinger RB. Renal coccidiosis caused by *Eimeria gavial* n. sp. in a common loon. Avian Dis 1978;22(4):809–14.
20. Oksanen A. Mortality associated with renal coccidiosis in juvenile wild greylag geese. J Wildl Dis 1994;30(4):554–6.
21. Helman RG, Jensen JM, Russell RG. Systemic protozoal disease in zebra finches. J Am Vet Med Assoc 1984;185(11):1400–1.
22. Randall CJ. Renal and nasal *Cryptosporidium* in a junglefowl. Vet Rec 1986; 119(6):130–1.
23. Gardiner CH, Imes GD. *Cryptosporidium* sp. in the kidneys of a black-throated finch. J Am Vet Med Assoc 1984;185(11):1401–2.
24. Barton CE, Phalen DN, Snowden KF. Prevalence of microsporidian spores shed by asymptomatic lovebirds: evidence for a potential emerging zoonosis. J Avian Med Surg 2003;17(4):197–202.
25. Rotstein DS, Flowers JR, Wolfe BA, et al. Renal trematodiasis in captive double-toothed barbets (*Lybius bidentatus*). J Zoo Wildl Med 2005;36(1):124–6.
26. Luppi MM, de Melo AL, Motta ROC, et al. Granulomatous nephritis in psittacines associated with parasitism by the trematode *Paratanasia* spp. Vet Parasitol 2007; 146:363–6.
27. Chandra M, Singh B, Singh N, et al. Hematological changes in nephritis in poultry induced by diets high in protein, high in calcium, containing urea or deficient in vitamin A. Poult Sci 1984;63:710–6.
28. Chandra M, Singh B, Gupta PP, et al. Clinicopathological, hematological and biochemical studies in some outbreaks of nephritis in poultry. Avian Dis 1985; 29:590–600.
29. Siller G. Renal pathology of the fowl: a review. Avian Pathol 1981;10:187–262.
30. Styles DK, Phalen DN. Clinical avian urology. Sem Avian Exot Pet Med 1998;7(2): 104–13.
31. Degernes L, Frank RK, Freeman ML, et al. Lead poisoning in trumpeter swans. In: Association of Avian Veterinarians Annual Conference Proceedings. Seattle (WA); 1989. p. 144–55.

32. Kowalczyk D. Clinical management of lead poisoning. J Am Vet Med Assoc 1984; 184(11):858–60.
33. Redig PT, Arent LR. Raptor toxicology. Vet Clin North Am Exot Anim Pract 2008; 11:261–82.
34. Flammer K, Clark C, Drewes L, et al. Adverse effects of gentamicin in scarlet macaws and galahs. Am J Vet Res 1990;51(3):404–7.
35. Frazier DL, Jones MP, Orosz SE. Pharmacokinetic considerations of the renal system in birds: part II. Review of drugs excreted by renal pathways. J Avian Med Surg 1995;9(2):104–21.
36. Hussain I, Khan Z, Khan A, et al. Toxicological effects of diclofenac in four avian species. Avian Pathol 2008;37(3):315–21.
37. Pereira ME, Wether K. Evaluation of the renal effects of flunixin meglumine, ketoprofen and meloxicam in budgerigars (Melopsittacus undulatus). Vet Rec 2007; 160:844–6.
38. Klein PN, Charmatz K, Langenberg J. The effect of flunixin meglumine (Banamine) on the renal function of northern bobwhite quail (Colinus virginiatus): an avian model. In: Association of Avian Veterinarians Annual Conference Proceedings. Boca Raton (FL): Association of Avian Veterinarians; 1994. p. 128–31.
39. Manning RO, Wyatt RD. Toxicity of Aspergillus ochraceus contaminated wheat and different chemical forms of ochratoxin A in broiler chicks. Poult Sci 1984; 63(3):458–65.
40. Pegram RA, Wyatt RD. Avian gout caused by oosporein, a mycotoxin produced by Chaetomium trilaterale. Poult Sci 1981;60(11):2429–40.
41. Neumann U, Kummerfeld N. Neoplasms in budgerigars (Melopsittacus undulatus): clinical, pathological and serological findings with special consideration of kidney tumours. Avian Pathol 1983;12:353–62.
42. Tudor DC. Congenital defects of poultry. Worlds Poult Sci J 1979;35:20–6.
43. Cowen BS, Wideman RF, Rothenbacher H, et al. An outbreak of avian urolithiasis on a large commercial egg farm. Avian Dis 1987;31:392–7.
44. Dennis PM, Bennett A. Ureterotomy for removal of two ureteroliths in a parrot. J Am Vet Med Assoc 2000;217(6):865–8.
45. Machado C, Mihm F, Buckley DN, et al. Disintegration of kidney stones by extracorporeal shockwave lithotripsy in a penguin. In: Proceedings of the First International Conference on Zoological and Avian Medicine. Oahu (HI); 1987. p. 343–9.
46. Marshall K, Craig LE, Jones MP, et al. Quantative renal scintigraphy in domestic pigeons (Columba livia domestica) exposed to toxic doses of gentamicin. Am J Vet Res 2003;64(4):453–62.
47. Wilson HR, Miles RD. Plasma uric acid of broiler breeder and leghorn male chickens: effect of feeding time. Poult Sci 1988;67:345–7.
48. Kolmstetter CM, Ramsay EC. Effects of feeding plasma uric acid and urea concentration in blackfooted penguins (Spheniscus demersus). J Avian Med Surg 2000;14(3):177–9.
49. Lumeij JT, Remple JD. Plasma urea, creatinine and uric acid concentrations in relation to feeding on peregrine falcons (Falco peregrinus). Avian Pathol 1991; 20:79–83.
50. Angel R, Ballam G. Dietary protein effect on parakeet plasma uric acid, reproduction and growth. In: Association of Avian Veterinarians Annual Conference Proceedings. Philadelphia; 1995. p. 27–32.
51. Harper EJ, Skinner ND. Clinical nutrition in small psittacines and passerines. Sem Avian Exot Pet Med 1998;7(3):116–27.

52. Koutsos EA, Smith J, Woods LW, et al. Adult cockatiels (*Nymphicus hollandicus*) metabolically adapt to high protein diets. J Nutr 2001;131(7):2014–20.
53. Laverty G, Skadhauge E. Adaptive strategies for post-renal handling of urine in birds. Comp Biochem Physiol A Physiol 2008;149:246–54.
54. Halsema WB, Alberts H, De Bruijne JJ, et al. Collection and analysis of urine in racing pigeons (*Columba livia domestica*). Avian Pathol 1988;17(1):221–5.
55. Tschopp R, Bailey T, Di Somma A, et al. Urinalysis as a noninvasive health screening procedure in Falconidae. J Avian Med Surg 2007;21(1):8–12.
56. Harr KE. Diagnostic value of biochemistry. In: Harrison GH, Lightfoot TL, editors. Clinical avian medicine. Palm Beach (FL): Spix Publishing; 2006. p. 611–30.
57. Forman MF, Beck MM, Kachman SD. *N*-Acetyl-beta-D glucosaminidase as a marker for renal damage in hens. Poult Sci 1996;75:1563–8.
58. Wimsatt J, Canon N, Pearce R, et al. Assessment of novel avian renal disease markers for the detection of experimental nephrotoxicosis in pigeons (*Columba livia*). J Zoo Wildl Med 2009;40(3):487–94.
59. Lierz M. Diagnostic value of endoscopy and biopsy. In: Harrison GH, Lightfoot TL, editors. Clinical avian medicine. Palm Beach (FL): Spix Publishing; 2006. p. 631–52.
60. Suedemeyer KW, Bermudez A. A new approach to renal biopsy in birds. J Avian Med Surg 1996;10(3):179–86.
61. Pollock CG, Carpenter JW, Antinoff N. Birds. In: Carpenter JW, editor. Exotic animal formulary. 3rd edition. St. Louis (MO): Elsevier Saunders; 2005. p. 135–344.
62. Grauer GF, Greco DS, Behrend EN, et al. Effects of dietary *n*-3 fatty acid supplementation versus thromboxane synthetase inhibition on gentamicin-induced nephrotoxicosis in healthy male dogs. Am J Vet Res 1996;57(6):948–56.
63. Lumeij JT, Sprang PM, Redig PT. Further studies on allopurinol-induced hyperuricaemia and visceral gout in red-tail hawks (*Buteo jamaicensis*). Avian Pathol 1998;27:390–3.

Advanced Diagnostic Approaches and Current Management of Avian Hepatic Disorders

Vanessa L. Grunkemeyer, DVM

KEYWORDS

• Avian • Hepatic • Liver • Bile acid • Hepatoprotectant

GROSS ANATOMY OF THE AVIAN LIVER

The normal adult avian liver is a dark red-purple color and is composed of right and left lobes, with the right lobe being larger in most species (**Fig. 1**). The lobes are enclosed in a thin capsule of connective tissue and joined along the cranial midline.[1,2] In various species, the lobes are subdivided into ventral and dorsal segments, and intermediate processes project from the ventral hilar region. The cranioventral aspects of the lobes surround the apex of the heart and the visceral surface of the liver is in contact with the proventriculus, ventriculus, and spleen. Ventrally the liver is in contact with the sternum and, in most avian species, the liver lobes do not extend beyond the caudal aspect of the sternum.[2]

Bile is drained from both lobes of the liver by the right and left hepatic ducts. The hepatic ducts fuse to form the common hepatoenteric duct, which empties in the distal end of the ascending duodenum.[3,4] When present, the gallbladder is found along the visceral surface of the right liver lobe. The size of the gallbladder can vary significantly between species, with a long gallbladder present in toucans, woodpeckers, and barbets.[1] A branch of the right hepatic duct forms the hepatocystic duct that drains bile to the gallbladder. The cystoenteric duct carries bile from the gallbladder to the duodenum.[3,4] Psittacine species, most species of pigeons, and ostriches do not have gallbladders.[1,2] In these species, the branch of the right hepatic duct forms the right hepatoenteric duct that empties directly into the duodenum.[4]

The liver receives its blood supply from the left and right hepatic arteries, which are branches of the celiac artery, and the hepatic portal veins.[2] The left and right hepatic

Avian and Zoological Medicine Service, Department of Small Animal Clinical Sciences, University of Tennessee College of Veterinary Medicine, 2407 River Drive, C247, Knoxville, TN 37996, USA
E-mail address: vgrunkem@utk.edu

Vet Clin Exot Anim 13 (2010) 413–427
doi:10.1016/j.cvex.2010.05.005
1094-9194/10/$ – see front matter © 2010 Elsevier Inc. All rights reserved.

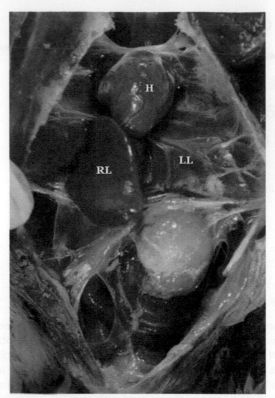

Fig. 1. Normal adult African gray parrot celomic cavity at the time of necropsy. The bird is in dorsal recumbency. A ventral midline incision has been made in the celomic cavity and the sternum has been removed to visualize the internal organs, including the heart (H), right liver lobe (RL), and left liver lobe (LL). (*Courtesy of* Cheryl B. Greenacre, DVM, DABVP [Avian and Small Mammal Specialties], Knoxville, TN.)

portal veins drain the proventriculus, ventriculus, large and small intestines, spleen, and pancreas.[5,6] Blood is drained from the liver by the left and right hepatic veins that join in the liver to form the caudal vena cava.[2]

FUNCTIONS OF THE LIVER

The avian liver performs numerous essential metabolic functions, which include the synthesis, storage, filtration, and excretion of various nutrients and chemicals. Bile acids, which aid in digestion through the emulsification of lipids and the activation of pancreatic enzymes, are synthesized in the liver from cholesterol.[3] Because birds produce little to no biliverdin reductase, hemoglobin is incompletely metabolized to biliverdin in the liver. Thus, unlike in mammals where bilirubin is the primary bile pigment, biliverdin is the primary bile pigment in avian species. This pigment gives the bile a characteristic green color.[4,6] Glycogen is produced by hepatic carbohydrate metabolism and stored in the liver along with iron and lipid-soluble vitamins. The liver is also the site of plasma protein, clotting factor, cholesterol, urea, and uric acid synthesis, and it functions in drug metabolism and excretion.[3,6] In addition, the macrophages in hepatic sinusoids (Kupffer cells) assist in clearing microorganisms from the portal blood.[6]

The liver has a sizeable capacity for regeneration and a large functional reserve. The destruction of hepatic tissue results in regeneration, fibrosis, and/or biliary hyperplasia. Hepatocytes are continually replaced until only one-twelfth of the cells remain undamaged.[7,8] Thus, the diagnosis of liver disease is particularly challenging because up to 80% of liver tissue must be compromised before hepatic dysfunction becomes clinically evident.[3,9]

DIAGNOSING HEPATIC DYSFUNCTION IN THE AVIAN PATIENT

The diagnosis of liver disease is made based on a constellation of supportive evidence from the clinical history, physical examination, clinical pathologic testing, imaging studies, and histopathologic examination of biopsy specimens. Although multiple tests are designed to indicate hepatocellular destruction and to measure hepatic function, these tests often give no indication as to the viability of the remaining hepatic tissue or the inciting cause of the damage.[6,7] Specific testing such as bacterial and fungal cultures, viral polymerase chain reactions, and heavy metal blood levels should be pursued to determine the inciting cause of the hepatic damage.

Patient History and Clinical Signs

Because hepatic dysfunction can result from various insults, the patient's history and clinical signs at the time of presentation are highly variable. The collection of a detailed anamnesis may provide information as to the duration, severity, and cause of the liver disease, and is essential to the complete evaluation of any avian patient. Information gathered about the patient should include, but is not limited to: signalment, history of ownership, diet, reproductive status, habitat design and maintenance, exposure to other animals including both captive and wild birds, health status of other animals in the house/aviary, current medications and supplements, potential toxin exposure, and details regarding the onset and progression of the clinical signs of the bird.[9]

Unfortunately, there are no pathognomonic clinical signs of avian liver disease. Nonspecific signs associated with liver disease in birds include anorexia, lethargy, weakness, dehydration, weight loss, obesity, regurgitation, vomiting, polydipsia, tachycardia, tachypnea, dyspnea, and sudden death.[7,9–11] Birds with hepatic dysfunction can also have a range of integumentary problems including overgrowth and flaking of the beak and nails, abnormal molting, poor feather quality with a darkening of the feather pigment, pruritus, and feather picking.[9,10] Abnormal bruising or bleeding of skin can occur in cases where hepatic failure results in a coagulopathy.[7] Icterus of the skin and sclera (hyperbilirubinemia) is rare in avian patients because of their previously described lack of bilirubin production.[11] Diarrhea, melena, and hematochezia can occur with hepatic disease, and birds that are anorexic for any reason can pass green feces due to an increase in fecal biliverdin. Hepatic dysfunction can also result in polyuria and biliverdinuria, which is a green or yellow coloration of the urine and urates.[7,12,13] Although the presence of biliverdinuria is highly suggestive of liver disease, hemolysis can also result in an increased biliverdin concentration in urates and urine.[12,14] Hepatomegaly and ascites can be associated with liver disease and can result in celomic distension and respiratory compromise (**Fig. 2**).[7,11] Neurologic signs such as tremors, seizures, and paresis can occur in cases with an encephalopathy secondary to hepatic disease.[9,11]

Clinical Pathologic Analysis

Complete blood counts (CBCs), biochemistry profiles, protein electrophoresis, bile acid levels, and plasma dye clearance tests can all provide evidence to support

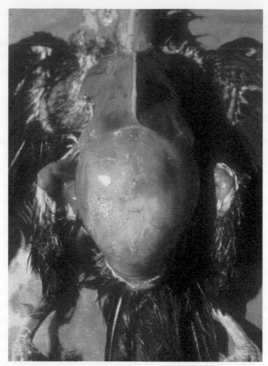

Fig. 2. Celomic distension due to hepatomegaly in a deceased myna bird (*Acridotheres* spp). The bird is in dorsal recumbency with the cranial aspect of the patient toward the top of the image, and the skin has been removed from the bird's ventrum. (*Courtesy of* Edward C. Ramsay, DVM, DACZM, Knoxville, TN.)

a diagnosis of liver pathology and its secondary complications. However, it is important to understand the sensitivity and specificity of these results when evaluating a patient and designing an appropriate treatment plan.

CBC abnormalities in avian patients with liver disease are nonspecific, but they may give an indication as to the chronicity and underlying pathologic condition of the disease process. Anemia can occur in these cases as a result of coagulopathies, hepatic trauma, hemochromatosis, and bone marrow suppression caused by hepatic infection, inflammation, or neoplasia. A leukocytosis may be present with infectious or inflammatory liver disease, especially when it is caused by *Chlamydophila*, *Mycobacterium*, or *Aspergillus*.[15] Examination of blood or buffy coat smears may reveal parasites that can cause hepatic damage such as *Atoxoplasma* spp, *Leukocytozoon* spp, and *Plasmodium* spp.[16]

The results of a biochemistry profile may indicate a loss of the liver's synthetic capabilities, hepatocellular damage, and systemic changes secondary to hepatic disease. As discussed earlier, the liver is responsible for synthesizing plasma proteins, cholesterol, and urea, and has a major role in carbohydrate metabolism. Thus hypocholesterolemia, hypouricemia, hypoglycemia, and hypoproteinemia can all occur with hepatic failure.[17] Hypercholesterolemia can occur in cases of hepatic lipidosis and bile duct obstruction.[18] Although a decrease in total protein levels due to a decrease in plasma albumin can develop as a result of liver disease, this abnormality can result from a multitude of other factors. These factors include overhydration, decreased availability and absorption of protein from the diet, and loss of protein from the gastro-intestinal tract or kidneys. By contrast, patients with infectious or inflammatory hepa-titis may have a hyperproteinemia characterized primarily by a hyperglobulinemia caused by stimulation of the immune system.[19] Protein abnormalities can be further investigated with electrophoresis to determine the relative changes in each protein fraction. Although normal electrophoretic reference ranges have not been determined for all avian patients, characteristic changes in the electrophoretogram may assist in the diagnosis and monitoring of diseases such as chronic active hepatitis.[9,20]

Increases in plasma enzyme activities can indicate the presence of hepatocellular damage and enzyme leakage. Enzyme activity profiles can vary significantly depend-ing on the severity of disease, the species being tested, and concurrent damage to other organ systems. It is best to analyze enzyme activities for patterns of elevation among a profile of enzymes and in repeated blood samples over time to avoid over-interpreting a single enzyme value. Furthermore, normal enzyme activities should not be interpreted as equating to normal hepatic function, but rather as indicating the lack of current detectable hepatocellular damage.[21]

Aspartate aminotransferase (AST), lactate dehydrogenase (LDH), creatinine kinase (CK), and alanine aminotransferase (ALT) have been analyzed in various avian species with hepatic damage. AST is a sensitive indicator of hepatic disease. However, because AST is present in liver tissue and all muscle types, an elevation in AST activity usually indicates either liver or muscle damage.[17,21] LDH is not specific or sensitive for liver damage because it is present in various tissues including liver, muscle, kidney, bone, and erythrocytes.[19] However, LDH has a very short plasma half-life with eleva-tions in this enzyme indicating recent tissue damage.[21] Increases in AST and LDH activity should be interpreted in conjunction with CK, which is a muscle-specific enzyme. When there is a concurrent elevation in CK activity, increases in AST and LDH are more likely caused by muscle damage. However, because AST has a longer plasma half-life than CK and LDH; an elevation in AST but not CK or LDH can indicate muscle or liver damage.[9,21] Decreases in AST and LDH activities can indicate a severe loss of hepatocellular mass.[21] Interpretation of ALT activity has limited diagnostic value in birds because this enzyme is present in almost all tissues, and ALT activity in some healthy avian patients is less than the sensitivity of many analyzers.[19] Hemo-lysis of the blood sample can result in a significant increase in LDH with lesser effects on AST, ALT, and CK.[21]

Gamma-glutamyltransferase (GGT) and glutamyl dehydrogenase (GLDH) are specific indicators of avian liver disease.[21] Increases in plasma GGT activity occur with biliary damage or obstruction, and marked elevations in this enzyme have been noted in cases of avian bile duct carcinoma.[17] GLDH is present within the mitochon-dria of numerous tissues including the liver. Elevations in GLDH have been associated with severe hepatic damage with cellular necrosis, such as occurs with Pacheco disease.[10] Neither of these enzymes is a sensitive indicator of avian liver disease, and normal reference intervals are available for only a few avian species.[19,21]

Hepatic, renal, intestine, and bone isoenzymes of alkaline phosphatase (ALP) have been identified in avian species. However, unlike in mammals where elevations in ALP activity are frequently associated with biliary disease, only very low ALP levels have been identified in the avian liver, and significant elevations in this enzyme have not been associated with hepatic disease.[17]

As discussed earlier, bile acids and bile salts are produced by the liver and secreted into the duodenum through the biliary ducts. Through enterohepatic circulation, more than 90% of the bile acids are reabsorbed in the distal small intestine and extracted from the portal blood by hepatocytes. If the liver is damaged, bile acids are not appropriately extracted, conjugated, and secreted.[21] Thus, the measurement of the bile acid concentration in plasma provides a sensitive and specific indication of hepatic function.[10] In a study where protein electrophoresis, bile acid levels, and enzyme levels including AST, CK, LDH, and GGT were analyzed in 442 psittacine plasma samples, elevated bile acid levels had the highest correlation with histologically confirmed hepatic disease. Nevertheless, bile acid levels were low or normal in 26% of the cases of confirmed hepatic disease and elevated in 18% of the nonhepatic cases in this study.[22]

Assays to measure bile acid concentrations are available in most veterinary laboratories. The clinician should be aware that both radioimmunoassay (RIA) and enzymatic assays are used to determine bile acid concentrations. Because the enzymatic assay measures a wider spectrum of bile acids, the reference values for that test tend to be higher than those for the RIA.[19,21] Unlike the enzymatic assay, the results of RIA performed on avian plasma samples in one study were not affected by lipemia, hemolysis, or elevated LDH concentrations.[23] Ideally, assay-specific and species-specific reference intervals provided by the laboratory where the test was performed should be used for interpretation. Although significant postprandial elevations in bile acids have been noted in pigeons, mallards, and peregrine falcons, other studies investigating fasting and postprandial elevations in avian bile acids have produced inconsistent results.[23–26] Because elevations with hepatobiliary disease are typically much greater than postprandial elevations, many investigators recommend only a single nonfasted sample in birds.[10,21]

Measurement of the clearance of exogenous dyes or sugars injected intravenously can also be used to assess hepatic function. The use of clearance tests involving indocyanine green, sulfobromophthalein, and galactose has been reported in avian species.[9] Studies performed in galahs (*Eolophus roseicapilla*) found that galactose clearance may be a more sensitive indicator of hepatic function than plasma bile acid assays.[27] However, the availability and clinical application of these tests are currently limited, and further research is necessary to assess the value of clearance tests in the diagnosis of avian hepatic disease.[9,17]

Imaging

Radiography and ultrasonography are commonly used to evaluate avian patients with suspected hepatic disease. Additional imaging studies including contrast radiography, computed tomography (CT), magnetic resonance imaging (MRI), and nuclear medicine scans may be used in select cases to provide further diagnostic and prognostic information.

Appropriately positioned, whole body radiographs can be used to assess hepatic size. On a ventrodorsal radiograph, the normal liver silhouettes with the heart to form an "hourglass" shape and it does not extend laterally beyond a line drawn from the scapula to the acetabulum. The normal liver does not extend beyond the caudal aspect of the sternum on a lateral radiograph.[10] Apparent microhepatica of unknown clinical significance is frequently observed on radiographs of macaws and cockatoos.[11] Hepatomegaly may result in widening of the cardiohepatic waist, compression of the abdominal air sacs, rounding of the liver margins, extension of the liver beyond the previously noted margins, cranial displacement of the heart, dorsal displacement of the proventriculus, and caudodorsal displacement of the ventriculus (**Fig. 3**).[28] Summation of an enlarged proventriculus with the liver can cause an apparent enlargement of the hepatic silhouette, and can be differentiated from true hepatomegaly using gastrointestinal contrast radiography or fluoroscopy.[11,28] Other pathologies including cardiomegaly, splenomegaly, air sac disease,

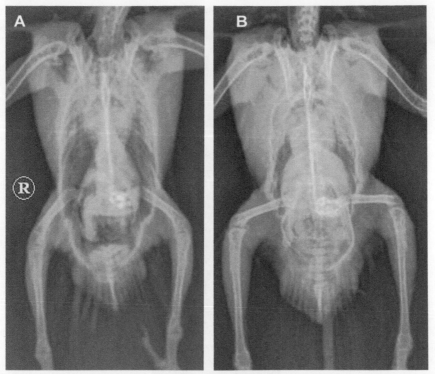

Fig. 3. (A) Ventrodorsal radiograph of a normal adult cockatiel. (B) Ventrodorsal radiograph of an obese adult cockatiel with a history of elevated bile acids, AST, ALT, and hyperuricemia. This radiograph shows a widening of the hepatic silhouette and a loss of the cardiohepatic waist.

and ascites can result in a widening of the cardiohepatic waist and can be further investigated with ultrasonography or other advanced imaging modalities.

Ultrasonography of the avian celomic cavity can be challenging because of the small size of the patient and interference from the air sacs. However, in the patient with hepatic disease, image clarity may be increased by the presence of ascites and the compression of air sacs by organomegaly.[29,30] A fast of 2 to 3 hours before ultrasonography should be adequate to empty the gastrointestinal tract in most avian species. However, some investigators have suggested up to a 2-day fast in carnivorous species to facilitate visualization of the gallbladder.[31] General anesthesia is rarely necessary for ultrasonography, and positioning the patient in dorsal recumbency with cranial aspect of the body elevated at a 30° angle may facilitate the visualization of celomic structures.[29] In cases of avian hepatobiliary disease, ultrasonographic evaluation may detect ascites, changes in the size and normal homogenous echogenicity of the liver, congestion of the hepatic vasculature, and rare pathologic changes in the gallbladder.[31] Centesis of celomic fluid, fine-needle aspiration of liver parenchyma, and hepatic biopsy can all be performed with ultrasonographic guidance. The details of how to obtain these samples are beyond the scope of this article, but these techniques have been described in greater detail by other investigators.[31–33]

The application of CT and MRI in cases of avian hepatic disease has been infrequently reported (**Fig. 4**). However, the high-resolution images acquired with these

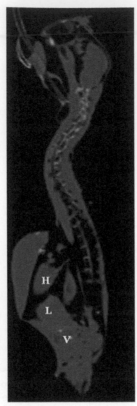

Fig. 4. Sagittal CT image of a Moluccan cockatoo (*Cacatua moluccensis*) with no known liver pathology. The cranial aspect of the patient is toward the top of the image. The heart (H), liver (L), and ventriculus (V) are all noted.

modalities are particularly useful in the precise anatomic localization of masses identified with radiography. In addition, the information provided by these imaging modalities can be useful in staging neoplastic processes and in planning accurate surgical intervention.[29] Drawbacks of CT and MRI include the need to place a potentially compromised patient under general anesthesia to acquire diagnostic images, the increased costs associated with these scans, and the need for a referral to a specialty hospital in most cases.

The use of nuclear medicine technologies has also been rarely reported in cases of avian hepatic disease. Nuclear medicine scans, which include hepatobiliary scintigraphy and positron emission tomography (PET), detect and map the distribution of radiopharmaceuticals that have been administered to a patient in order to diagnose and monitor disease processes. Hepatobiliary scintigraphy is used in mammalian patients to evaluate hepatic function and morphology, and the patency of the biliary tract. In avian medicine, quantitative hepatobiliary scintigraphy using the radiopharmaceutical ^{99m}Tc-mebrofenin has been used to evaluate hepatic function in pigeons before and after exposure to ethylene glycol. A correlation between histologic damage in the liver and scintigraphic measures of hepatic function has been found. However, further research is necessary to determine the clinical applications of this imaging modality in diagnosing and monitoring clinical patients with hepatic disease.[34] PET scans are routinely obtained in human oncology patients for diagnosis and therapeutic monitoring. ^{18}F-Fluorodeoxyglucose (FDG), a glucose analogue labeled with a positron-emitting radionuclide, is the most common radiopharmaceutical used for these scans. FDG-PET scans map the accumulation of FDG within cells with active glucose metabolism such as those of the brain, liver, inflammatory lesions, and neoplastic tissue.[35,36] The FDG-PET scans of 16 healthy Hispaniolan Amazon parrots (*Amazona ventralis*) showed increased radioactivity in the heart, brain, eyes, kidneys, segments of the gastrointestinal system, and some skeletal muscle (**Fig. 5**) (Marcy Souza, DVM, MPH, DABVP (Avian), personal communication, January 2010).[37] Fusion PET/CT scanners are also available, and the integration of these scans allows for the precise anatomic localization of lesions with increased uptake of the radionuclide.[35] To the author's knowledge, neither PET nor PET/CT imaging have been used in the evaluation of avian patients with proven hepatic disease. However, these imaging modalities may have an application in the diagnosis and posttherapeutic monitoring of primary and metastatic hepatic neoplasia in avian species. The drawbacks of nuclear medicine scans are similar to those of CT and MRI, with the additional negative aspect of exposure of the patient and the clinical staff to even higher doses of radiation.

Hepatic Biopsy

Biopsy of the liver is often required to definitively diagnose and appropriately characterize hepatic disease. The diagnostic and prognostic value of a hepatic biopsy is dependent on many factors, including the stage and cause of disease, method of biopsy collection, and tissue handling.[9,38] A hepatic biopsy specimen can be obtained by blind percutaneous techniques, with ultrasonographic guidance, with endoscopic visualization, or surgically. Because there are risks associated with each of these biopsy techniques, the clinician should have a high index of suspicion for the presence of hepatic disease before performing a biopsy. Risks of obtaining a hepatic biopsy

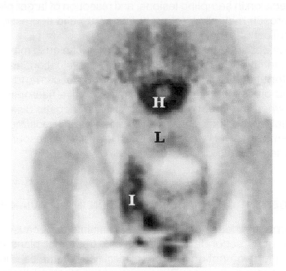

Fig. 5. A 2-deoxy-2-[^{18}F]fluoro-D-glucose (FDG) positron emission tomography scan of a healthy Hispaniolan Amazon parrot (*Amazona ventralis*). The cranial aspect of the patient is toward the top of the image. Increased radioactivity in the heart (H) and intestines (I) is evident, with subjectively less FDG uptake apparent in the liver (L). (*Courtesy of* Marcy J Souza, MPH, DVM, DABVP [Avian Specialty], Knoxville, TN.)

include severe hemorrhage, perforation of other internal organs, asphyxiation secondary to leakage of ascitic fluid into iatrogenically ruptured air sacs, and the associated risks of general anesthesia in a potentially compromised patient.[9] Because coagulopathies can develop secondary clotting factor deficiencies in cases with hepatic dysfunction, the patient's clotting potential should be assessed before obtaining a biopsy specimen. Thrombocytopenia and prolongation of the cutaneous bleeding time, whole blood clotting time, or prothrombin time may indicate decreased coagulation function in the avian patient. However, accurate interpretation of these tests may be complicated by the lack of normal reference values for most avian species.[39] To help prevent aspiration of ascitic fluid, the fluid can be aspirated prior to the anesthetic event and the patient can be positioned in an upright position while under anesthesia.[9]

Endoscopic examination allows for minimally invasive visualization of intracelomic structures and targeted sampling of identified lesions. As with ultrasonography, a preanesthetic fast of at least 3 hours can aid in visualization of organs during the procedure. However, the most common impediment to organ visualization is intracelomic fat in obese patients.[38] A ventral midline approach just caudal to the sternum allows for direct access into the ventral hepatoperitoneal cavities. With this approach, the liver lobes can be visualized and sampled. A lateral approach through either the left or right caudal thoracic air sac can also be used to access the liver. However, because a connection between the caudal thoracic air sacs and the ventral hepatoperitoneal cavities will be made via this approach, it is contraindicated in patients with ascites.[38,40] The reader is referred to other resources for descriptions of the necessary endoscopic instrumentation, specific biopsy techniques, and ideal tissue handling.[38,40,41]

Surgical approaches for hepatic biopsy can include a small keyhole incision or a longer celiotomy incision. For a keyhole hepatic biopsy, a skin incision is made on the ventral midline just caudal to the sternum and the caudal margin of the liver is visualized and biopsied through this incision. A celiotomy allows for greater visualization of the liver, more precision in sampling lesions, and resection of larger pieces of tissue. In addition, this approach may allow for more immediate and aggressive intervention in the event of complications.[9]

Hepatic samples obtained by any of these biopsy techniques may be prepared and submitted for bacterial and fungal culture, cytologic evaluation, and histopathologic examination. Unfortunately, diagnosis of the specific cause and evaluation of the severity of hepatic disease may not be determined until a necropsy is performed. In aviary situations where an infectious or toxic cause of hepatic disease is suspected, it is often beneficial for the flock health to sacrifice a bird for postmortem examination and diagnostic sampling. The reader is referred to additional resources for pathologic descriptions of avian hepatic disorders.[2,42]

MEDICAL MANAGEMENT OF HEPATIC DYSFUNCTION IN THE AVIAN PATIENT

Because avian hepatic disease can result from a multitude of causes and the patient can experience various secondary complications, treatment plans are varied. If the cause of the hepatic dysfunction has been identified, therapies should be directed at treating the diagnosed disease. Discussion of the targeted therapeutic plans for hepatic disorders such as infectious hepatitis, hemochromatosis, hepatic lipidosis, heavy metal toxicosis, and hepatic neoplasia is outside the scope of this article. The reader is referred to additional resources wherein the specific treatments for these diseases are detailed.[11,43,44] Therapies can also be directed at remediating secondary complications of hepatic dysfunction and supporting the remaining cellular function and regeneration.

Secondary complications of hepatic disease can include weakness, respiratory distress, dehydration, anorexia, emaciation, encephalopathy, anemia, or ascites. General supportive care includes providing a quiet, warm environment with oxygen therapy for patients with respiratory compromise. Formulation of an appropriate fluid therapy plan should take into consideration the patient's hydration status, general organ function including noted cardiac and renal disease, and ongoing fluid losses. Fluids should be warmed and dextrose can be added to isotonic crystalloid fluids for hypoglycemic patients.[43]

Nutritional recommendations to support birds with hepatic disease vary because patients can range in body condition from obese to emaciated, and they can have a normal appetite or be anorexic. Diets that contain only 8% protein with low levels of aromatic amino acids and higher levels of branched chain amino acids have been recommended to reduce the hepatic workload in patients with liver disease.[45] However, some investigators have countered that dietary protein should not be restricted in patients with hepatic dysfunction that are not showing signs of encephalopathy.[6] The diet offered to avian patients with hepatic dysfunction should have easily metabolized energy sources such as carbohydrates and fats, and be high in soluble fiber. Vitamin supplementation, such as the use of the antioxidant vitamin E in cases of inflammatory hepatitis, may be of benefit.[7] A patient's dietary requirements can vary significantly with the specific cause of the hepatic disease, especially in cases of hemochromatosis and hepatic lipidosis. In addition, gavage feeding of lique-fied diets may be necessary in anorexic patients.

Hepatic encephalopathy, an alteration in brain function secondary to the accumulation of unfiltered metabolic products, is a poorly documented syndrome in avian species. In mammalian species, hepatic encephalopathy typically occurs in cases of portosystemic shunting or liver failure, and is positively correlated with increased blood ammonia levels.[10,21] Lactulose, a synthetic disaccharide derivative of lactose that is minimally digested and absorbed by the mammalian gastrointestinal system, is commonly prescribed in cases of hepatic encephalopathy. Lactulose helps to lower blood ammonia levels through acidification of colonic contents, stimulation of an osmotic diarrhea, and increasing nitrogen fixation by bacteria in the gastrointestinal tract.[46,47] A positive correlation between elevated blood ammonia levels and encephalopathy has not been identified in avian patients.[10,21] In addition, it is unknown whether lactulose is digested, absorbed, and results in acidification in the avian gastrointestinal tract as it does in mammals. Nevertheless, lactulose is frequently prescribed in birds with hepatic dysfunction with anecdotal evidence of clinical improvement. Few adverse effects have been associated with its administration.[47,48]

Patients with hepatic disease can develop anemia through several pathophysiologic mechanisms including gastroduodenal ulcerations and coagulopathies. Gastrointestinal ulcerations can be treated with various protectants including sucralfate and H_2 receptor antagonists, such as cimetidine.[7,48] Coagulopathies have been previously discussed and can be treated with vitamin K supplementation. In addition, avian patients with anemia secondary to hepatic disease may benefit from vitamin B supplementation, iron dextran administration, and even whole blood transfusions depending on the severity of the anemia. Iron supplementation should not be administered in patients suspected of having hemochromatosis.[43]

If ascitic fluid is present, it can be aspirated from the celomic cavity with or without ultrasonographic guidance. The needle should be inserted on midline through the body wall and directed toward the right side of the celomic cavity to avoid the ventriculus.[49] The sample can be submitted for cytologic analysis, which should include evaluation of the color, character, specific gravity, total solid concentration, and cellularity of the aspirated fluid. A cytologic preparation of the fluid should be microscopically evaluated and, if a bacterial cause is suspected, the fluid should be cultured.[11,50] If an effusion develops with severe hepatic dysfunction, it is typically a transudate that results from the decrease in oncotic pressure that occurs with hypo-albuminemia. Transudate effusions are usually clear with a low specific gravity, total protein concentration, and cellularity.[50] Because the removal of a large volume of ascitic fluid can result in severe protein loss, the volume of fluid aspirated from the celomic cavity should be restricted to only that required to relieve respiratory compro-mise.[7,43] Diuretic therapy may be instituted to help promote fluid excretion in patients with ascites.[43]

The use of nutraceuticals, such as milk thistle and S-adenosylmethionine (SAMe), as adjunctive treatments of hepatic dysfunction in veterinary patients is becoming increasingly commonplace. The medicinal extract from the milk thistle plant (*Silybum marinum*) is silymarin, and the active component of silymarin is silybin. Silymarin is thought to assist in the treatment of liver disease through its antioxidant properties, stabilization of cell membranes, regulation of cell permeability, and promotion of DNA, RNA, and protein synthesis.[46,51,52] Although it is often prescribed to avian patients with hepatic diseases, with anecdotal evidence of clinical improvement, only a small number of studies have investigated the efficacy of this compound in ameliorating avian liver dysfunction. Two avian studies, one using pigeons and the other using broiler chicks, have investigated the hepatoprotective effects of silymarin in experimentally induced cases of aflatoxicosis. Although the conclusions of these studies were conflicting in their assessment of silymarin efficacy, this may have been the result of differences in the silymarin and aflatoxin doses.[51,52] Side effects of silymarin administration are rarely reported, but can include nausea and diarrhea.[46] SAMe, a glutathione precursor that is normally produced by the liver, is most commonly prescribed in mammalian patients as a supplemental treatment for hepatic diseases including chronic hepatitis, hepatic lipidosis, and acute hepatotoxicosis.[7,46] To the author's knowledge, no research has been published on the efficacy of SAMe as an adjunctive treatment of avian hepatic diseases. Anecdotal evidence exists that supports the use of therapeutics to promote choleresis, such as ursodiol (ursodeox-ycholic acid) and dandelion, in cases of avian liver disease with cholestasis.[6,7,53] However, as with SAMe, no controlled studies have been performed to demonstrate the efficacy and safety of these compounds in avian patients. In addition, because many of the previously mentioned therapeutics are not available in formulations that have been approved by the Food and Drug Administration, clinicians must be aware that the potency, purity, and safety of available formulations may vary significantly among manufacturers.[46,54]

SUMMARY

The diagnosis of avian hepatic disease should be made based on the results of multiple diagnostic tests including physical examination, clinicopathologic testing, imaging studies, and hepatic biopsy. An understanding of the anatomy and function of the avian liver is essential for the proper interpretation of diagnostic findings related to hepatic disease. The diagnostic plan should be designed to investigate the severity and under-lying cause of the hepatic disease so that a treatment plan that includes both targeted and supportive therapies can be implemented. Patients should be monitored for their response to treatment by periodically repeating the tests that were used to diagnose the hepatic disease. The intervals at which these tests are repeated will depend on many factors including the specific cause of the disease, the treatments being used, the invasiveness of the tests, and the owner's commitment to pursuing these tests.

REFERENCES

1. King AS, McLelland J. Digestive system. In: Birds their structure and function. 2nd edition. Philadelphia: Baillière Tindall; 1984. p. 84–109.
2. Schmidt RE, Reavill DR, Phalen DN. Liver. In: Pathology of pet and aviary birds. Ames (IA): Blackwell Publishing; 2003. p. 67–93.
3. Hoefer HL, Orosz S, Dorrestein GM. The gastrointestinal tract. In: Altman RB, Clubb SL, Dorrestein GM, et al, editors. Avian medicine and surgery. Philadelphia: WB Saunders Co; 1997. p. 412–53.
4. Denbow DM. Gastrointestinal anatomy and physiology. In: Whittow GC, editor. Sturkie's avian physiology. 5th edition. San Diego: Academic Press; 2000. p. 299–321.
5. King AS, McLelland J. Cardiovascular system. In: Birds their structure and function. 2nd edition. Philadelphia: Baillière Tindall; 1984. p. 214–28.
6. Doneley B. Treating liver disease in the avian patient. Semin Avian Exotic Pet Med 2004;13(1):8–15.
7. Hochleithner M, Hochleithner C, Harrison LD. Evaluating and treating the liver. In: Harrison GJ, Lightfoot TL, editors. Clinical avian medicine. Palm Beach: Spix Publishing, Inc; 2006. p. 441–9.
8. Hochleithner C, Hochleithner M. Innovative approach to liver and kidney disease in psittacine birds. Exotic DVM 2000;2(3):84–7.
9. Jaensch S. Diagnosis of avian hepatic disease. Semin Avian Exotic Pet Med 2000;9(3):126–35.
10. Lumeij JT. Hepatology. In: Ritchie BW, Harrison GJ, Harrison LR, editors. Avian medicine: principles and application. Lake Worth (FL): Wingers Publishing, Inc; 1994. p. 640–72.
11. Lawrie A. Systemic non-infectious disease. In: Harcourt-Brown N, Chitty J, editors. BSAVA manual of psittacine birds. 2nd edition. Quedgeley, Gloucester England: British Small Animal Veterinary Association; 2005. p. 245–65.
12. Harrison GJ, Ritchie BW. Making distinctions in the physical examination. In: Ritchie BW, Harrison GJ, Harrison LR, editors. Avian medicine: principles and application. Lake Worth (FL): Wingers Publishing, Inc; 1994. p. 144–75.
13. Dorrestein GM, de Wit M, Schmidt V. Pathology as a base for clinical understanding [abstract 630]. In: Proceedings of the Annual Conference and Expo, Association of Avian Veterinarians. Savannah (GA), August 11–14, 2008. p. 207–15.
14. Johnston MS, Son TT, Rosthenthal KL. Immune-mediated hemolytic anemia in an eclectus parrot. J Am Vet Med Assoc 2007;230:1028–31.
15. Campbell TW, Ellis CK. Hematology of birds. In: Avian & exotic animal hematology & cytology. 3rd edition. Ames (IA): Blackwell Publishing; 2007. p. 3–50.
16. Davies RR. Avian liver disease: etiology and pathogenesis. Semin Avian Exotic Pet Med 2000;9(3):115–25.
17. Harr KE. Diagnostic value of biochemistry. In: Harrison GJ, Lightfoot TL, editors. Clinical avian medicine. Palm Beach (FL): Spix Publishing, Inc; 2006. p. 611–29.
18. Rupley AE. Manual of avian practice. Philadelphia: WB Saunders Co; 1997.
19. Hochleithner M. Biochemistries. In: Ritchie BW, Harrison GJ, Harrison LR, editors. Avian medicine: principles and application. Lake Worth (FL): Wingers Publishing, Inc; 1994. p. 223–45.

20. Cray C, Tatum LM. Applications of protein electrophoresis in avian diagnostics. J Avian Med Surg 1998;12(1):4–10.

21. Fudge AM. Avian liver and gastrointestinal testing. In: Fudge AM, editor. Laboratory medicine, avian and exotic pets. Philadelphia: WB Saunders Co; 2000. p. 47–55.

22. Cray C, Gautier D, Harris D, et al. Changes in clinical enzyme activity and bile acid levels in psittacine birds with altered liver function and disease. J Avian Med Surg 2008;22(1):17–24.

23. Cray C, Andreopoulos A. Comparison of two methods to determine plasma bile acid concentrations in healthy birds. J Avian Med Surg 2003;17(1):11–5.

24. Lumeij JT. Fasting and postprandial plasma bile acid concentrations in racing pigeons (*Columba livia domestica*) and mallards (*Anas platyrhynchos*). J Assoc Avian Vet 1991;5(4):197–200.

25. Lumeij JT, Remple JD. Plasma bile acid concentrations in response to feeding in peregrine falcons (*Falco peregrinus*). Avian Dis 1992;36:1060–2.

26. Battison AL, Buckzowski S, Archer FJ. Plasma bile acid concentration in the cockatiel. Can Vet J 1996;37:233–4.

27. Jaensch SM, Cullen L, Raidal SR. Assessment of liver function in galahs (*Eolophus roseicapillus*) after partial hepatectomy: a comparison of plasma enzyme concentrations, serum bile acid levels, and galactose clearance tests. J Avian Med Surg 2000;14(3):164–71.

28. McMillan MC. Imaging techniques. In: Ritchie BW, Harrison GJ, Harrison LR, editors. Avian medicine: principles and application. Lake Worth (FL): Wingers Publishing, Inc; 1994. p. 246–326.

29. Helmer P. Advances in diagnostic imaging. In: Harrison GJ, Lightfoot TL, editors. Clinical avian medicine. Palm Beach (FL): Spix Publishing, Inc; 2006. p. 653–9.

30. Pees M, Kiefer I, Krautwald-Junghanns ME, et al. Comparative ultrasonographic investigations of the gastrointestinal tract and the liver in healthy and diseased pigeons. Vet Radiol Ultrasound 2006;47(4):370–5.

31. Krautwald-Junghanns ME, Zebisch K, Enders F, et al. Diagnosis of liver disease in birds by radiography and ultrasonography: under special consideration of ultrasound-guided liver biopsies. Semin Avian Exotic Pet Med 2001;10(4):153–61.

32. Zebisch K, Krautwald-Junghanns ME, Willuhn J. Ultrasound-guided liver biopsy in birds. Vet Radiol Ultrasound 2004;45(3):241–6.

33. Nordberg C, O'Brien RT, Paul-Murphy J, et al. Ultrasound examination and guided fine-needle aspiration of the liver in Amazon parrots (*Amazona* species). J Avian Med Surg 2000;14(3):180–4.

34. Hadley TL, Daniel GB, Rotstein DS, et al. Evaluation of hepatobiliary scintigraphy as an indicator of hepatic function in domestic pigeons (*Columba livia*) before and after exposure to ethylene glycol. Vet Radiol Ultrasound 2007;48(2):155–62.

35. LeBlanc AK, Daniel GB. Advanced imaging for veterinary cancer patients. Vet Clin Small Anim 2007;37:1059–77.

36. Souza MJ, Greenacre CB, Jones MP. Clinical uses of microPET and CT imaging in birds [abstract 220]. In: Proceedings of the Annual Conference and Expo, Association of Avian Veterinarians. San Antonio (TX), August 7–10, 2006. p. 13–6.

37. Souza MJ, Wall JS, Daniel GB. Positron emission tomography in normal Hispaniolan Amazon parrots (Amazona ventralis) [abstract 800]. In: Proceedings of the Annual Conference and Expo, Association of Avian Veterinarians. Milwaukee (WI), August 10–13, 2009. p. 301–2.

38. Taylor M. Endoscopic examination and biopsy techniques. In: Ritchie BW, Harrison GJ, Harrison LR, editors. Avian medicine: principles and application. Lake Worth (FL): Wingers Publishing, Inc; 1994. p. 327–54.

39. Morrisey JK, Paul-Murphy K, Fialkowski JP, et al. Estimation of prothrombin times of Hispaniolan Amazon parrots (*Amazona ventralis*) and umbrella cockatoos (*Cacatua alba*). J Avian Med Surg 2003;17(2):72–7.
40. Hernandez-Divers SJ, Hernandez-Divers SM. Avian diagnostic endoscopy. Compend Contin Educ Pract Vet 2004;26(11):839–52.
41. Lierz M. Diagnostic value of endoscopy and biopsy. In: Harrison GJ, Lightfoot TL, editors. Clinical avian medicine. Palm Beach (FL): Spix Publishing, Inc; 2006. p. 631–52.
42. Rae MA. Diagnostic value of necropsy. In: Harrison GJ, Lightfoot TL, editors. Clinical avian medicine. Palm Beach (FL): Spix Publishing, Inc; 2006. p. 661–78.
43. Redrobe S. Treatment of avian liver disease. Semin Avian Exotic Pet Med 2000; 9(3):136–45.
44. Lierz M. Systemic infectious disease. In: Harcourt-Brown N, Chitty J, editors. BSAVA manual of psittacine birds. 2nd edition. Quedgeley, Gloucester England: British Small Animal Veterinary Association; 2005. p. 155–69.
45. Roudybush TE. Psittacine nutrition. Vet Clin Exot Anim 1999;2(1):111–25.
46. Plumb DC. Veterinary drug handbook. 5th edition. Ames (IA): Blackwell Publishing; 2005.
47. Jankowski G. Lactulose. J Exot Pet Med 2009;18(2):156–9.
48. Pollack C, Carpenter JW, Antinoff N. Birds. In: Carpenter JW, editor. Exotic animal formulary. 3rd edition. St Louis: Elsevier/Saunders; 2005. p. 135–344.
49. Campbell TW. Cytology. In: Ritchie BW, Harrison GJ, Harrison LR, editors. Avian medicine: principles and application. Lake Worth (FL): Wingers Publishing, Inc; 1994. p. 199–222.
50. Campbell TW, Ellis CK. Comparative cytology. In: Avian & exotic animal hematology & cytology. 3rd edition. Ames (IA): Blackwell Publishing; 2007. p. 139–222.
51. Grizzle J, Hadley TL, Rotstein DS, et al. Effects of dietary milk thistle on blood parameters, liver pathology, and hepatobiliary scintigraphy in white carneaux pigeons (*Columba livia*) challenges with B_1 aflatoxin. J Avian Med Surg 2009; 23(2):114–24.
52. Tedesco D, Steidler S, Galletti S, et al. Efficacy of silymarin-phospholipid complex in reducing the toxicity of aflatoxin B_1 in broiler chicks. Poult Sci 2004;83: 1839–43.
53. Orosz SE. Common herbs and their use in avian practice [abstract 670]. In: Proceedings of the Annual Conference and Expo, Association of Avian Veterinarians. San Antonio (TX), August 7–10, 2006. p. 79–84.
54. Orosz SE, Johnson-Delaney CA, Echols S. Application of nutritional supplements and herbs in avian practice [abstract 630]. In: Proceedings of the Annual Conference and Expo, Association of Avian Veterinarians. Providence (RI), August 6–9, 2007. p. 175–89.

Management of Common Psittacine Reproductive Disorders in Clinical Practice

Tarah L. Hadley, DVM, DABVP (Avian)

KEYWORDS

- Chronic egg laying • Dystocia • Prognosis • Psittacine

The reproductive organs play a key role in the maintenance of normal homeostasis in psittacine birds. For this reason, sex determination should be part of the baseline data collected on every avian patient. Disorders of the psittacine reproductive tract can have a negative effect on the function of other organ systems in the body. Reproductive organs may be plagued by a multitude of problems ranging from infection and neoplasia to inflammation and idiopathic issues that affect fertility. Detection of reproductive problems may require the use of a variety of modalities. The ability to treat these problems often depends on the presenting complaint as well as the clinical condition of the avian patient. Improvement in detection and treatment of reproductive conditions will occur as new information is presented through publication of research and clinical cases.

REVIEW OF FEMALE REPRODUCTIVE ANATOMY

The reproductive tract of all psittacine birds is present only on the left side of the bird. During embryonic growth of the female, a right gonad does exist for a brief period before its development is arrested. From this point on, the left-sided organs become the dominant reproductive organs.

From the cranial to the caudal aspect, the reproductive tract of the mature hen consists of the follicle-containing ovary, an infundibulum, the magnum, the isthmus, the uterus (also known as the shell gland), and the vagina. The size of the follicles in the breeding hen tends to vary from small to very large, giving the appearance of a large cluster of grapes. At this stage of development, the follicles may occupy a larger part of the cranial aspect of the reproductive tract. In the mature, nonbreeding hen or

Atlanta Hospital for Birds and Exotics, Inc, 2274 Salem Road, #106-149, Conyers, GA 30013, USA
E-mail address: drtarah@atlantabirdsandexotics.com

Vet Clin Exot Anim 13 (2010) 429–438
doi:10.1016/j.cvex.2010.05.006
1094-9194/10/$ – see front matter © 2010 Elsevier Inc. All rights reserved.

the immature hen, the follicles are regressed in appearance and tend to be tiny to small in size.

The infundibulum, which represents the first part of the left oviduct, serves a key function that requires successful capture of the oocyte in its funnel-like cup. The second part or tubular region of the infundibulum is the likely site for fertilization of the oocyte by the spermatozoon.

The magnum with its thick mucosal folds and coiled regions follows the infundibulum. After the magnum, a short isthmus is followed by the uterus. In general, it may be difficult to grossly distinguish the boundaries between the magnum, the isthmus, and the uterus. The uterus is the primary site for formation of the shell of the egg. It is also the primary place in the oviduct where the egg spends most of its time during formation.

A vaginal sphincter abruptly marks the junction between the caudal aspect of the uterus and the cranial aspect of the vagina. The sphincter area of the vagina is where the storage of spermatozoa occurs. The main compartment of the vagina is characterized by a thick muscular wall. In general, it takes an egg about 25 hours to pass down the entire extent of the oviduct.[1,2]

FEMALE REPRODUCTIVE DISORDERS
Polyostotic Hyperostosis

Polyostotic hyperostosis is a normal physiologic process in which calcium is deposited into the nonpneumatic long bones of hens before the beginning of egg laying. Radiographically, this condition may be seen as increased calcium deposition in the bones of the radius, ulna, femur, tibiotarsus, or vertebrae.[3] A similar pathologic condition called osteomyelosclerosis may be seen in hens with disease of the reproductive tract, such as ovarian cysts or egg yolk peritonitis, or in males with gonadal tumors.[4] The cause of both these processes has not been fully determined, but reproductive hormones such as estrogen or testosterone are thought to play a role. The pathologic lesions associated with osteomyelosclerosis usually resolve with resolution of the disease process.[5,6]

Chronic Egg Production

Chronic egg laying is another common disorder seen in female birds. Species that tend to be overrepresented as chronic egg layers include parakeets (Melopsittacus undulatus), cockatiels (Nymphicus hollandicus), and lovebirds (Agapornis spp). In captivity, most normal egg layers lay no more than 2 to 3 clutches per year. A bird that lays eggs chronically may have multiple clutches per year—some as frequently as once monthly or every 2 months. Other chronic layers may lay more than the average 2 to 4 eggs per clutch. The cause of this condition may differ among individual birds. Suspected causes include increased photoperiod, increased temperature, bonding with a bird of either sex, bonding with a favorite toy, providing substrate in the cage that resembles nesting materials, or potentially abnormal bonding with the owner.[7,8]

One of the main risks of overproduction of egg in these birds is the potential to deplete calcium stores necessary to form a proper egg.[9] Initially, birds may lay calcified eggs, but as calcium stores decrease, the eggs produced may become thin or soft shelled. These birds are also susceptible to depletion of energy stores because of the constant egg laying and pathologic fractures. Such birds are the classic future candidates for dystocia. Management of these birds may include nutritional adjustment, such as oral calcium supplementation, and minimizing exposure to some of the potential environmental causes previously described.[7,8]

When these methods fail to control chronic egg laying, some birds may respond to hormone therapy. Leuprolide acetate, the superactive gonadotropin-releasing hormone agonist, has been used in these patients to attempt to control present or future episodes of egg overproduction.[10] In a crisis situation, a dose of leuprolide acetate of up to 800 μg/kg intramuscularly (IM) every 14 days for 3 doses followed by monthly maintenance of up to 800 μg/kg IM every 21 to 30 days has been successfully used in some patients by Mitchell.[10] However, the dose and frequency of doses needed to control ovulation varies between individual birds and should be considered on a case-by-case basis.[11] Some birds may need hormone therapy only at certain times of the year, whereas others may need it monthly throughout the year. In general, the prognosis for control of chronic egg laying is guarded to fair in these birds.

Birds in which chronic egg production cannot be adequately controlled may be candidates for surgery. A salpingohysterectomy is performed in chronic egg layers to prevent recurrence.[7,12–14] The inability to remove the left ovary may create a small risk, in that some birds may continue to be reproductively active and potentially ovulate into the coelomic cavity.

Dystocia

Dystocia, or delayed oviposition, is one of the most common female reproductive disorders seen in clinical practice. In psittacine birds, the normal length of time for egg production and the delivery of an egg through the reproductive tract as well as the total number of eggs produced in a clutch are dependent on the species of the bird. These reproductive functions represent dynamic processes that are also affected by influences such as health status, temperature, presence or absence of a mate, hormones, photoperiod, season of the year, nutrition, and other related environmental stressors that captivity may bring. Eutocia occurs when all of these influences come together to create normal delivery of an egg without a negative effect on the hen. Under circumstances of dystocia, there is some interference with the hen's ability to undergo a normal egg delivery. Abnormal egg delivery may also result from or be a cause of concurrent health issues in the hen.

Dystocia clinical signs

Clinical symptoms of dystocia in a hen include fluffed feathers that give the bird a puffy appearance, open-mouth breathing, decreased to scant to absent droppings, watery droppings that contain little or no feces, and a coelomic cavity enlarged with fluid or of a firm circular structure.[15] Other signs include weakness or paresis of the left leg, a decreased appetite that may progress to anorexia, regurgitation, vomiting, and straining to defecate or pass an egg. Decreased function of the left leg may be a direct result of egg pressure on the nearby left sciatic nerve. Prolapse of the cloaca or oviduct, which has a cobblestone appearance to the mucosa, is also commonly seen. Avian species commonly seen in dystocia include budgerigars (*M undulatus*), lovebirds (*Agapornis* spp), cockatiels (*N hollandicus*), cockatoos (*Cacatua* spp), and Amazon parrots (*Amazona* spp).[16]

A bird in dystocia may appear completely normal at the onset of this syndrome. In some of these birds, the only clinical signs may be that the egg can be palpated by the owner for more than 24 hours and mild straining. For this reason, it is vital to obtain a complete and thorough history from the owner to aid in appropriate assessment of the bird's condition. Other birds in dystocia may run the gamut of health from mild to moderate to severe illness characterized by a combination of the clinical symptoms previously described. Severely ill birds tend to be extremely lethargic and stay only in the bottom of the cage. These birds may have difficulty breathing and may also be exhausted from occasional attempts to push the egg out of their bodies. Some of these birds exhibit continual winking of the vent, which is an outward sign that lower coelomic muscles are constantly working to push out an egg.

Diagnosis, assessment, and therapy of dystocia

Initial assessment of the clinical condition of a hen in dystocia is the key to determining the prognosis as well as the best initial treatment needed to stabilize the bird. Assessment of preliminary blood work, such as a complete blood count and chemistry profile, may provide information on kidney function, total white cell count, and differential white cell count. A cloacal culture and sensitivity may be needed to rule out the presence of infection. Direct palpation may reveal an egg that is located very high in the coelomic cavity or just cranial to the pelvis. In a more distally located egg, slight manipulation of the external skin of the vent during the physical examination may reveal the egg's chalky white shell.

If more certainty regarding the location of the egg is needed, a radiograph may be the most logical next step. A ventrodorsal or standing radiograph may provide more specific information about egg location than just palpation alone. Whether or not sedation is used should be based on the general condition of the patient. Some very critical hens may not survive sedation in part due to renal shock caused by direct pressure of the egg on the left kidney. Palpation or radiography may reveal an egg of either normal diameter or overlarge diameter that is too big to fit across the pelvic canal.

A mildly ill hen in dystocia for 24 hours or less may initially require parenteral fluid therapy (100–125 mL/kg/d of a balanced electrolyte solution divided into twice or thrice daily treatments), application of a water-based lubricant to the inside of the vent area and possibly surrounding the egg itself, a warm incubator heated up to 85°F to 90°F, and parenteral calcium therapy (100 mg/kg IM once). In many situations, this minimal treatment may be all that is needed to help the bird facilitate the passage of the egg. The prognoses in these cases tend to be fair to good.

Use of a broad-spectrum antibiotic medication at this stage may not be required and is at the discretion of the clinician. Possible pain and inflammation associated with dystocia may be relieved with an antiinflammatory medication such as meloxicam, 0.1 to 1.0 mg/kg. An opioid medication such as butorphanol (1–4 mg/kg IM) may also help ease pain.[11] In cases of suspected renal compromise, care should be taken to avoid high doses of nonsteroidal antiinflammatory medications. Leuprolide acetate (800 µg/kg IM) or the luteinizing hormone activity of chorionic gonadotropin have also been used in an attempt to prevent further egg laying in the near future; however, this may not prevent oviposition in the current clutch.[17] Published or commonly used doses of these and other medications are available.[11]

Oxytocin (5–10 IU/kg IM) or prostaglandin $F_{2\alpha}$ (0.02–0.1 mg/kg IM) may also be used to facilitate egg laying. Use of either drug is contraindicated if the vaginal sphincter is constricted or if uterine adhesions exist. A prostaglandin E_2 gel (0.02–0.1 mg/kg applied topically) may induce relaxation of the vaginal sphincter. Parenteral calcium administration should also precede oxytocin use.[11]

More immediate and invasive initial steps may be needed for a bird that is moderately to severely ill. The birds that fall in this category have usually been trying to pass an egg for more than 24 to 48 hours. These birds may be extremely critical metabolically, and actions should be taken to immediately relieve the pressure created by the egg on their left kidney as well as their left sciatic nerve. That is why it is vital to obtain as thorough a history as possible. Some of the initial treatment may resemble what was previously described for mildly affected birds.

These critical birds may also require invasive methods to deflate or remove the egg. One common procedure performed involves aspiration of the egg. A 20- or 22-gauge needle attached to a 12-mL or 20-mL syringe is directly inserted into the egg via a vent approach, if the egg can be grossly visualized or via a transcutaneous approach, if the egg is located higher in the coelomic cavity. Care must be taken to insert the needle cleanly so that a good seal is created between the egg and the needle. When the needle bevel is near the center of the egg the contents may be aspirated. Aspiration should enable collapse of the egg and facilitate easy exit from the coelomic cavity as long as no adhesions already exist between the egg and the oviduct. Sedation of birds for this procedure, particularly to minimize pain and movement, is recommended, except in critically ill birds for which anesthesia is precluded. In either situation, use of parenteral antiinflammatory and analgesic medications helps mediate any discomfort. The collapsed egg may be manually removed from the vent or is usually found in the droppings within 1 to 2 days postcollapse (**Fig. 1**).

Another possible complication in hens with delayed oviposition is that a second or third egg may start to work its way down the oviduct before the original problematic egg is removed. This complication usually occurs when adhesions have formed between the original egg and the oviduct (**Fig. 2**). In most cases, surgery is needed to remove the eggs from the oviduct. If the oviductal tissue damage is severe and the tissue cannot be saved, a salpingohysterectomy may be performed.[12] A procedure for minimally invasive endoscopic surgery has been developed in birds.[13,14] The tissue removed during this procedure should be submitted for histopathology to aid with diagnosis and to rule out neoplasia. The prognosis for complete recovery in critical birds is guarded. Assessment of other complicating factors, such as cloacal prolapse, is warranted to determine whether additional treatments are needed. Many other clinical symptoms seen early in the course of assessment, such as difficulty breathing and weakness of the hind limbs, may resolve over time with resolution of the dystocia.

Soft- or thin-shelled eggs may be palpated but not always easily visualized radiographically. These eggs are more likely to form when the bird's calcium stores have become depleted due to chronic egg laying and poor calcium content in the diet or when the eggs are unable to reach the uterus for calcium deposition due to a blockage near the uterus. Such eggs may also play a role in dystocia, if they are too large or form adhesions with the oviduct. Rupture of eggs may occur because of rough handling of the bird, when an egg has been in the oviduct too long and starts to break down, or secondary to straining on the part of the bird to pass the egg. Ruptured eggs with secondary oviductal adhesions or related infection carry a guarded to poor prognosis for survival.

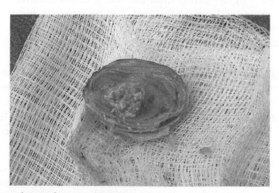

Fig. 1. Part of collapsed egg of parrot. (*Courtesy of* Dr Kemba Marshall, DVM, Phoenix, AZ, USA.)

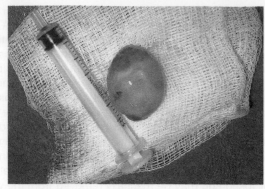

Fig. 2. Surgically removed parrot egg with evidence of adhesions. (*Courtesy of* Dr Kemba Marshall, DVM, Phoenix, AZ, USA.)

Oviductal Prolapse

Prolapse of the left oviduct may occur under several scenarios. It may occur as part of normal egg laying or as part of a disease process in which the differentials include infection or inflammation of the oviductal tissue, neoplasia, or behavioral causes.[7] Dystocia is one of the most common causes of oviductal prolapse. Inflammation, irritation, and eventual prolapse are likely sequelae when a bird struggles to pass an egg. Many birds are exhausted by the time a prolapse has occurred. Both infection and inflammation secondary to uterine adhesions from ruptured eggs may occur. A complete blood count, chemistry profile, whole body radiography, cloacal endoscopy, and culture and sensitivity of the prolapsed tissue may be obtained for a more thorough patient evaluation.

A prolapse of the oviduct may be grossly distinguishable from a cloacal prolapse by the corrugated or cobblestone appearance of the oviductal mucosa. The prolapse may be resolved by successfully treating the inciting cause. Prolapsed tissue should be addressed immediately to prevent dessication. Topical water-based lubricants may be applied to the tissue until medical intervention is possible. The patient must also be discouraged from causing any mutilation of the tissue. If needed, an Elizabethan collar may be placed around the bird's neck to prevent access to that area.

Many cases require surgery to resolve the prolapse. Parenteral antibiotic, analgesic, and antiinflammatory medications should be considered. Under general anesthesia, the prolapsed tissue may be gently cleaned with a dilute chlorhexidine solution and rinsed with saline. A water-based lubricant may be applied and the cleaned tissue may be removed with a cotton-tipped applicator using gentle inward pressure. Vent sutures may be applied to the mucosa of the vent using 3-0 or 4-0 monofilament sutures.

In general, prognosis for resolution of the prolapse is fair. However, birds may chronically prolapse if the underlying problem is not adequately addressed. Behavioral causes tend to be difficult to pinpoint and treat and may worsen the prognosis. Administration of psychotropic medications is helpful in some situations.[11] Birds in which the cause of prolapse is not determined have a guarded to poor prognosis for recovery.

Oviductal Impaction

Impaction of the oviduct most commonly occurs secondary to dystocia or inflammation. In dystocia, hens with delayed oviposition may continue to ovulate, causing inflammation and swelling of the reproductive tract. The swelling may become grossly visible as abdominal swelling. Many of these patients may be lethargic, have decreased droppings, and have difficulty breathing due to pressure placed on the surrounding air sacs. Serious concern should also be given to the potential effect of pressure and infectious material on the nearby kidney and sciatic nerves. Continual insult to the kidneys likely results in shock to the patient and eventual death.

Diagnosis of impaction may be based on results of radiography or ultrasonography, although laparoscopy may be helpful. Aspiration of a swollen abdomen may reveal egg yolk material; however, there is a risk of seeding egg contents and other potentially infectious material from the interior of the reproductive tract into the coelomic cavity. After a period of time, the eggs inside an impacted oviduct will likely form adhesions with the mucosal tissue and require surgery to remove either the eggs or the entire reproductive tract in severe situations.[12,18] These patients tend to be moderately to severely ill and the prognosis is guarded. Antiinflammatory and long-term antibiotic medications may help reduce inflammation and infection. Administration of high-dose hormone therapy, such as leuprolide acetate, may prevent the onset of future reproductive activity.

Oviductal or Uterine Rupture

Rupture of the oviduct or uterus is a potential outcome of dystocia, especially when a hen has been struggling to pass an egg for a long period. Necrotic tissue, which is prone to rupture, may develop as a result of adhesions between the egg and reproductive tract. Ruptures may also occur secondary to neoplasia.[4] Administration of hormones such as oxytocin or prostaglandin in the face of adhesions is contraindicated and likely to cause a rupture and possible death of the bird. Clinical signs of rupture may be nonspecific, including lethargy, abdominal swelling, an increased respiratory rate, an elevated heart rate, anorexia, and regurgitation.

Diagnosis is based on ultrasonography or laparoscopy. The prognosis for survival may be guarded to poor. Emergency exploratory surgery, which likely involves a salpingohysterectomy and gentle, copious flushing with a warm balanced electrolyte solution, may provide the best outcome. Care must be taken during flushing to avoid the air sacs so that the bird does not drown. The presence of a large amount of egg contents or other inspissated material in the coelomic cavity increases the likelihood of development of coelomitis and systemic infection and worsens the patient's prognosis. These patients may require an extensive hospital stay, frequent testing of cultures and blood parameters, and improvement in clinical condition before they are considered healthy.

Salpingitis and Metritis

Salpingitis and metritis refer to inflammation or infection of the oviduct and uterus, respectively. Possible causes of salpingitis and metritis include inflammation secondary to dystocia or ruptured eggs, ascending infections, or inflammation and infection from surrounding tissues, such as the liver or air sacs. Clinical signs in mild to moderately affected patients may be subtle and nonspecific and include some of those signs discussed previously, such as difficulty breathing, lethargy, fluffed feathers, or changes in the appearance of the droppings.[6]

Patients with suspected disease may be evaluated based on blood work, radiographs, culture, and laparoscopy. In more serious situations, such as ruptured eggs, exploratory surgery may be needed for proper assessment and treatment of damaged tissue. Broad-spectrum antibiotic and antiinflammatory medications as well as fluid therapy and recovery in a warm incubator may help improve the outcome in this condition. Any additional treatment, such as oxygen therapy, may be based on the clinical signs observed.

Neoplasia of the Ovary and Oviduct

Neoplasia of the reproductive tract may occur more commonly in the ovary when compared with the oviduct, and some avian species, such as the budgerigar and cockatiel, tend to be more represented than others.[7] Clinical signs include difficulty breathing, fluid in the coelomic cavity, abdominal enlargement, fluffed feathers, lameness, lethargy, and anorexia.[15] In budgerigars, female birds may show a change in the color of the cere in the presence of reproductive tract neoplasia. The types of reproductive neoplasia previously identified included hemangiosarcoma, adenocarcinoma, adenoma, and carcinomatosis.[4,7,19]

Diagnosis of neoplasia may be difficult to obtain with radiographs, because it may be difficult to distinguish normal enlargement of the reproductive tract from neoplastic causes. Other diagnostic tools to consider include ultrasonography, laparoscopy, and histopathology of suspected lesions. Treatment depends on the type and location of the neoplasia and the clinical signs of the patient. In some early tumors of the oviduct, for instance, surgical excision may be curative. Other tumors may be treated with chemotherapy, but the lack of extensive case studies makes it difficult to understand what the tumor response will be. Overall, the prognosis for patients with neoplasia is guarded to poor.

REVIEW OF MALE REPRODUCTIVE ANATOMY

The testes are located on the right and left sides of the coelomic cavity near the caudal border of the respective lungs and the cranial border of the kidneys (**Fig. 3**). The testes, which are circular to oval in shape, are small in the reproductively inactive male and grow to a large size in the reproductively active male.

The outer layer of the testis is covered by a thin tunic. The internal portion of the testis contains thousands of seminiferous tubules. The seminiferous tubules connect to straight tubules where sperm formation occurs. Sperm formation, or spermatogenesis, occurs in 3 steps with the final step resulting in the formation of the spermatozoa. The mature spermatozoa travel from the straight tubules into the rete testis. Although the rete testis is present in some birds, it is not clear whether it is present in all psittacines.

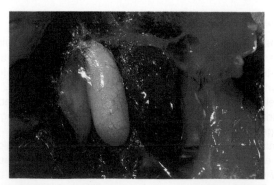

Fig. 3. Left testicle (center) located adjacent to left kidney and right testicle. (*Courtesy of* Dr Kemba Marshall, DVM, Phoenix, AZ, USA.)

Channels in the rete testis, through which sperms travel, normally connect to the epididymis along the medial surface of the testis. The epididymis makes a connection to the efferent ductules and smaller ductules, which eventually open into the very straight epididymal duct. The epididymal duct runs directly into the deferent duct. In the sexually active male chicken, spermatozoa may be found from the epididymal duct to the deferent duct. In general, it takes the spermatozoa about 1 to 4 days to travel from the rete testis to the deferent duct.[1,2]

MALE REPRODUCTIVE DISORDERS
Orchitis

Orchitis can occur from infection and less likely from primary inflammation. Infection may come from a variety of sources including nearby infected organs, an ascending infection, or secondary to a systemic infection. The most commonly cultured bacteria include *Escherichia coli* and *Salmonella* spp.[7] Clinical signs may be vague and nonspecific, although orchitis should be a serious consideration when infertility is suspected. Evaluation of baseline blood work may be the first step toward identification of an infection or other organ changes, but testing for other specific diseases that may affect the testes should not be overlooked. Radiographs may show enlargement of testes; however, normal testicular enlargement may be difficult to distinguish from enlargement due to an infection. Laparoscopy or ultrasonography may also demonstrate gross changes in the appearance of the testes. Culture and histopathology of the affected testicle, culture and cytology of the semen, or culture of the cloaca likely aids the diagnosis.[7,20] Medical treatment should be based on the results of antimicrobial sensitivity testing.

Testicular Neoplasia

Neoplasia of the testicles is commonly diagnosed in male budgerigars. Similar to female budgerigars with neoplasia of the reproductive tract, males may also show changes in the color of the cere. The most dramatic clinical signs may include behavioral changes, such as increased aggressiveness or feminization, and an enlarged coelomic cavity in advanced scenarios. One or both testes may be affected. Although seminomas represent the most commonly diagnosed testicular tumor, Sertoli and interstitial cell tumors have also been diagnosed. Surgical removal of testes, which may be challenging to perform under most circumstances, may be curative. However, severely enlarged tumors tend to be difficult to resect. The prognosis for return to normal testicular function is poor, whereas the prognosis for overall survival is guarded.[7]

REFERENCES

1. King AS, McLelland J. Birds their structure and function. Philadelphia: Bailliere Tindall; 1984.
2. Johnson AL. Reproduction in the female. In: Whittow GC, editor. Sturkie's avian physiology. 5th edition. San Diego (CA): Academic Press; 1999. p. 569–96.
3. Bowles HL. Reproductive diseases of pet bird species. Vet Clin North Am Exot Anim Pract 2002;5(3):489–506.
4. Carleton RE, Garner MM. Oviductal adenocarcinoma with osseous and myeloid metaplasia associated with sternal hyperostosis in a cockatiel (*Nymphicus hollandicus*). J Avian Med Surg 2002;16(4):309–13.
5. Orosz S, Dorrestein GM, Speer BL. Urogenital disorders. In: Altman RB, Clubb SL, Dorrestein GM, et al, editors. Avian medicine and surgery. Philadelphia: WB Saunders Company; 1997. p. 614–44.

6. Bowles HL. Evaluating and treating the reproductive system. In: Harrison GJ, Lightfoot TL, editors, Clinical avian medicine, vol. 2. Palm Beach (FL): Spix Publishing; 2006. p. 519–40.

7. Romagnano A. Reproduction and paediatrics. In: Harcourt-Brown N, Chitty J, editors. BSAVA manual of psittacine birds. 2nd edition. Gloucester (UK): British Small Animal Veterinary Association; 2005. p. 222–33.

8. Van Sant F. Problem sexual behaviors of companion parrots. In: Luescher A, editor. Manual of parrot behavior. Ames (IA): Wiley-Blackwell; 2006. p. 233–45.

9. Bowles H, Lichtenberger M, Lennox A. Emergency and critical care of pet birds. Vet Clin North Am Exot Anim Pract 2007;10(2):345–94.

10. Mitchell M. Leuprolide acetate. Sem Avian Exotic Pet Med 2005;14(2):153–5.

11. Pollock C, Carpenter JW, Antinoff N. Birds. In: Carpenter JW, editor. Exotic animal formulary. 3rd edition. Philadelphia: Elsevier Saunders; 2005.

12. Echols S. Surgery of the avian reproductive tract. Sem Avian Exotic Pet Med 2002;11(4):177–95.

13. Hernandez-Divers SJ. Minimally invasive endoscopic surgery of birds. J Avian Med Surg 2005;19(2):107–20.

14. Pye GW, Bennett RA, Plunske R, et al. Endoscopic salpingohysterectomy of juvenile cockatoos. J Avian Med Surg 2001;15(2):90–4.

15. De Matos R, Morrisey JK. Emergency and critical care of small psittacines and passerines. Sem Avian Exotic Pet Med 2005;14(2):90–105.

16. Clayton LA, Ritzman TK. Egg binding in a cockatiel (Nymphicus hollandicus). Vet Clin North Am Exot Anim Pract 2006;9(3):511–8.

17. Pollock CG. Avian reproductive anatomy, physiology, and endocrinology. Vet Clin North Am Exot Anim Pract 2002;5(4):441–74.

18. Reisinho A. Salpingohysterectomy in a female budgerigar (Melopsittacus undulatus) due to oviduct impaction. Revista Lusofona de Ciencia e Medicina Veterinaria 2008;2:17–20.

19. Mickley K, Boute M, Kiupel M, et al. Ovarian hemangiosarcoma in an orange-winged Amazon parrot (Amazona amazonica). J Avian Med Surg 2009;23(1): 29–35.

20. Crosta L, Gerlach H, Burkle M, et al. Endoscopic testicular biopsy technique in Psittaciformes. J Avian Med Surg 2002;16(2):106–10.

Advanced Diagnostic Approaches and Current Medical Management of Insulinomas and Adrenocortical Disease in Ferrets (*Mustela putorius furo*)

Sue Chen, DVM, DABVP (Avian)

KEYWORDS

• Ferret • Insulinoma • Adrenocortical disease

Large-scale studies documenting the types of neoplasms seen in the domestic ferret (*Mustela putorius furo*) have found that endocrine neoplasms are the most common type reported, with islet cell tumors and adrenocortical tumors making up a large percentage of the neoplasms diagnosed.[1,2] Both of these tumors are commonly seen in middle-aged to older ferrets, although increasing numbers of younger ferrets are being diagnosed. An exception is the black-footed ferret (*Mustela nigripes*), an endangered and genetically distinct species in the United States, that is not plagued by insulinomas and adrenocortical neoplasms despite having a high incidence of neoplastic disease.[3] Although surgical excision is still considered by most practitioners as the treatment of choice for insulinomas and adrenocortical neoplasia, practitioners should be cognizant of the medical therapies available for ferrets when surgery is not an option. This article discusses the proposed causes, current diagnostics, and the medical management of insulinomas and adrenocortical disease.

INSULINOMA

Pancreatic islet beta-cell tumor, more commonly known as insulinoma, is a well-documented neoplasm that produces its effects through the overproduction of insulin.[1,2,4–8] This neoplasm is commonly seen in middle-aged to older ferrets, with a reported incidence of approximately 25% of the neoplasms diagnosed.[1] These

Gulf Coast Avian & Exotics, Gulf Coast Veterinary Specialists, 1111 West Loop South, Suite 110, Houston, TX 77027, USA
E-mail address: drchen@gcvs.com

Vet Clin Exot Anim 13 (2010) 439–452
doi:10.1016/j.cvex.2010.05.002
1094-9194/10/$ – see front matter © 2010 Elsevier Inc. All rights reserved.

tumors secrete insulin indiscriminately and are not responsive to inhibitory stimuli such as hypoglycemia and hyperinsulinemia. In addition, rapidly increasing glucose levels, even in the presence of low blood glucose concentration, can stimulate excessive insulin release from these tumors, causing a profound rebound hypoglycemia. Although local tumor recurrence in the pancreas is a common feature, there is a low rate of metastasis to other organs; with the regional lymph nodes, liver, and spleen being the most commonly reported sites.[9,10] In contrast, insulinomas in dogs are usually malignant and have a high rate of gross metastasis at the time of diagnosis.[11] At present, it is thought that there is a genetic cause for the predisposition of insulinomas in ferrets. It has also been theorized that excessive carbohydrate intake may play a role in the development of this disease.[1,4,12] Both sexes are represented, but there are conflicting reports on whether males are slightly overrepresented.[1,8] Most ferrets begin exhibiting clinical signs around 4 years of age, although a functional insulinoma has been reported in a ferret as young as 2 weeks.[2]

Clinical signs include mental dullness, irritability, stargazing, hindlimb weakness, and ataxia. Other common signs noted in ferrets include ptyalism or pawing at the mouth secondary to presumed nausea. Ferrets with severe hypoglycemia may exhibit generalized seizures, which is the most common clinical finding in dogs with insulinomas. The relatively low frequency of generalized seizures in ferrets compared with dogs may be due to the fact that most ferrets are fed ad libitum and have a low-activity lifestyle associated with cage restriction.[11,13] Clinical signs are often episodic, but the severity and frequency of clinical signs often progress if left untreated. Prolonged episodes of severe hypoglycemia can result in neuronal glucose deprivation and cerebral hypoxia, leading to subsequent lesions in the cerebral cortex.[14]

Diagnostics

A presumptive diagnosis of insulinoma is made in ferrets when they demonstrate a fasting blood glucose level lower than 70 mg/dL in the presence of neurologic symptoms that cease after a feeding or intravenous administration of glucose.[8,15] Other causes of hypoglycemia such as sepsis, starvation, hepatic disease, and laboratory artifact should be systematically ruled out. Immediate evaluation of freshly drawn blood with a handheld glucometer provides a quick relative assessment of the blood glucose status. However, most handheld point-of-care glucometers are not validated for ferrets and may report values that are 10 to 20 mg/dL lower than actual glucose levels.[8] If a sample is to be sent to a diagnostic laboratory, immediately centrifuge the collected blood to separate the plasma to minimize artifactual decreases through red cell metabolism. In patients in whom an insulinoma is suspected but the blood glucose is within normal limits (90–125 mg/dL), a carefully monitored 3- to 4-hour fast may be required to confirm hypoglycemia.[8]

Hyperinsulinism can be documented by submitting plasma or serum to laboratories that have validated assays for ferrets. An elevated insulin level with concurrent hypoglycemia is consistent with and supports the diagnosis of an insulinoma. However, normal insulin levels (5–35 μU/mL; 36–251 pmol/L) with concurrent hypoglycemia do not rule out the presence of an insulinoma since there may be erratic production and secretion of insulin by some beta-cell tumors.[8,16,17] Insulin to glucose ratios are no longer recommended because of their high incidence of false positives.[8,17] Studies investigating fructosamine and glycosylated hemoglobin show a direct relationship with serum glucose levels in people and dogs, and studies for their use in ferrets are warranted.[18,19] Nonspecific elevations in alanine aminotransferase and aspartate aminotransferase are sometimes noted and may reflect the presence of hepatic lipidosis from chronic hypoglycemia.[8] Other changes in blood work are usually unremarkable, and if present may be a result of concurrent disease.

Diagnostic imaging is usually unrewarding, because most insulinomas are only a few millimeters in diameter and may even be microscopic in size. However, rare cases of pancreatic tumors as large as 1 cm in diameter have been observed in the author's practice and could be visualized on ultrasonographic examination. The use of intraoperative ultrasonography of the pancreas has been described in dogs to identify pancreatic nodules, but the result is highly dependent on operator experience.[14,17]

A small clinical study in dogs showed the use of intravenous 1% methylene blue, which is preferentially absorbed by hyperfunctional pancreatic tumors, to enhance visualization of the neoplastic nodules during a laparotomy. Adverse clinical signs in some of the study subjects included pseudocyanosis from damage and lysis of red blood cells.[20] The use of methylene blue has not been investigated in ferrets.

Histologic examination of surgical biopsies is required for definitive diagnosis, and lesions can range from hyperplasia to adenomas to carcinomas, or have a combination of any of these processes. Most insulinomas consist of cords and nests of eosinophilic polyhedral cells on a fine fibrovascular stroma. Although most tumors are usually well encapsulated, some tumors can be infiltrative or unencapsulated (**Fig. 1**). Immunohistochemistry can be used to further characterize pancreatic neoplasms and any metastatic nodules in the surrounding organs. Most pancreatic islet cell tumors express strong immunoreactivity for insulin, although immunostaining for peptide hormones such as glucagon, somatostatin, and pancreatic polypeptide has been occasionally noted. The neuroendocrine markers chromogranin A and neuron-specific enolase are also effective immunocytochemical markers for islet cell tumors in ferrets, and could be used to characterize poorly differentiated pancreatic tumors or metastasis in distant organs that may be insulin negative.[21]

Therapeutics

Management of a hypoglycemic episode

Advise owners on the clinical signs of hypoglycemia and on what measures to take during a hypoglycemic episode. If mild clinical signs such as lethargy or excessive salivation are noted, owners should provide a feed to abate the clinical sign. If

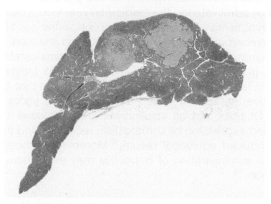

Fig. 1. Subgross view of a pancreatic limb from a ferret with an encapsulated (*left*) and unencapsulated (*right*) pancreatic islet cell tumors, more commonly referred to as insulinomas. These tumors are often found in multiples less than 1 mm in diameter or up to several millimeters in size. (*Courtesy of* Catherine M. Pfent, DVM, College Station, TX.)

the ferret is nonresponsive or exhibiting seizures, owners should drip Karo syrup or honey on the mucous membranes to provide temporary relief from the hypoglycemia until the ferret can be transported to a veterinary facility for supportive care.

If a ferret is comatose or seizuring on presentation, quickly check the blood glucose level for hypoglycemia. If hypoglycemic, place an intravenous catheter for a slow bolus of 50% dextrose (0.25–2 mL) and titrate to effect.[8] Once the seizures have ceased, the patient should be maintained on continuous-rate infusion of fluids supplemented with 5% dextrose. The ferret should be gradually weaned off the dextrose, and maintenance fluids administered during the following 12 to 24 hours. Medications to help maintain their blood glucose levels should also be administered so that clinical signs do not return.

Palliative therapy

Glucocorticoids such as prednisone and prednisolone increase the blood glucose level by increasing hepatic gluconeogenesis, decreasing glucose uptake by peripheral tissues, and inhibiting insulin binding to insulin receptors.[22] Doses of 0.25 to 2 mg/kg by mouth every 12 hours have been used.[8,23] Start at a low dose and increase in small increments as needed to control clinical symptoms and to approach normoglycemia. The blood glucose level should be rechecked within 5 to 7 days to assess if any dose adjustments are needed, and should be rechecked every 2 to 3 months thereafter. Ferrets are relatively resistant to the immunosuppressive effects of prednisolone; however, some ferrets on long-term glucocorticoid therapy may gain weight in the abdominal region and have slow or impaired hair growth in shaved areas.

Diazoxide (Proglycem; Baker Norton), a nondiuretic benzothiadiazide, directly inhibits pancreatic insulin secretion by decreasing the intracellular release of ionized calcium, which subsequently prevents the release of insulin from the insulin granules. In addition, by stimulating the release of epinephrine, diazoxide promotes hepatic gluconeogenesis and glycogenolysis, and decreases the cellular uptake of glucose.[8,22] This medication can be used as the initial palliative therapy in lieu of prednisolone, but is considerably more expensive. Diazoxide can also be used in combination with prednisolone when glucocorticoids alone cannot control clinical symptoms. Recommended dosing starts at 5 to 10 mg/kg by mouth every 12 hours and can be gradually increased to a maximum of 30 mg/kg every 12 hours if lower doses do not control signs adequately.[8,23] Adverse side effects typically include anorexia, vomiting, and diarrhea, but may be abated by administering the medication with food. This medication should be used cautiously in patients with renal disease or congestive heart failure because the conditions can be exacerbated through sodium and fluid retention.[11,22]

Octreotide is a synthetic, long-acting analogue of somatostatin that inhibits the secretion of insulin, glucagon, secretin, gastrin, and motilin. Limited use of this drug has been reported in ferrets, but it may be useful in patients that are not responding to traditional palliative therapy. Reported dosage is 1 to 2 μg/kg every 8–12 hours subcutaneously.[24] Of note, not all insulinomas are responsive to this medication because of the varied expression of somatostatin receptors and the sporadic use of octreotide have produced equivocal results.[8] Moreover, if somatostatin receptors are not present, the administration of octreotide may exacerbate hypoglycemia by suppressing glucagon.[24]

Diet modification

A rapid increase of blood glucose from the ingestion of simple sugars can induce a rebound release of insulin from an insulinoma, thus triggering a hypoglycemic episode.[8,25] Therefore, it is important to instruct owners to discontinue all treats that are high in simple sugars, including raisins, peanut butter, and any ferret supplements containing corn syrup or other sugar products. A high-protein, low-carbohydrate kibble may be beneficial in decreasing the consumption of simple carbohydrates. Changes should be made gradually to make sure that the ferret is accepting the new diet. Kibble should be available at all times, and multiple feeding stations are recommended so that it is easily accessible. It has been suggested that the development of insulinomas may be prevented by switching to a diet high in protein and fats and low in carbohydrates and fiber.[12] However, studies supporting this theory are currently lacking and further scientific investigations are warranted before specific recommendations can be made.

Definitive treatment of insulinomas

The aforementioned therapeutics only manage the clinical symptoms and do not have any antineoplastic properties. Doxorubicin has been used safely in ferrets as part of chemotherapy protocols for the treatment of lymphoma, and its use for the treatment of insulinomas could be considered.[10] Proposed dosing of doxorubicin for the treatment of insulinomas is 30 mg/m^2 every 3 weeks intravenously, and the cumulative dose should stay below 240 mg/m^2.[14,22] Administration of doxorubicin requires precise venipuncture because inadvertent extravasation can result in severe tissue necrosis. Other reported side effects include bone marrow suppression, gastroenteritis, nephrotoxicity, and cardiac toxicity.[22] Investigational studies in dogs have shown that the chemotherapeutic drugs streptozotocin and alloxan also have direct toxic effects on pancreatic beta cells; however, their use in ferrets has not been evaluated and because of their many toxic side effects, further studies are needed before their use can be recommended.[10,14]

Surgical excision is considered as the treatment of choice for greater clinical resolution and longer survival times. Although an ideal goal would be for patients to be normoglycemic after surgery, some may remain hypoglycemic and many will have recurrence of clinical signs due to tumor metastasis. Case studies have demonstrated that as many as 52% (26 out of 50) of ferrets remained hypoglycemic after surgery, and the reported disease-free intervals have ranged from 0 to 23.5 months.[7,8,26] Because of the likely recurrence of signs, owners should be advised that surgery should not be considered to be curative, but rather may temporarily stop or slow the progression of disease for a longer disease-free interval.

ADRENOCORTICAL NEOPLASIA

In ferrets, the associated syndrome is a type of hyperadrenocorticism and is more commonly known as adrenal disease. Neoplasms of the adrenal cortex have the potential to overproduce one or more of the steroids (glucocorticoids, mineralcorticoids, androgens) that the adrenal gland normally produces. Practitioners should be aware that the clinical disease seen in ferrets is not Cushing disease as seen in dogs when cortisol levels are elevated due to a pituitary tumor. Instead, neoplasms of the adrenal cortex in ferrets usually overproduce one or more of the sex hormones estradiol, androstenedione, or 17α-hydroxyprogesterone.[8,27] Overproduction of the sex hormones (hyperandrogenism) is the most commonly seen disease syndrome, although overproduction of cortisol (hypercortisolism) or aldosterone (hyperaldosteronism) concurrently with the sex hormones has been reported.[28,29] Also in contrast to Cushing disease, the contralateral adrenal gland usually does not atrophy in ferrets with adrenocortical disease.

In a large retrospective study, adrenocortical cell tumors had an incidence of 25% (380 of 1525) of neoplasms identified. In addition to these neoplasms, hyperplasia of the adrenal cortex was also commonly seen (29%; 439 of 1525) and caused similar clinical signs as adrenocortical neoplasms.[1] The prevalence of lesions may be increasing, as one pathologist has noted some degree of adrenal pathology in 95% of the ferrets necropsied, although not all the ferrets were exhibiting clinical signs at the time of death (Catherine M. Pfent, College Station, TX, personal communication, January 2010). Unilateral disease is noted in approximately 85% of ferrets with adrenocortical disease, whereas the remaining 15% have bilateral disease.[30,31] In cases of unilateral disease the left adrenal gland seems to be more commonly affected, although this may be a factor of the right adrenal gland being more difficult to locate because of its dorsal position over the vena cava. Different histopathologic lesions may be present concurrently in each adrenal gland or within a single adrenal gland. Histopathologic lesions range from hyperplasia to adrenocortical adenoma to adrenocortical carcinomas (**Fig. 2**). Metastasis to other organs is uncommon.[1]

Adrenocortical disease most commonly affects ferrets around 4 years of age and both sexes are represented.[8,30,32] The incidence of adrenal tumors is higher in sterilized ferrets compared with those kept sexually intact, which has led to the theory that the practice of early sterilization may play a role in the development of these tumors.[1,2] This finding is supported by studies where mice that have undergone early-age gonadectomy developed adrenocortical hyperplasia or tumors. Removal of the gonads at a young age removes negative feedback to the hypothalamus, resulting in increased concentrations of gonadotropins. It is theorized that the elevations in gonadotropins in turn persistently stimulate small nests of undifferentiated gonadal cells that may rest under the capsule of the adrenal gland.[8,33] One study showed that regardless of age, gonadectomy in general may predispose ferrets to development of adrenocortical disease. Ferrets in the Netherlands, which are typically castrated or spayed at 1 year of age, seem to develop adrenocortical disease around 3.5 years after sterilization.[34] Another important consideration is that clinical cases in intact ferrets are likely underreported because some of the clinical signs (ie, swollen vulva, aggressive sexual behavior) may be mistaken as normal changes in intact ferrets during the breeding season. Prolonged photoperiods are also thought to play a role in the development of adrenocortical disease. Ferrets kept indoors under artificial lighting are subjected to unnatural prolonged periods of "daylight" (>8 hours), which is thought to deplete the body's store of melatonin. As the concentration of this

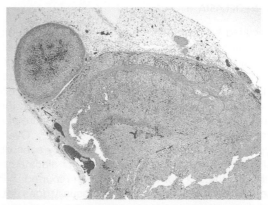

Fig. 2. Low power magnification (2×) of the adrenal gland from a ferret with marked adrenocortical hyperplasia and an extracapsular adenoma. (*Courtesy of* Catherine M. Pfent, DVM, College Station, TX.)

antigonadotropic hormone in blood decreases, there is an increase in gonadotropin-releasing hormone (GnRH) and luteinizing hormone (LH) synthesis and release.[35,36] Finally, a genetic component may also play a role in the development of this disease, especially considering the limited gene pool used in North America resulting in a highly inbred population.[1,4]

Varying degrees of alopecia is the most commonly noted sign, with an incidence of up to 90% in some reports (**Fig. 3**).[8] The hair epilates easily, and the loss is usually symmetric and progressive. Pruritus that may or may not be associated with the alopecia is sometimes noted. Excoriations and erythema may be noted in ferrets with unrelenting pruritus. Vulvar swelling is also commonly noted in more than 70% of the affected female ferrets (**Fig. 4**).[32] Male ferrets may display signs of stranguria due to urethral compression by an enlarged prostate caused by prostatitis or prostatic cysts.[37] Aggressive behavior, which is normal in intact male ferrets during the breeding season, may be observed in sterilized ferrets with adrenocortical disease. Bone marrow toxicity caused by prolonged hyperestrogenism can result in a rare but severe anemia (<15%) with diffuse petechia and ecchymotic lesions in both male and female ferrets. The overproduction of estrogen by the tumor mimics the pancytopenia seen in unbred, intact jills that are in constant estrus.[35]

Diagnostics

Ultrasonographic examination of the adrenal glands allows for evaluation of the size, shape, and structure of each adrenal gland. To look for the left adrenal gland, first obtain a sagittal view of the left kidney. With the cranial pole of the left kidney at the center of the image, angle the transducer gradually from a vertical to horizontal plane to fan the image toward midline until the left adrenal gland is located. The transducer may then need to be slightly rotated to acquire a longitudinal image of the adrenal gland. Images of the right adrenal gland are obtained by scanning the caudal vena cava along the longitudinal plane right where the vessel enters the liver. The right adrenal gland is located dorsal to the caudal vena cava. An alternative technique first scans the liver in a transverse plane to identify the aorta, caudal vena cava, and portal vein. The transducer is then angled in a craniocaudal direction and the caudal vena cava is gradually scanned in a caudal direction until the right adrenal gland is located.[38] Normal adrenal glands can vary greatly in length, but should not vary

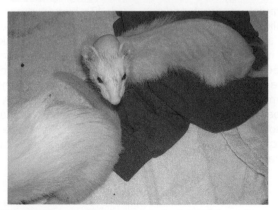

Fig. 3. Symmetric hair loss usually starts at the tail and tail base but can progress to the entire body if left untreated.

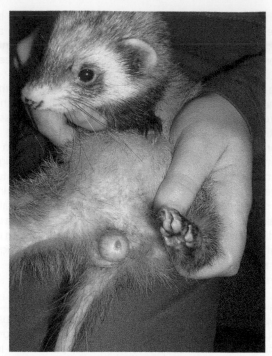

Fig. 4. Engorged, swollen vulvas are commonly seen in spayed female ferrets with adrenocortical disease. This clinical sign resembles the enlarged vulvas of jills in estrus.

much in thickness. The left adrenal gland on average measures from 5.4 to 9.8 mm in length and ranges 2.3 to 3.6 mm in thickness. The right adrenal gland size ranges from 5.8 to 10.5 mm in length and 2.2 to 3.8 mm in width. Abnormalities can include increased widths of more than 3.9 mm, a rounded appearance, asymmetric poles, increased echogenicity, and mineralization.[38] Color flow Doppler is useful in evaluating the compression of or invasion into the caudal vena cava by the right adrenal gland. Concurrent pathology secondary to adrenocortical disease such as prostatomegaly in male ferrets may also be noted on ultrasonographic examination.

Levels of estradiol, androstenedione, and 17α-hydroxyprogesterone can be measured by a validated sex steroid serum panel available through the Clinical Endocrinology Service at the University of Tennessee (http://www.vet.utk.edu/diagnostic/endocrinology/). These androgens are normally found in minute quantities in neutered ferrets, but may be pathologically elevated in ferrets with adrenocortical disease. A seasonal influence to the hormone cycle has been observed, so that fluctuations in androgen levels may be noted depending on the time of year.[4] A complete blood count should be performed to check for nonregenerative anemia that may be related to an estrogen-induced pancytopenia. Serum biochemistry profiles do not usually have any specific changes, but are important in screening for other common diseases such as insulinoma.

Therapeutics

Most of the medical therapies for hyperadrenocorticism are aimed at controlling the clinical signs through manipulation of hormonal effects. It is important to recognize that most medications currently in use do not treat the neoplasm, and in many cases the neoplasms continue to grow. The medical options detailed here are good alternatives for most nonsurgical candidates or if there is a recurrence of clinical signs after an adrenalectomy.

Leuprolide acetate (Lupron; Abbott Laboratories) is a long-acting GnRH agonist used for the treatment of prostate and testicular cancer in men and endometriosis in women. When administered at sufficiently high levels for a prolonged period, this GnRH agonist desensitizes GnRH receptors at the pituitary to downregulate the release of gonadotropins follicle-stimulating hormone (FSH) and luteinizing hormone (LH). Current dosing recommendations range from 100 to 200 μg/kg intramuscularly every 4 to 8 weeks and should be tailored by how the ferret is responding to the hormone.[23] Improvement of clinical signs, such as decreased vulvar swelling, decreased pruritus, and decreased aggression is usually noted within 2 weeks. Resolution of dysuria is usually noted within a few days. Hair growth typically occurs within 4 to 8 weeks. The average time to recurrence of clinical signs after administration of one dose of leuprolide acetate (100 μg intramuscularly) is around 3 months (range 1.5–8 months).[39] Most of the controlled studies were performed using the monthly depot form, which should not be confused with the once-a-day injectable or 3- and 4-month depot formulations. The 3- and 4-month formulations anecdotally do not seem to have the expected duration of action, and further clinical studies are recommended.[40] A 1-year leuprolide implant (Viadur; Bayer AG) has been manufactured for the palliative treatment of advanced prostate cancer in humans.[4] However, the amount of leuprolide acetate in this implant (72 mg) is more than 720 times the typical 100-μg dose currently used in ferrets, and toxicologic studies on ferrets should be conducted before the use of the implant can be recommended. Leuprolide acetate is not curative for adrenal neoplasia, and there are conflicting reports on whether or not tumor size is affected. Some of the largest tumors in the author's practice have been in ferrets that have been managed long term (>2 years) with leuprolide acetate. It is thought that some tumors may become autonomous and nonresponsive to the effect of the leuprolide acetate, especially after prolonged therapy.

Deslorelin acetate (Suprelorin; Peptech) is a synthetic analogue of gonadorelin. Deslorelin acetate stimulates LH and FSH secretion that desensitizes the pituitary by downregulating GnRH receptors, which in turn effectively stops the release of gonadotropins. Ferrets receiving a single 3-mg implant had improved clinical signs within 2 weeks, and plasma hormone concentrations remained decreased until recurrence of clinical signs were noted 8.5 to 20.5 months later (mean 13.7 months). Although this hormone is effective in controlling the clinical signs of adrenocortical disease, like Lupron it does not seem to deter tumor growth or metastasis.[41]

Melatonin is low in ferrets exposed to prolonged photoperiods (>8 hours). Oral supplementation of this antigonadotropic hormone at 0.5 mg once a day temporarily improved clinical signs and decreased androgen levels. However, recurrence of clinical signs and elevated androgen levels were noted at an 8-month recheck.[42] Anecdotal oral dosing is recommended at 0.5 to 1.0 mg once a day, 8 to 9 hours after sunrise.[22,23] Melatonin supplements are readily available at most health food stores, but as with any nutraceutical there are no regulations for quality control or false labeling. Melatonin implants are used in the mink and fox pelt industry to promote the development of a thick winter haircoat. In one clinical trial, 5.4-mg implants for mink (Neo Dynamics LLP, Lake Delton, WI, USA) were implanted subcutaneously into ferrets; findings included resolution of vulvar swelling in 1 to 2 weeks and hair growth by 6 to 8 weeks. Lethargy in the first 3 to 5 days after injection was the only side effect noted. The ferrets were only followed for 3 to 4 months, and long-term studies are needed to determine the duration of efficacy.[36] At present, a 5.4-mg implant (Ferretonin; Melatek LLC, Middleton, WI) is being marketed for ferrets, with good anecdotal results, but studies evaluating the long-term efficacy have not yet been published.[4]

The following drugs have been used anecdotally to help shrink enlarged prostates more quickly while waiting for leuprolide acetate to become effective, but controlled studies have not been conducted on their safety and efficacy in ferrets. Bicalutamide (Casodex; AstraZeneca) and flutamide (Eulexin; Schering-Plough) are androgen receptor blockers used to treat prostate hyperplasia and prostate cancer in men and in ferrets, and have had some anecdotal benefit for severe prostate cases and for aggression in ferrets. Anastrozole (Arimidex; AstraZeneca), a drug used to treat breast cancer in humans, inhibits the synthesis of estradiol and estrogen by inhibiting the catalytic enzyme aromatase. This drug may be useful in ferrets with elevated estradiol levels. Finasteride (Proscar/Propecia; Merck) is an antiandrogen used in men for the treatment of benign prostatic hyperplasia, prostate cancer, and male pattern baldness. It prevents the conversion of testosterone to dihydrotestosterone, and has been used in ferrets in combination with leuprolide acetate without any reported side effects.[4,8,40]

The aforementioned therapies are aimed at controlling the clinical signs through suppression of hormone production, release, or binding to receptor sites, but do not appreciably treat the diseased adrenal tissue. Mitotane (Lysodren; Bristol-Myers Squibb) has been used to chemically debulk the adrenal gland, but has fair to poor efficacy, depending on the type of tumor involved. The chemical debulking is not specific to the zona reticularis, where androgens are produced. This drug can be especially detrimental if the ferret has a concurrent insulinoma, because it decreases the level of circulating cortisol and may precipitate a hypoglycemic episode. Reported dosing consists of 50 mg every 24 hours for a week, followed by maintenance dosing of 50 mg every 48 to 72 hours. Resolution of clinical signs is highly variable, and the clinical signs often recur once the medication is discontinued.[4,8,22,23]

Adrenalectomy of diseased adrenal glands alleviates clinical signs in most ferrets and carries a good long-term prognosis. In one study the 1- and 2-year survival rates were 98% and 88%, respectively. The same study also found that the survival time was not significantly affected by the type of tumor involved or if unilateral or bilateral disease was present.[43] Although surgical resection of diseased adrenal gland is the treatment of choice for many practitioners, recurrence of disease after adrenalectomy is possible.[44] Various surgical techniques for the removal of adrenal glands have been reviewed thoroughly in the literature.

Management of Conditions Secondary to Adrenocortical Disease

Male ferrets with adrenocortical disease may present on emergency for urinary obstruction secondary to prostatomegaly. Urethral catheterization with a 3.5F red rubber catheter, tomcat catheter, or "slippery sam" catheter is indicated for relief of the obstruction (Fig. 5). Under sedation, the penis is exposed from the prepuce by placing gentle but cranially directed pressure at the base of the os penis. Once exposed, gauze can be hooked at the curved end of the os penis to keep the penis exposed. The opening to the urethra can be located just lateral to the tip of the penis. Leuprolide acetate should be administered immediately to help decrease the size of the prostate within a few days. Multiple antiandrogens have been anecdotally used to treat prostatic enlargement, but controlled studies have not been conducted to confirm if the antiandrogens have any additional benefit in comparison with giving leuprolide acetate alone. Any effects from postrenal azotemia should also be immediately

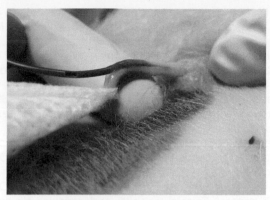

Fig. 5. Male ferrets with prostatomegaly are at risk of obstruction of their urinary tract. Urinary catheterization can be performed in cases of urinary tract obstruction. Gauze can be hooked at the curved end of the os penis to keep the penis exposed. The opening of the urethra is just lateral to the tip of the exposed penis.

addressed. Placement of a temporary tube cystostomy has been described in cases when the maintenance of a urethral catheter had failed.[45]

Pancytopenia secondary to hyperestrogenism is a rare life-threatening condition that requires intensive supportive care. Affected ferrets are severely anemic (<15%), and may have petechia or ecchymotic lesions caused by thrombocytopenia. In the author's practice, ferrets presenting with these clinical signs have failed to respond to leuprolide acetate. If surgical excision of the estrogen-producing tumor is to be attempted, multiple transfusions may be required preoperatively, perioperatively, and postoperatively. Hospitalization for intravenous fluids, blood transfusions, and supportive care is often required until the bone marrow can regenerate after the source of excess estrogen production has been removed. Owners should be advised that these ferrets have a poor prognosis, especially in cases where the adrenal neoplasm is nonresectable.

SUMMARY

At present, insulinomas and adrenocortical disease are the 2 most commonly seen neoplasms that affect middle-aged and older ferrets. A thorough understanding of the diagnostics and treatment options of both these diseases is important to appropriately manage their medical conditions. Although surgical excision is still a good treatment option for most ferrets with insulinomas and adrenocortical neoplasia, appropriate medical management can provide a good quality of life for ferrets when surgery is not an option.

REFERENCES

1. Willams BH, Weiss CA. Ferret neoplasia. In: Quesenberry KE, Carpenter JW, editors. Ferrets, rabbits, and rodents: clinical medicine. 2nd edition. St. Louis (MO): Saunders; 2003. p. 91–106.
2. Li X, Fox JG, Padrid PA. Neoplastic diseases in ferrets: 574 cases (1968–1997). J Am Vet Med Assoc 1998;212(9):1402–6.

3. Lair S, Barker IK, Mehren KG, et al. Epidemiology of neoplasia in captive black-footed ferrets (Mustela nigripes), 1986–1996. J Zoo Wildl Med 2002;33(3):204–13.

4. Lewington JH. Endocrine diseases. In: Lewington JH, editor. Ferret husbandry, medicine & surgery. 2nd edition. Edinburgh (UK): Elsevier Science Limited; 2007. p. 346–79.

5. Jergens AE, Shaw DP. Hyperinsulinism and hypoglycemia associated with pancreatic islet cell tumor in a ferret. J Am Vet Med Assoc 1989;94(2):269–71.

6. Luttgen PJ, Storts RW, Rogers KS, et al. Insulinoma in a ferret. J Am Vet Med Assoc 1986;189(8):920–1.

7. Caplan ER, Petereon ME, Mullen HS, et al. Diagnosis and treatment of insulin-secreting pancreatic islet cell tumors in ferrets: 57 cases (1986–1994). J Am Vet Med Assoc 1996;209(10):1741–5.

8. Quesenberry KE, Rosenthal KL. Endocrine diseases. In: Quesenberry KE, Carpenter JW, editors. Ferrets, rabbits, and rodents: clinical medicine and surgery. 2nd edition. St. Louis (MO): Saunders; 2003. p. 79–90.

9. Fix AS, Harms CA. Immunocytochemistry of pancreatic endocrine tumors in three domestic ferrets (Mustela putorius furo). Vet Pathol 1990;27:199–201.

10. Antinoff N, Hahn K. Ferret oncology: diseases, diagnostics, and therapeutics. Vet Clin North Am Exot Anim Pract 2004;7(3):579–625.

11. Elie MS, Zerbe CA. Insulinoma in dogs, cats, and ferrets. Compend Contin Educ Pract Vet 1995;17(1):51–9.

12. Finkler MR. A nutritional approach to the prevention of insulinomas in the pet ferret. Exotic Mam Med Surg 2004;2(2):1–4.

13. Marini RP, Ryden EB, Rosenblad BS, et al. Functional islet cell tumor in six ferrets. J Am Vet Med Assoc 1993;202(3):430–4.

14. Meleo KA, Caplan ER. Treatment of insulinoma in the dog, cat, and ferret. In: Bonagura JD, editor. Current veterinary therapy XIII. Philadelphia: WB Saunders; 1999. p. 357–61.

15. Ehrhart N, Withrow SJ, Ehrhart EJ, et al. Pancreatic beta cell tumor in ferrets: 20 cases (1986–1994). J Am Vet Med Assoc 1996;209(10):1737–40.

16. Antinoff N. Neoplasia in ferrets. In: Bonagura JD, editor. Current veterinary therapy XIII. Philadelphia: WB Saunders; 1999. p. 1149–52.

17. Lurye JC, Behrend EN. Endocrine tumors. Vet Clin North Am Small Anim Pract 2001;33(5):1083–110.

18. Elliott DA, Nelson RW, Feldman EC, et al. Glycosylated hemoglobin concentrations in the blood of healthy dogs and dogs with naturally developing diabetes mellitus, pancreatic beta-cell neoplasia, hyperadrenocorticism, and anemia. J Am Vet Med Assoc 1997;211(6):723–7.

19. Loste a, Marca MC, Unzueta A. Clinical value of fructosamine measurements in non-healthy dogs. Vet Res Commun 2001;25:109–15.

20. Fingeroth JM, Smeak DD. Intravenous methylene blue infusion for intraoperative identification of pancreatic islet-cell tumors in dogs. Part II: clinical trials and results in four dogs. J Am Anim Hosp Assoc 1988;24(2):175–82.

21. Andrews GA, Myers NC. Immunohistochemistry of pancreatic islet cell tumors in the ferret (Mustela putorius furo). Vet Pathol 1997;34(5):387–93.

22. Plumb DC. Plumb's veterinary drug handbook. 5th edition. Stockholm (WI): Blackwell; 2005.

23. Gamble C, Morrisey JK. Ferrets. In: CarpenterJW, editor. Exotic animal formulary. 3rd edition. Philadelphia: WB Saunders; 2004. p. 447–76.

24. Usukura M, Yoneda T, Oda N, et al. Medical treatment of benign insulinoma using octreotide LAR: a case report. Endocr J 2007;54(1):95–101.

25. Rosenthal KL. Feeding the hypoglycemic ferret. In: Proceedings for North American Veterinary Conference. Orlando (FL), January 7–11, 2006. p. 1766.
26. Weiss CA, Willams BH, Scott MV. Insulinoma in the ferret: clinical findings and treatment comparison of 66 cases. J Am Anim Hosp Assoc 1998;34(6):471–5.
27. Schoemaker N. New developments in research on hyperadrenocorticism in ferrets. Exotic DVM 2000;2(3):81–3.
28. Schoemaker NJ, Kuijten AM, Galac S. Luteinizing hormone-dependent Cushing's syndrome in a pet ferret (Mustela putorius furo). Domest Anim Endocrinol 2008; 34:278–83.
29. Desmarchelier M, Lair S, Dunn M, et al. Primary hyperaldosteronism in a domestic ferret with an adrenocortical adenoma. J Am Vet Med Assoc 2008;233(8): 1297–301.
30. Schoemaker NJ, Hawkins MG. Hyperadrenocorticism in ferrets: clinical updates. In: Proceedings of the Association of Avian Veterinarians with AEMV. Providence (RI); August 4–9, 2007. p. 79–84.
31. Weiss CA, Scott MV. Clinical aspects and surgical treatment of hyperadrenocorticism in the domestic ferret: 94 cases (1994–1996). J Am Anim Hosp Assoc 1997;33:487–93.
32. Rosenthal KL, Peterson ME, Quesenberry KE, et al. Hyperadrenocorticism associated with adrenocortical tumor or nodular hyperplasia in ferrets: 50 cases (1987–1991). J Am Vet Med Assoc 1993;203:271–5.
33. Bielinska M, Kiiveri S, Parviainen J, et al. Gonadectomy-induced adrenocortical neoplasia in the domestic ferret (Mustela putorius furo) and laboratory mouse. Vet Pathol 2006;43:97–117.
34. Schoemaker NJ, Schuurmans M, Moorman H, et al. Correlation between age at neutering and age at onset of hyperadrenocorticism in ferrets. J Am Vet Med Assoc 2000;216(2):195–7.
35. Schoemaker NJ, Lumeij JL, Rijnberk A. Current and future alternatives to surgical neutering in ferrets to prevent hyperadrenocorticism. Vet Med 2005;100(7): 484–96.
36. Murray J. Melatonin implants: an option for use in the treatment of adrenocortical disease in ferrets. Exotic Mam Med Surg 2005;3(1):1–6.
37. Coleman GD, Chavez MA, Williams BH. Cystic prostatic disease associated with adrenocortical lesions in the ferret (Mustela putorius furo). Vet Pathol 1998;35: 547–9.
38. Kuijten AM, Schoemaker NJ, Voorhout G. Ultrasonographic visualization of the adrenal glands of healthy ferrets and ferrets with hyperadrenocorticism. J Am Anim Hosp Assoc 2007;43:78–84.
39. Wagner RA, Bailey EM, Schneider JF, et al. Leuprolide acetate treatment of adrenocortical disease in ferrets. J Am Vet Med Assoc 2001;218(8):1272–4.
40. Johnson-Delaney CA. Medical therapies for ferret adrenal disease. Semin Avian Exotic Pet Med 2004;13(1):3–7.
41. Wagner RA, Piché CA, Jöchle W, et al. Clinical and endocrine responses to treatment with deslorelin acetate implants in ferrets with adrenocortical disease. Am J Vet Res 2005;66(5):910–4.
42. Ramer JC, Benson KG, Morrisey JK, et al. Effects of melatonin administration on the clinical course of adrenocortical disease in domestic ferrets. J Am Vet Med Assoc 2006;229(11):1743–8.
43. Swiderski JK, Seim HB III, MacPhail CM. Long-term outcome of domestic ferrets treated surgically for hyperadrenocorticism: 130 cases (1995–2004). J Am Vet Med Assoc 2008;232(9):1338–43.

44. Weiss CA, Williams BH, Scott JB, et al. Surgical treatment and long-term outcome of ferrets with bilateral adrenal tumors or adrenal hyperplasia: 56 cases (1994–1997). J Am Vet Med Assoc 1999;215(6):820–3.
45. Nolte DM, Carberry CA, Gannon KM, et al. Temporary tube cystostomy as a treatment for urinary obstruction secondary to adrenocortical disease in four ferrets. J Am Anim Hosp Assoc 2002;38:527–32.

Advanced Diagnostic Approaches and Current Management of Internal Disorders of Select Species (Rodents, Sugar Gliders, Hedgehogs)

Erika E. Evans, DVM, MBA[a], Marcy J. Souza, DVM, MPH, DABVP-Avian[b],*

KEYWORDS

- Hedgehog • Sugar gliders • Rodents
- Diagnostics • Therapeutics

African pygmy hedgehogs (*Atelerix albiventris*) are unusual, but increasingly common pets. Due to strict regulations preventing importation of African pygmy hedgehogs into the United States, those in the pet trade are from captive bred populations. The European hedgehog (*Erinaceous europaeus*), although occasionally kept as a pet, is the most common British mammal seen in wildlife rescue and rehabilitation centers.[1] Both species are commonly kept as zoologic specimens.

Sugar gliders (*Petaurus breviceps*), marsupials native to Australia, Tasmania, New Guinea, and islands of Indonesia, are seen as pets in veterinary practices throughout the United States. These unique creatures are often presented for illness related to inadequate husbandry and/or nutrition. As clients become more educated about these animals, interest is being generated in finding increased levels of veterinary care.

Rodents such as rats (*Rattus norvegicus*), mice (*Mus musculus*), gerbils (*Meriones unguiculatus*), hamsters (*Mesocricetus auratus*), guinea pigs (*Cavia porcellus*), and chinchillas (*Chinchilla lanigera*) continue to be presented to veterinarians as pets and as collection species. There is a great deal of knowledge about these animals

a Department of Small Animal Clinical Sciences, University of Tennessee College of Veterinary Medicine, Knoxville, TN 37996, USA
b Department of Comparative Medicine, University of Tennessee College of Veterinary Medicine, Knoxville, TN 37996, USA
* Corresponding author.
E-mail address: msouza@utk.edu

Vet Clin Exot Anim 13 (2010) 453–469
doi:10.1016/j.cvex.2010.05.003
1094-9194/10/$ – see front matter © 2010 Elsevier Inc. All rights reserved.

vetexotic.theclinics.com

and their use as laboratory research species, but less is known about diagnosing and treating them as individual pets.

As their popularity increases, more and more practitioners are being asked to examine, diagnose, and treat these animals for a bevy of disorders and diseases. Many procedures and techniques used in both traditional small and large animal medicine are used for these species, with minor adaptations or considerations. This article examines available diagnostic tools and treatment methodologies for use in hedgehogs, sugar gliders, and selected rodents.

PHYSICAL EXAMINATION

Hedgehogs that are comfortable and accustomed to human contact can be examined with minimal restraint and the use of a clean towel or glove.[2] Physical examination in hedgehogs that are unaccustomed to handling or are nervous in an unusual situation can be a challenge. Therefore, an initial hands-off observation is a critical step to take note of any obvious abnormalities; this can often be accomplished by observing the hedgehog from a distance in a clear container.[3] The animal's carriage and ambulation status should be evaluated. When standing, hedgehogs should have a plantigrade stance with the body lifted off the substrate. There are several proposed techniques to encourage the hedgehog to not roll into a ball, including scruffing the hedgehog before it rolls into a ball, exposing it to water,[4] or placing it on a flat surface without handling for a few minutes.[5] However, these techniques even when safely performed rarely work well enough or long enough for a complete physical examination and assessment to be performed. Isoflurane anesthesia is often used to facilitate a thorough physical examination (**Fig. 1**). Particular attention should be paid to areas prone to disease in hedgehogs. Commonly seen diseases and disorders of pet hedgehogs include, but are not limited to, oral masses, periodontal disease, pneumonia, cardiomyopathy, trauma, and neoplasia.[3,5] Therefore, a thorough examination should include a complete examination of the oral cavity and mucous membranes, auscultation of heart and lung sounds, dermatologic assessment, abdominal palpation, visualization and assessment of the reproductive organs, and close inspection of the limbs and feet.

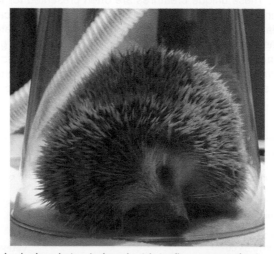

Fig. 1. An African hedgehog being induced with isoflurane anesthesia.

As with hedgehogs, sugar gliders are often best first examined with a hands-off approach to assist the clinician in evaluating for signs of respiratory distress, neurologic deficits, or evidence of trauma. Handling can be accomplished manually by holding the individual in cupped hands or while supporting the body, restraining the head at the mandibular joint.[6] Restraint by the tail is not recommended. The use of anesthesia is encouraged to perform a full physical examination.[7] Conditions seen in sugar gliders include, but are not limited to, problems associated with inadequate husbandry/nutrition, dental disease, and trauma. Therefore, complete visual examination and palpation of the sugar glider in addition to obtaining a weight, body condition score, temperature, pulse, and respiratory rate is appropriate.

Rodents differ greatly in their receptiveness to manual restraint and examination because of species differences, familiarity with being handled, and presence and severity of illness.[8] Rodents that are accustomed to handling may allow an examination without chemical restraint. However, even rodents accustomed to handling may become panicked due to the unfamiliar location and/or an underlying disease. Brief periods of gas anesthesia are often worth the risk in order to reduce stress for a physical examination. Review of individual species susceptibility to and prevalence of disease may help guide a thorough physical examination of the rodent. Observation of the rodent in the cage is an appropriate starting point for an examination, and allows evaluation of the respiratory rate and character, locomotion ability, and overall demeanor of the animal.[9] Rodents such as guinea pigs and chinchillas that are prone to dental disease may benefit from having the oral cavity examined at the end rather than the beginning of the examination.

Based on the history, initial observation, and physical examination, a problem-oriented approach may be used to define identified problems, determine appropriate diagnostic tests, establish treatment, educate clients, and monitor patient progress.[10] Diagnostic testing should be aimed at proving likely items or disproving unlikely items on a differential diagnostic list. Published research on diagnostic testing with information regarding test accuracy for the appropriate species should be used when available. However, many problem-specific diagnostic tests are not validated in exotic species. The use of a clinically healthy animal as a comparison can provide data that, although not statistically significant, can still aid in developing an index of support for a particular diagnosis. The diagnostician should keep in mind that many examinations and tests will need to be performed with the use of anesthesia.[11] Therefore, planning ahead to minimize the number of times an animal is subjected to anesthetic episodes is advised.

DIAGNOSTIC PROCEDURES
Venipuncture

A safe sample volume of blood in small exotic mammals is often estimated to be 1% of lean body mass.[12] If the animal sampled is geriatric, suspected to be anemic, hypoproteinemic, or otherwise compromised, smaller amounts of blood should be collected. Continued loss of blood through hematoma formation also needs to be considered. Limiting the blood collected to 0.5% of the animal's body weight is appropriate in ill or otherwise debilitated animals,[13,14] Techniques for collecting blood are often similar to those used in cats and dogs because the vascular anatomy is often comparable.[12] The challenge often stems from the small size of the vessels and the change in approach that is often required to access different vessels.

Obtaining blood from hedgehogs, sugar gliders, or rodents without the use of chemical restraint or anesthesia is typically only possible if the animal is severely debilitated.[15,16] Isoflurane is frequently used for anesthesia. Small amounts of blood (even as small as one drop) are often worth the effort of collection.[11] In a hematocrit tube, blood volumes this minute can still provide indispensable information such as a blood glucose level, a blood smear for a differential, or a packed cell volume and total solids.

In hedgehogs, up to 0.5 mL of blood can be taken from the lateral saphenous and cephalic veins.[3,12] The lateral saphenous vein is often best sampled just below the stifle.[2] These vessels can be difficult to visualize and are prone to collapse.[12] Different techniques have been described to avoid the common complications of venous collapse and sample clotting.[5] These techniques include collecting the blood in a 25-gauge needle hub and then collecting the blood from the hub with a microhematocrit tube or by using a preheparinized tuberculin syringe outfitted with a 25- or 27-gauge needle. The femoral vein can be used for blood collection of up to 1 mL in hedgehogs. However, due to its anatomic location, care must be taken to not lacerate the closely approximated femoral artery.

Unlike hedgehogs, sugar gliders have cephalic, lateral saphenous, and femoral veins that are typically easily visualized.[7] As in hedgehogs these tiny vessels are easily collapsed, and the use of an insulin syringe with a 27-gauge needle is recommended for collection. These animals also have a ventral tail vein; warming the animal is recommended to aid in vasodilatation of this vessel.[12] A maximum of 0.1 to 0.25 mL may be obtained from each of the previously described venipuncture sites. Sugar gliders also have a medial tibial artery, which is readily visualized and from which 0.5 mL of blood may be collected. However, this vessel is very mobile and tends to roll, making successful bleeding difficult. Digital pressure should be applied immediately after drawing from the artery to aid in avoiding the formation of a hematoma.[6]

Small amounts of blood may be obtained from most rodents seen in clinical practice by use of the lateral saphenous veins.[12] In mice, venipuncture of the submandibular vein at the junction where it meets the jugular vein behind the mandibular joint has been described. Small amounts may also be collected from the cephalic vein of guinea pigs, hamsters, chinchillas, and other larger rodents. In almost all cases, the use of anesthesia to minimize stress and reduce complications associated with the blood draw is indicated.[13] Blood collection without the use of anesthesia from the dorsal tail vein of rats has been described.[17] Rats were preconditioned to handling and crawling in a towel with their tail gently extended for 2-minute periods 4 to 5 days before the actual collection. A small incision was made about 15 mm from the distal end of the tail and digital pressure was applied proximal to the incision while blood was collected in a microhematocrit tube. Venipuncture of the lateral tail veins of rats has also been described without the use of anesthesia.[12] However, venipuncture using manual restraint has been shown to interfere with a rat's ability to thermoregulate for up to 30 hours after sampling, and in venipuncture taking longer than 2 to 3 minutes, blood corticosterone levels were increased, indicating high levels of stress.

Complete blood cell counts, chemistry panels, and other more focused testing will require larger volumes of blood than can be gained from the techniques previously described.[11] The jugular vein is of sufficient size in hedgehogs to collect a diagnostic blood sample.[3] This vessel may be difficult to visualize, particularly in obese hedgehogs, but it runs between the ramus of the mandible and the point of the shoulder as in other small mammals.[12] To access the vessel, the hedgehog may be held in ventrodorsal recumbency with the legs stretched caudally, as described in ferrets. The authors have also had success with positioning the hedgehog in dorsoventral recumbency with the legs stretched caudally over the end of a table, as is typically used to bleed the jugular of domestic cats and some ferrets. A 22- to 25-gauge needle on a 1- to 3-mL syringe may be used to collect this sample.

Approximately 0.5 to 1 mL of blood can be collected from the jugular vessel of a sugar glider.[12] The use of a 25- to 27-gauge needle on a 1-mL syringe is recommended for collection. Rodents, due to size and species variation, will differ somewhat with regard to the appropriate size of needle and syringe as well as the amount of blood that can successfully be drawn from the jugular.

A peripheral vessel not typically used in blood draws for cats and dogs, but used with some frequency in exotic small mammal practice, is the cranial vena cava. The internal and external jugular veins join into the cranial vena cava, which unites with the subclavian vein before it empties into the right atrium of the heart.[18] Venipuncture technique for accessing this vessel will differ slightly between species of varying size and anatomic diversity, but all will likely require the use of general anesthesia.[13] Possible risks associated with collecting a sample from the cranial vena cava include hemorrhage, hemothorax, penetration of the heart, and hemopericardium.

In species the size of a hedgehog, chinchilla, guinea pig, or rat, a 1- to 3-mL syringe and 25- to 27-gauge needle are appropriate for sampling.[12] In animals of smaller stature such as sugar gliders, mice, and hamsters, a 1-mL syringe with a 27-gauge needle or tuberculin syringe with a 30-gauge needle may be needed.[18] Individuals should be placed in ventrodorsal recumbency with the front limbs placed to the respective sides of the thoracic cavity.

Rats, mice, hamsters, and gerbils have well-developed clavicles that articulate between the sternum and the scapular-humeral junction.[18] Methods described for accessing the cranial vena cava of the rat are often also successful in hedgehogs.[12] A 0.5-inch length needle is inserted cranial to the clavicle and angled 45° toward the opposite leg.[14] Positioning the needle caudal to the clavicle and cranial to the first rib will force the needle into a more lateral position and makes successful venipuncture difficult.

In guinea pigs and chinchillas, the clavicle is not as well developed, and a needle (five-eighths-inch length) should be placed cranial to the manubrium and first rib.[14] Techniques used to successfully sample guinea pigs have been found to be successful in sugar gliders.[12] The needle should not be advanced more than 1 to 1.5 cm into the thoracic cavity (**Fig. 2**). If no blood is aspirated into the syringe when negative pressure is applied, the needle should be slightly retracted and redirected toward midline.

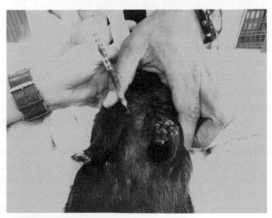

Fig. 2. Venipuncture of the cranial vena cava in a guinea pig.

Hematology and Immunoassay

More advanced hematologic testing, such as blood cultures, serology, antigen detection, and virus isolation, may be performed to further evaluate for evidence of disease.[16] Many diagnostic laboratories that assist with handling of laboratory animal specimens are also willing to run samples on individual pet animals, and most can run serology (immunofluorescent antibody [IFA] and enzyme-linked immunosorbent assay [ELISA]) on small amounts of blood (0.1 mL or less). Antigen detection via polymerase chain reaction (PCR) can also be performed on various samples including blood, nasal swabs, tracheal swabs, and fecal samples. Individual laboratories should be contacted in regard of their specific sample handling and shipping requirements. It is noteworthy that for some common microbes that infect small exotic mammal patients, such as *Mycoplasma* spp, culture results may be negative in infected animals.[19] In these animals, additional serologic testing such as ELISA or IFA in combination with PCR is often indicated. Providing the diagnostic agency with information regarding the disease process or processes you suspect may aid their recommendations for which tests or test packages to perform.

Many viral infections in small exotic mammals are asymptomatic unless further complicated via secondary bacterial infection.[20] Therefore, most diagnoses of viral infections in pets are based on clinical signs rather than serologic identification. Serologic testing for an individual is often not warranted because antibodies are often only present after clinical signs are abating. For households with multiple pets or that allow breeding, serologic testing to allow for disease prevention may be appropriate. Mice, rats, and guinea pigs are common laboratory species and, as such, microbial testing is readily available for these species. Hedgehogs and chinchillas have had reports of suspected infection with herpes simplex virus, but given their minimal representation as laboratory animals, additional hematologic testing is not routinely performed.[5] Gerbils and sugar gliders have no current reports of naturally occurring viral diseases and therefore routine serologic testing is also not commonly performed.[20] Serologic testing is available for select fungal[21] and parasitic organisms, and should be pursued when appropriate. For instance, sugar gliders have been shown to be highly susceptible to toxoplasmosis, and testing via ELISA or IFA may be indicated.[6,22]

Fecal Analysis

Fresh fecal samples can be evaluated via cytology and culture. Swabbing the rectum of small mammals gently with a culturette will supply a sample appropriate for fecal culture.[23] Anesthesia should be used for this procedure to decrease the likelihood of contamination of the sample and to decrease the risk of perforation. Suspected pathogens should be communicated to the diagnostic laboratory to aid in identification.[16] Some organisms, such as *Salmonella* spp, require different media for successful culture and are a potential zoonosis.

Fecal floatation and a direct smear are often sufficient in identifying most problematic parasites.[16] An anal tape test can also be employed to identify pin worms. Although rodents are often forthcoming with fecal samples, many species such as guinea pigs and chinchillas experience minor constipation within novel environments such as a veterinary hospital.[23] Hedgehogs also are often not forthcoming with fecal samples in a clinical setting.[2] Therefore, fresh fecal samples should be collected by owners whenever possible. If there is a delay between collection of the fecal sample and the transportation of the sample to the veterinarian, the sample should be kept refrigerated away from any human food items.

Urinalysis

Urinalysis can help identify urinary and reproductive tract disease. Collecting a free catch urine sample from a hedgehog may be attempted by placing the hedgehog in a clean plastic or stainless steel container.[5] Obtaining a sample appropriate for culture can be obtained via ventral percutaneous cystocentesis (ultrasound guided) or through sterile placement of a small flexible catheter.[2] Both procedures should be attempted only with appropriate anesthesia. Although urinalysis parameters have not been established for use in hedgehogs, neoplastic cells, crystals, white blood cells, and red blood cells may be considered abnormal findings depending on the collection method.[5] Urine test strips, although not verified in these species, can often be used successfully to help determine if a red hue observed in free catch urine is due to porphryin pigment or blood. A urine antigen test performed by MiraVista Diagnostics (Indianapolis, IN, USA) is also available for histoplasmosis, a fungal disease recently reported in an African pygmy hedgehog[24] and sugar gliders[11]; 2 mL of urine is requested by the company for antigen testing. However, analysis may be completed on a urine volume as small as 600 µL (Wheat LJ, MiraVista Diagnostics, Indianapolis, IN, personal communication, 2010). Multiple urine samples from one individual may be collected and refrigerated for up to 3 to 5 days to obtain sufficient sample size. However, the longer the delays in sample analysis, the higher the risk for contamination of other fungal growths that may cross-react and result in false positives. Other urine antigen tests are available for blastomycosis, aspergillosis, and coccidioidomycosis.

Cystocentesis can often be attempted in larger rodents such as guinea pigs, rats, and chinchillas, as described for the hedgehog.[23] Urine collection in sugar gliders and other common rodents can be difficult due to their small size. Sugar glider urine and fecal collection are further complicated by their unique anatomic composition. The urinary ducts, gastrointestinal tract, and genital ducts empty into a common cloaca.[25] Some species such as the gerbil are physiologically programmed to conserve water, and therefore only small amounts of highly concentrated urine are typically available.[23] These animals are often too small to safely perform cystocentesis or atraumatic urinary catheterization, and free catch samples should be collected when appropriate.

Cytologic Sampling

Additional and more advanced diagnostics are often pursued based on the clinician's assessment and localization of the disease process. Fluid in the thorax or abdomen can be collected via thoracocentesis or abdominocentesis (**Fig. 3**), respectively. The use of a 25-gauge butterfly catheter with a 3- or 6-mL syringe to perform thoracocentesis has been described in rodents.[14] Performing these procedures with ultrasound guidance is recommended. In addition to its potentially therapeutic value, the fluid removed can then be evaluated for protein levels, possible etiologic agents, cell population, and morphology. Samples should also be submitted for culture and sensitivity.

Although respiratory disease is often diagnosed on clinical suspicion and treated empirically, individuals that fail to respond to initial therapy often require additional diagnostics. The use of cytology with culture and sensitivity is often used to identify possible respiratory pathogens. Nasal swabs are used frequently and carry little risk to the individual, but these swabs are contaminated samples and do not accurately assess disease occurring in the lower airways. In stable patients, culture of samples collected via tracheal or bronchoalveolar lavage is recommended.[14] A method for endoscopic assisted tracheal aspiration in guinea pigs has been described.[26] The

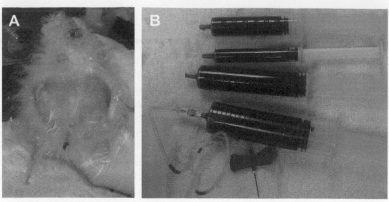

Fig. 3. (A) This hamster presented with severe abdominal distension. (B) Abdominocentesis was performed and cytology performed on the resulting fluid.

focus is on minimizing the fluid needed for sampling (approximately 0.5 mL), by positioning the guinea pig in sternal recumbency with the thoracic inlet lower than the remainder of the body.

Cytologic evaluation of the reproductive tract may also aid in diagnosis. Pouch infections have been documented with some frequency in captive female marsupials including the sugar glider.[25] The pouch should be swabbed and checked for yeast and bacteria.[27] Culture is recommended in addition to cytology. Males presenting with stranguria, hematuria, or penile trauma should be evaluated for prostatitis and involvement of the paracloacal glands common to both genders.[25] In hedgehogs, the predominant cause of abnormal vaginal discharge is reported to be neoplasia, but pyometra and metritis have also been reported.[3] Infection and inflammation of the uterus, testicles, vagina, epididymis, and mammary glands have been reported in rodents.[28] Cytologic evaluation with culture and sensitivity of any discharge or milk should be completed to determine etiology.[28]

Neoplasia is common in hedgehogs, sugar gliders, and rodents.[15] As a result, these animals are often presented for oncologic evaluation. Fine-needle aspiration, as in other species, is of minimal risk, but often the quantity and quality of cells evaluated is poor.[29] Aspiration is often completed with a 22- or 25-gauge needle for most sites and ultrasound guidance is used when appropriate. Biopsies, both incisional and excisional, are options that increase the likelihood of diagnosis (**Fig. 4**). Samples can be evaluated via cytology and histopathology. Additional stains and immunohistochemistry may also be completed depending on the index of suspicion for a particular diagnosis.

Evaluation of the bone marrow may be completed if neoplasia is suspected or for malignancy staging.[13] Other indications for bone marrow examination include hematologic disorders, anemia, thrombocytopenia, gammopathies, and lymphoproliferative disorders. The most common site for bone marrow aspiration and biopsy in small exotic mammals is the proximal femur. Other locations that may be used are dependent on the size of the patient but include the proximal tibia, proximal humerus, and the ileum. General anesthesia and infiltration of the area to be sampled with a local anesthetic, such as lidocaine, is recommended. After surgical preparation of the site, a small skin incision should be made and a spinal needle with stylet advanced into the medullary cavity. Once the stylet is removed, negative pressure is applied via the syringe until blood is seen and marrow has been aspirated. The use of excessive

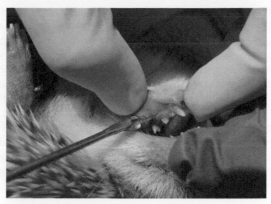

Fig. 4. Biopsy of a gingival mass in an African hedgehog.

negative pressure should be avoided because it can contaminate the sample with peripheral blood artifact, which hinders interpretation. Bone biopsy has been described with the use of an 18- and 20-gauge spinal needle.[29] Due to the small size of these pets, penetration of both cortices and exiting the skin through the opposite side may be attempted to preserve the core. The stylet can then be reintroduced before the needle is removed to push the sample out through the bottom of the needle (**Fig. 5**).

Radiographs

As with most of the previously described diagnostic techniques, taking diagnostic quality radiographs in all but the most severely ill hedgehogs, sugar gliders, and rodents will require the use of sedation and/or anesthesia.[30,31] Manual restraint may be attempted in animals that are critically ill and are at high anesthetic risk, but the stress induced from handling often limits its sole use. The use of anesthesia also lessens the likelihood that images will need to be repeated because it allows for correct patient positioning and greatly reduces the probability that the patient will move at an inopportune time.

Total body projections including the skull, extremities, and tail are the views taken most often for the species discussed here. Radiolucent tape is often used to

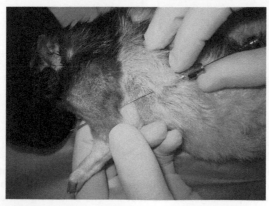

Fig. 5. Bone marrow biopsy of rat humerus using a 20-gauge spinal needle with stylet.

appropriately position limbs and anesthetic face masks when needed. Ventrodorsal and lateral projections are the most commonly taken views. When evaluating for diseases localized to the head including dental disease, multiple projections of the head including lateral, oblique, ventrodorsal, and rostrocaudal are needed.[32,33]

As with small animals, systematic evaluation of the thoracic and abdominal cavities is indicated. Comparing radiographs of patients with those taken of clinically unremarkable animals is one of the most beneficial ways to identify abnormalities (**Fig. 6**). Collections of radiographs featuring these species have been published demonstrating examples of both healthy and ill individuals.[15,30,31] Radiographs provide valuable, noninvasive supporting evidence for disease conditions commonly seen in these species including, but not limited to, respiratory disease, fractures, luxations, neoplasia, gastric distention, and impaction (**Fig. 7**). Radiographs are also beneficial in evaluating the urinary and reproductive tracts (**Fig. 8**).

Contrast Radiography

Contrast radiography may help identify and localize disease conditions of the gastrointestinal tract, urinary tract, and reproductive tract. The use of barium as a contrast agent has been described as a method to successfully evaluate gastrointestinal motility in the guinea pig.[34] Fluoroscopy may also be used for this purpose. Gastrointestinal-positive contrast studies with barium have been completed in multiple rodents including guinea pigs, rats, chinchillas, and hamsters.[31] In mammals, the uterus lies in close proximity to the colon, dorsal to the bladder, and when enlarged due to pregnancy or pyometra, can be difficult to distinguish from the colon (**Fig. 9**). A small amount of air or barium carefully injected into the colon can help differentiate between the terminal colon and reproductive tract. This technique is not recommended in sugar gliders because the gastrointestinal and urogenital systems have a common exit point.

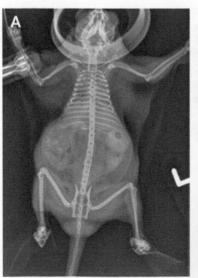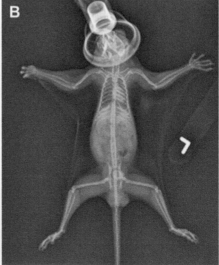

Fig. 6. Ventrodorsal radiographs of 2 sugar gliders. (*A*) Gastric and intestinal dilation is shown in this clinically ill animal. (*B*) A sugar glider with an unremarkable gastrointestinal tract, missing the distal phalanges of the first 2 digits of the right manus is offered for comparison.

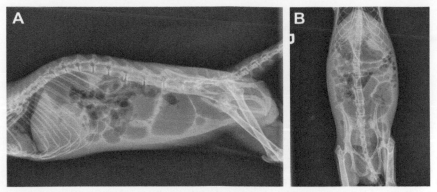

Fig. 7. Lateral (*A*) and ventrodorsal (*B*) radiographs of a chinchilla that show marked gas and fluid distention of the cecum as well as gas and fluid noted throughout the gastrointestinal structures.

Urinary tract disease is also common in these species and although plain radiographs are often sufficient to identify the presence and probable location of calculi, additional studies such as contrast cystography, urethrography, or intravenous pyelography may be indicated to evaluate for bladder wall integrity, concurrent disease conditions, and renal function.[35] In most cases, the small size of these patients makes these procedures technically difficult and time consuming. As a result, these diagnostics are rarely performed in private practice.

Another form of contrast radiography, myelography, is used in addition to survey films to more fully evaluate the spinal cord.[36] An example of successful myelography

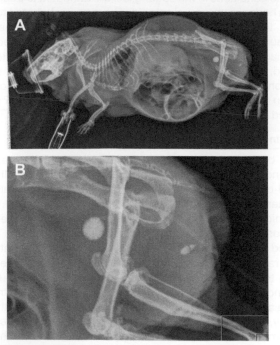

Fig. 8. (*A*) Right lateral radiograph of female guinea pig with urethral and urinary bladder stone. (*B*) Magnified image showing urethral and urinary bladder stone.

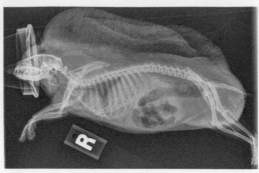

Fig. 9. A lateral radiograph of a female hedgehog 3 days postpartum with either dilated gastrointestinal loops or a gas-filled uterus. Additional diagnostics including contrast radiography or ultrasound are recommended.

in a clinically unremarkable guinea pig has been published.[31] Indications for completing a myelogram include trauma (luxation or fracture), suspect neoplasia, or other potential compression or space occupying lesion(s) affecting the brain or spinal cord.[36] Collection of cerebrospinal fluid to evaluate for inflammation, infection, or neoplasia may also be indicated and should be done before injection of contrast material. Although myelography and cerebrospinal fluid collection are relatively inexpensive, completing the procedures in extremely small patients can be technically challenging, and the potential disadvantages can include exacerbation of neurologic signs leading to seizures, paralysis, and death.

Most neurologic conditions in the sugar glider are attributed to trauma or inadequate nutrition.[7,11,15] In hedgehogs, neurologic signs have been attributed to multiple causes including trauma, toxins, infection, and malnutrition.[3,5] Wobbly hedgehog syndrome is a progressive neurologic disease that presents with ataxia followed by paresis and paralysis. This diagnosis is made either by clinical signs or via histologic evaluation of the spinal cord, brain, and peripheral nerves. Reports of clinical signs and pathologic changes consistent with intravertebral disc disease have also been described recently in African hedgehogs.[37] No reports of myelography in sugar gliders or hedgehogs are reported in the literature.

Magnetic Resonance Imaging

A less invasive, but more expensive method for imaging the neurologic system, including brain and spinal cord, is magnetic resonance imaging (MRI). In addition to providing clinical data to support neurologic diagnoses, MRI has also proven useful in evaluating other soft tissues within the thoracic and abdominal cavities. Despite its promising clinical use, there are no current reports of MRI used in a veterinary setting for diagnoses of pet rodents, sugar gliders, or hedgehogs. There is a report of MRI performed in Sprague-Dawley rats to determine appropriate techniques for evaluation of the rat brain and abdomen.[38] Multiple MRI studies have been completed in rodent models to research human disease conditions such as multiple sclerosis in mice[39] and pulmonary lesions from infection with *Mycobacterium tuberculosis* in guinea pigs.[40] Disadvantages of MRI usage in a clinical setting with these pets include lack of availability, cost, length of anesthesia time in animals prone to hypothermia, and lack of documented use in pets. It is hoped that as the breadth of usage of MRI in laboratory animal medicine is published, examples of clinically healthy species will be made more readily available to clinical practitioners focused on the care of pets.

Computed Tomography

Computed tomography (CT) has proven useful in evaluating the skull and vertebral column of exotic mammals.[36] Perhaps most promising is the use of CT as a modality for accessing rodents with dental disease.[41] CT enables the clinician to assess multiple slices of tissue, minimizing the effects of superimposition of bony and soft tissue structures seen in traditional radiographs. This modality allows for more thorough assessment of bone loss and osteomyelitis. CT is routinely used at the authors' facility for evaluating the extent of soft tissue and bony involvement of facial and/or tooth root abscesses (**Fig. 10**). In addition, the use of microCT has been reported to evaluate a tooth root abscess and osteomyelitis in a guinea pig.[42] MicroCT scanners offer superior resolution compared with conventional CT. However, microCT scanners are not readily available in clinical settings, aside from veterinary research facilities.

Ultrasound

Another imaging modality used with increasing frequency in small animal exotic practices and in the authors' facility is ultrasound. In many cases ultrasound is used instead of contrast procedures. Indications for abdominal ultrasound include palpable masses, fluid, or systemic disease to which a cause cannot be readily identified. Ultrasound provides greater imaging detail than that of contrast procedures for abdominal neoplasms and urogenital abnormalities.[14] Ovarian cysts (**Fig. 11**), dystocias, reproductive tract neoplasias, and urinary tract calculi are well visualized via ultrasound.[43] Pleural effusion, pulmonary pathology, and mediastinal masses may also be evaluated via thoracic ultrasound.[44] Cardiac structure and function may be examined via ultrasound in rodents.[45]

Endoscopy

Endoscopy has multiple uses with exotic mammal and marsupial medicine, but actual use is dependent on clinical signs and limited to some extent by the size of the patient.[46] The most common uses for endoscopy in these small patients are assisted tracheal intubation and oral examination. The ability to appropriately diagnosis and

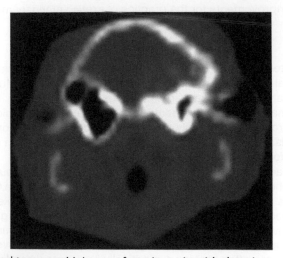

Fig. 10. A computed tomographic image of a guinea pig with chronic severe left-sided otitis media/interna and osteomyelitis.

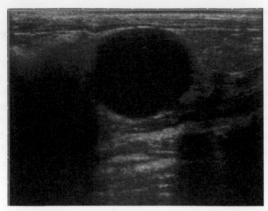

Fig. 11. Ultrasound of a guinea pig showing polycystic ovarian disease.

determine the extent of dental disease and associated pathology is greatly enhanced by endoscopy because of focal illumination and magnification. The use of the endoscope may also aid in biopsies and foreign body retrieval, and serve as a surgical aid in the oral and paranasal cavities. The use of endoscopy to identify and take samples of pathology of the distal urogenital tract has also been described for use in larger rodents such as guinea pigs.[47]

Necropsy

A final and very valuable diagnostic method is necropsy. Although every effort is made to prolong a high quality of life, individuals that have succumbed to disease present a unique opportunity to learn valuable information. Much of our understanding in these species has been gained from necropsy reports that have given us valuable information regarding commonality and pathology of certain disease processes. As we learn more about the disorders and diseases that incapacitate these animals, our ability to accurately diagnose and identify appropriate treatments continues to improve. The pairing of this knowledge with the ever increasing medical technological advances promises great improvements for the practice of exotic veterinary medicine.

THERAPEUTICS

Although many dosages and delivery methods currently used in these animals are anecdotal, clinical improvement is noted in many individuals. Multiple resources have published data on drug usage in hedgehogs and sugar gliders.[15,16,48] However, most of the information lacks pharmacokinetic and pharmacodynamic backing. Pharmaceutical research is more readily available for rodent species commonly kept as laboratory animals. However, much work remains for determination of pharmaceuticals appropriate for rodents kept as pets.

Subcutaneous administration of medication and fluids is typically successfully delivered in the hedgehog.[5] However, due to the large amount of adipose tissue present in the subcutaneous layer, there may be decreased or delayed uptake or distribution. Subcutaneous medications are also easily administered in sugar gliders and most rodents.[11,14] Intravenous medications can be difficult in these small animals, and venous catheters are dislodged when hedgehogs roll into a defensive position. Intraosseous catheters are often preferred in critically ill patients when fluids, colloids, or intravenous antibiotics are indicated. Oral medications work well in patients that are

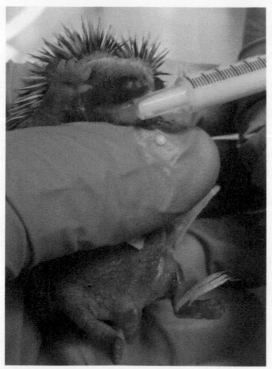

Fig. 12. Oral antibiotic administration in a young hoglet.

stable and interested in food (**Fig. 12**). Many veterinarians advocate mixing oral medication with small amounts of juice or a favorite food such as banana or peanut butter, and report clinical improvement using this method.[5] However, studies are lacking that identify what effect, if any, mixing the various drugs with foods and liquids of varying pH and chemical composition has on the activity and bioavailability of different drugs.

Therapeutics should be based on results of a thorough diagnostic evaluation. In more critically ill animals or those with significant financial limitations, empirical supportive care may be initiated with regard to background information about the species being treated and the clinical signs of the individual animal.[10] Despite some of the current challenges in diagnosing and treating pet sugar gliders, hedgehogs, and rodents, increasing experience with examining and caring for these animals is furthering veterinarians' ability to provide quality medical care to these beloved and special pets.

REFERENCES

1. Stocker L. Practical wildlife care. Ames (IA). 2nd edition. Oxford (UK): Blackwell Pub; 2005.
2. Simone-Freilicher EA, Hoefer HL. Hedgehog care and husbandry. Vet Clin North Am Exot Anim Pract 2004;7(2):257–67, v.
3. Ivey E, Carpenter JW. African hedgehogs. In: Quesenberry KE, Carpenter JW, editors, Ferrets, rabbits, and rodents clinical medicine and surgery, vol. 2. St. Louis (MO): Saunders; 2004. p. 339–53.

4. Conn M. Mammals—how to unball a Hedgehog. Exotic DVM 2001;3(5):10.
5. Heatley JJ. Hedgehogs. In: Mitchell MA, Tully TN Jr, editors. Manual of exotic pet practice. St. Louis (MO): Saunders; 2009. p. 433–55.
6. Gamble KC. Marsupial care and husbandry. Vet Clin North Am Exot Anim Pract 2004;7(2):283–98, vi.
7. Ness RD, Booth R. Sugar gliders. In: Quesenberry KE, Carpenter JW, editors, Ferrets, rabbits, and rodents clinical medicine and surgery, vol. 2. St. Louis (MO): Saunders; 2004. p. 330–8.
8. Brown CJ, Donnelly TM. Rodent husbandry and care. Vet Clin North Am Exot Anim Pract 2004;7(2):201–25, v.
9. Donnelly TM, Brown CJ. Guinea pig and chinchilla care and husbandry. Vet Clin North Am Exot Anim Pract 2004;7(2):351–73, vii.
10. Gibbons PM. Problem-oriented exotic companion animal practice. Journal of Exotic Pet Medicine 2009;18(3):181–6.
11. Lennox AM. Emergency and critical care procedures in sugar gliders (*Petaurus breviceps*), African hedgehogs (*Atelerix albiventris*), and prairie dogs (*Cynomys* spp). Vet Clin North Am Exot Anim Pract 2007;10(2):533–55.
12. Joslin JO. Blood collection techniques in exotic small mammals. Journal of Exotic Pet Medicine 2009;18(2):117–39.
13. Pilny AA. Clinical hematology of rodent species. Vet Clin North Am Exot Anim Pract 2008;11(3):523–33, vi–vii.
14. Hawkins MG, Graham JE. Emergency and critical care of rodents. Vet Clin North Am Exot Anim Pract 2007;10(2):501–31.
15. Quesenberry KE, Carpenter JW. Ferrets, rabbits and rodents: clinical medicine and surgery. 2nd edition. St. Louis (MO): Saunders; 2004.
16. Mitchell MA, Tully TN Jr. Manual of exotic pet practice. St. Louis (MO): Saunders; 2009.
17. Fluttert M, Dalm S, Oitzl MS. A refined method for sequential blood sampling by tail incision in rats. Lab Anim 2000;34(4):372–8.
18. Capello V. Application of the cranial vena cava venipuncture technique to small exotic mammals. Exotic DVM 2006;8(3):51–5.
19. Donnelly TM. Application of laboratory animal immunoassays to exotic pet practice. Exotic DVM 2006;8(4):19–26.
20. Kashuba C, Hsu C, Krogstad A, et al. Small mammal virology. Vet Clin North Am Exot Anim Pract 2005;8(1):107–22.
21. Lane RF. Diagnostic testing for fungal diseases. Vet Clin North Am Exot Anim Pract 2003;6(2):301–14, v.
22. Barrows M. Toxoplasmosis in a colony of sugar gliders (*Petaurus breviceps*). Vet Clin North Am Exot Anim Pract 2006;9(3):617–23.
23. Klaphake E. Common rodent procedures. Vet Clin North Am Exot Anim Pract 2006;9(2):389–413, vii–viii.
24. Snider TA, Joyner PH, Clinkenbeard KD. Disseminated histoplasmosis in an African pygmy hedgehog. J Am Vet Med Assoc 2008;232(1):74–6.
25. Johnson-Delaney CA. Reproductive medicine of companion marsupials. Vet Clin North Am Exot Anim Pract 2002;5(3):537–53, vi.
26. Johnson D. Endoscopic tracheal wash in two guinea pigs. Exotic DVM 2005;7(3):11–5.
27. Johnson-Delaney C. Medical update for sugar gliders. Exotic DVM 2000;2(3):91–3.
28. Bishop CR. Reproductive medicine of rabbits and rodents. Vet Clin North Am Exot Anim Pract 2002;5(3):507–35, vi.

29. Antinoff N. Oncologic diagnostic sampling for the general practitioner. Exotic DVM 2001;3(3):37–41.
30. Capello V, Lennox AM. Clinical radiology of exotic companion mammals. 1st edition. Ames (IA): Wiley-Blackwell; 2008.
31. Silverman S, Tell LA. Radiology of rodents, rabbits, and ferrets an atlas of normal anatomy and positioning. St. Louis (MO): Elsevier Saunders; 2005.
32. Capello V. Diagnosis and treatment of dental disease in pet rodents. Journal of Exotic Pet Medicine 2008;17(2):114–23.
33. Tell L, Silverman S, Wisner E. Imaging techniques for evaluating the head of birds, reptiles and exotic small mammals. Exotic DVM 2003;5(2):31–7.
34. Ruelokke ML, Arnbjerg J, Martensen MR. Assessing gastrointestinal motility in guinea pigs using contrast radiography. Exotic DVM 2004;6(1):31–6.
35. Fisher PG. Exotic mammal renal disease: diagnosis and treatment. Vet Clin North Am Exot Anim Pract 2006;9(1):69–96.
36. Knipe MF. Principles of neurological imaging of exotic animal species. Vet Clin North Am Exot Anim Pract 2007;10(3):893–907, vii.
37. Raymond JT, Aguilar R, Dunker F, et al. Intervertebral disc disease in African hedgehogs (*Atelerix albiventris*): four cases. Journal of Exotic Pet Medicine 2009;18(3):220–3.
38. Yamada K, Miyahara K, Sato M, et al. Optimizing technical conditions for magnetic resonance imaging of the rat brain and abdomen in a low magnetic field. Vet Radiol Ultrasound 1995;36(6):523–7.
39. Nesslen S, Boretius S, Stadelmann C, et al. Early MRI changes in a mouse model of multiple sclerosis are predictive of severe inflammatory tissue damage. Brain 2007;130(8):2186–98.
40. Kraft SL, Dailey D, Kovach M, et al. Magnetic resonance imaging of pulmonary lesions in guinea pigs infected with mycobacterium tuberculosis. Infect Immun 2004;72(10):5963–71.
41. Capello V, Cauduro A. Clinical technique: application of computed tomography for diagnosis of dental disease in the rabbit, guinea pig, and chinchilla. Journal of Exotic Pet Medicine 2008;17(2):93–101.
42. Souza MJ, Greenacre CB, Avenell JS, et al. Diagnosing a tooth root abscess in a guinea pig (*Cava porcellus*) using micro computed tomography imaging. Journal of Exotic Pet Medicine 2006;15(4):274–7.
43. Hochleithner C, Hochleithner M. Select exotic animal cases using ultrasound. Exotic DVM 2004;6(3):53–6.
44. Tell L, Wisner E. Diagnostic techniques for evaluating the respiratory system of birds, reptiles, and small exotic mammals. Exotic DVM 2003;5(2):38–44.
45. Johnson K. Introduction to rodent cardiac imaging. ILAR J 2008;49(1):27–34.
46. Hernandez-Divers S. Clinical technique: dental endoscopy of rabbits and rodents. Journal of Exotic Pet Medicine 2008;17(2):87–92.
47. Lennox AM. Endoscopy of the distal urogenital tract as an aid in differentiating causes of urogenital bleeding in small mammals. Exotic DVM 2005;7(2):43–7.
48. Carpenter JW. Exotic animal formulary. 3rd edition. St. Louis (MO): Elsevier Saunders; 2005.

Advanced Diagnostic Approaches and Current Management of Proventricular Dilatation Disease

Ady Y. Gancz, DVM, MSc, DVSc, DABVP (Avian Practice)[a,*],
Susan Clubb, DVM, DABVP (Avian Practice)[b],
H.L. Shivaprasad, BVSc, PhD, DACPV[c]

KEYWORDS

• Proventricular dilatation disease • Avian borna virus
• Management • Diagnosis

Proventricular dilatation disease (PDD; synonyms: proventricular dilatation syndrome, macaw wasting/fading syndrome, neuropathic gastric dilatation of Psittaciformes, psittacine encephalomyelitis, myenteric ganglioneuritis, infiltrative splanchnic neuropathy) is a fatal inflammatory disease that affects mainly, but not exclusively, psittacine birds (Order: Psittaciformes). The disease was first recognized in the 1970s in imported macaws (*Ara* sp) in Europe and North America,[1–7] but has since been reported from Australia,[8,9] the Middle East,[10–12] and South America.[13] PDD is also present in South Africa (Dr Emily Lane, BVSC, MPHIL, MRCVS, DACVP, personal communication, 2009).

PDD has been reported in more than 70 psittacine species.[6,14–16] These species include members of the most well-known parrot genera in both the Psittacidae and Cacatuidae families, such as macaws (*Ara* sp), African gray parrots (*Psittacus erithacus*), cockatoos (*Cacatua* sp), Amazon parrots (*Amazona* sp), conures (eg, *Aratinga* sp), and cockatiels (*Nymphicus hollandicus*) (**Table 1**). PDD has not been reported in the budgerigar (*Melopsittacus undulatus*), which may be resistant to the disease.[15,16]

In addition to Psittaciformes, pathologic findings identical to those seen in PDD have been reported in several captive and free-ranging birds representing at least 5

[a] The Exotic Clinic, 26 Ben Gurion Street, Herzliya 46785, Israel
[b] Rainforest Clinic for Birds and Exotics, 3319 East Road, Loxahatchee, FL 33470, USA
[c] Avian Pathology, California Animal Health and Food Safety Laboratory System–Tulare, University of California, Davis, 18830 Road 112, Tulare, CA 93274, USA
* Corresponding author.
E-mail address: ady@exoticdoc.co.il

Vet Clin Exot Anim 13 (2010) 471–494
doi:10.1016/j.cvex.2010.05.004
1094-9194/10/$ – see front matter © 2010 Elsevier Inc. All rights reserved.

vetexotic.theclinics.com

Table 1
Psittacine species that have been diagnosed with PDD[a]

Genus	Species	Origin
Family: Cacatuidae		
Nymphicus	hollandicus	A/P
Cacatua	alba, ducrops, galerita, goffini, haematuropygia, moluccensis, sanguine, sulphurea	A/P
Eolophus	roseicapillus	A/P
Calyptorhynchus	magnificus	A/P
Prosciger	atterimus	A/P
Family: Psittacidae		
Psittacula	alexandri, derbiana, eupatria, krameri	A/P
Eclectus	roratus	A/P
Trichoglossus	haematodus	A/P
Ara	ararauna, auricollis, chloroptera, glacogularis, macao, maracan, militarisa, nobilis, rubrogenys, severa, (+hybrids)	AM
Anodorhyncus	hyacinthinus	AM
Cyanopsitta	spixii	AM
Aratinga	acuticaudata, aurea, auricapilla, erythrogenys, finschi, guarouba, jandaya, solstitialis, weddellii	AM
Nandayus	nenday	AM
Cyanoliseus	patagonus	AM
Pyrrhura	molinae, rupicola	AM
Brotogeris	pyrrhopterus	AM
Rhynchopsitta	pachyrhynca	AM
Amazona	aestiva, albifrons, amazonica, auropalliata, autumnalis, leucocephala, ochrocephala, tucumana, xantholora	AM
Pionopsitta	pileata	AM
Pionus	chalcopterus, fuscus, mestruus, senilis	AM
Pionetes	leucogaster, melanocephala	AM
Deroptyus	accipitrinus	AM
Forpus	coelestris	AM
Psittacus	erithacus	AF
Poicephalus	guliemi, meyeri, rufiventris, senegatus	AF
Coracopsis	vasa	AF
Agaporis	personata, roseicollia	AF

Abbreviations: AF, African; AM, American; A/P, Asian/Pacific.
[a] Based on published[6,14–16] and unpublished data of S. Clubb and H.L. Shivaprasad, 1980–2010.

additional orders. These birds include canaries (*Serinus canaria*, order: Passeriformes), greenfinches (*Carduelis chloris*, order: Passeriformes), long-wattled umbrella birds (*Cephalopterus penduliger*, order: Passeriformes), Canada geese (*Branta canadensis*, order: Anseriformes), roseate spoonbills (*Ajaja ajaja*, order: Pelecaniformes), peregrine falcons (*Falco peregrinus*, order: Falconiformes), toucans (*Ramphastos* sp, order: Piciformes), and bearded barbets (*Lybius dubius*, order: Piciformes).[7,17–20]

Based on the occurrence of case clusters, PDD has been long considered an infectious disease[5]; however, under most circumstances the disease seems to spread slowly within aviaries. Outbreaks affecting dozens of birds during a short time period (eg, several weeks) have also been described.[10,21,22] Crowded indoor aviaries as well as nurseries where parrot chicks are being hand-fed seem to be at the highest risk for PDD outbreaks. Although most of the reported PDD cases are of adult birds,[6] birds as young as 5 weeks may be affected.[22] Female psittacines have previously been reported to be overrepresented in PDD cases at a ratio of 1:0.6 or more,[6,15] whereas in another study males were overrepresented at a ratio of 1:0.9.[14] Therefore, it is most likely that males and females are equally susceptible to PDD. Little is known about the occurrence of PDD in wild avian populations. No PDD cases have been reported to date in free-ranging parrots of any continent. PDD is considered the main threat to captive populations of the highly endangered Spix macaw (*Cyanopsitta spixii*), a species that is now extinct in the wild.[12]

ETIOLOGY

PDD has long been suspected to be a viral disease based on epidemiologic observations, its apparent infectious nature, the typical lesions associated with it, and by ruling out other possible causes.[5,14,15] Several researchers have attempted to identify the PDD virus using standard virological methods such as culture and electron microscopy (EM). Initially, a virus was recovered from macaws suffering from serositis, and that was later identified as the Eastern equine encephalitis virus, which was suggested to be the candidate causative agent of PDD.[23,24] However, further research did not support this hypothesis.[7,14] Pleomorphic virus-like particles of variable size (30–250 nm) have also been described in tissues of affected birds by EM.[25] These particles were suspected to be of the genus avian paramyxovirus (APMV); however, birds affected by PDD have been shown to lack antibodies against APMV of serotypes 1 to 4, 6, and 7, as well as against avian herpes viruses, polyomavirus, and avian encephalitis virus.[5,6] In studies from Germany, APMV-1, closely related to the Hitchner B1 vaccine strain, was isolated from the spinal cords of around 20% of patients with PDD; however, these isolates showed very low pathogenicity and failed to reproduce the disease in African gray parrots.[26,27] Other virus species that have been sporadically documented in tissues or excretions of affected birds include an adeno-like virus, enterovirus, coronavirus, and reovirus.[6,7,28,29]

More consistently, an unidentified, enveloped virus of about 80 nm in diameter has been demonstrated by EM in feces of affected birds, and a similar virus was isolated from tissues of affected birds using an embryonic cell culture of a macaw.[7,29–31] This virus was initially suspected to be an alphavirus, but further investigation has ruled out this possibility.[32] Tissue homogenates from an affected bird that contained this virus were used to inoculate and successfully reproduce the disease in several psittacine birds,[7,31] but despite this success and nearly 3 decades of PDD research, the identity of the PDD agent remains enigmatic, with some researchers suggesting an autoimmune rather than a viral cause.[15,33]

The major breakthrough in identifying what is now widely believed to be the causative agent of PDD only happened recently, when advanced molecular tools, such as panviral DNA microarrays and high-throughput sequencing, were used to test tissues of PDD-positive birds. In 2008, Kistler and colleagues[11] and Honkavuori and colleagues[34] independently reported on the recovery of a novel Bornavirus from birds with PDD from the United States and Israel. This virus is now designated avian Bornavirus (ABV). Based on 16 ABV isolates, 5 distinct genotypes were identified, each sharing only around 65% nucleotide sequence identity with previously known members of the Bornaviridae family (all originating from mammalian hosts), and around 85% with other ABV genotypes.[11]

Bornaviruses are negative-encoded, single-stranded, nonsegmented RNA viruses of the order Mononegavirales. The placement of Bornaviruses within a separate family (Bornaviridae) was based on several unique characteristics of their genome and mechanism of replication, most notably that they replicate in the host-cell nucleus rather than in its cytoplasm.[35–40] Before the discovery of ABV, the single known species within this family was the Borna disease virus (BDV). Borna disease is an encephalitic disease found in horses, sheep, and occasionally other domesticated mammals. The disease was first described in the early nineteenth century in Southeast Germany and has since remained endemic in that area. Many additional species, including the chicken (*Gallus gallus*), are susceptible to BDV infection under experimental conditions, with the outcome ranging from severe encephalomyelitis to persistent asymptomatic infection.[37] The lesions seen with BDV are the result of neural invasion by T CD8+ lymphocytes rather than virus-inflicted cellular damage.[38]

BDV is an enveloped, spherical, medium-sized virus, with most virions being in the range of 70 to 130 nm.[39] The approximately 8900 base-pair genome encodes 6 major genes, including a nucleoprotein (N), a nonstructural protein (P10), a regulatory phosphoprotein (P), a matrix protein (M), a membrane-bound glycoprotein (G), and an RNA-dependent RNA polymerase (L).[40] BDV strains show remarkable sequence homogeneity and are all derived from mammalian hosts.[11] There is only one report on the recovery of partial BDV RNA sequences from wild avian species.[41]

In the short time since the publication of the 2 pioneering efforts by Kistler and colleagues[11] and Honkavuori and colleagues,[34] 8 additional studies have reported detecting ABV in PDD-positive birds or in birds exposed to PDD cases originating from 4 continents.[20,22,42–47] A sixth ABV genotype has been described,[44] and ABV has been recovered from at least 28 psittacine species and 1 nonpsittacine species, a canary (*S canaria*) with typical PDD lesions. Partial sequence analysis has shown the canary ABV strain to be closely related to ABV5.[20] Although most of the recoveries of ABV so far have been from clinically affected birds, asymptomatic infection and long-term virus shedding have also been identified and likely play an important role in the epidemiology of PDD.[22,43,45,48]

PDD has been successfully reproduced in cockatiels (*N hollandicus*) inoculated with brain homogenate containing ABV4, and the presence of an ABV4, nearly identical to that of the inoculum, was demonstrated in various organs of the inoculees.[43] PDD has also been reproduced in cockatiels and Patagonian conures (*Cyanoliseus patagonus*) using cultured ABV, fulfilling Koch postulates.[47] The distribution of ABV in different tissues and organs of PDD-positive birds has been studied by several researchers, using immunohistochemical (IHC) staining, Western blot, and quantitative real-time reverse transcription-polymerase chain reaction (RT-PCR).[20,22,34,42–46] Clear tropism to nervous tissue was demonstrated; however, multiple additional tissue types were involved (see later discussion). The route of transmission of ABV is unknown, but is believed to be feco-oral. Although our understanding of ABV pathogenesis and epidemiology is still in its infancy, the studies published so far provide convincing direct and indirect evidence that the causative agent of PDD has finally been identified.

PATHOLOGY

Detailed macroscopic and microscopic lesions in birds with PDD have been described.[14–16] Grossly, many birds suffering from PDD can be dehydrated and mildly to severely emaciated. Atrophied pectoral muscles may especially be seen in birds with a prolonged history of regurgitation or passing of undigested seeds. The proventriculus may or may not be dilated in all birds suffering from PDD, but in nearly 70% of the cases the proventriculus can be distended with seeds and thin walled (**Fig. 1**). In some cases, the proventricular wall may rupture with spillage of food into the celomic cavity, resulting in peritonitis. The duodenum may also be distended and the adrenal glands may be enlarged. In occasional cases, a pale area may be seen on the epicardium. Occasionally, there may be no significant gross lesions in birds that die suddenly without any clinical signs of PDD.

Microscopic lesions can be found in various organs involving the gastrointestinal (GI) tract; central, peripheral, and autonomic nervous systems; heart; adrenal glands; and occasionally in the nerves and ganglia of various visceral organs. It should be pointed out that the lesions in various organs may or may not be present consistently in all birds suffering from PDD. In one study, cases were selected based on lesions in proventriculus and/or gizzard and compared with other organs. The adrenal gland was the second most frequently affected organ, in 89.3% of the psittacines examined, followed by intestine (86.5%), heart (79.3%), brain/spinal cord (78.8%), esophagus/crop (72.1%), peripheral nerves (71.4%), eye (66.7%), and skin (25.0%).[14]

The microscopic lesions consist of infiltration of the serosal nerves of the proventriculus and/or gizzard, duodenum, and other parts of the intestine by few to large numbers of lymphocytes mixed with some plasma cells (**Fig. 2**). Often in the

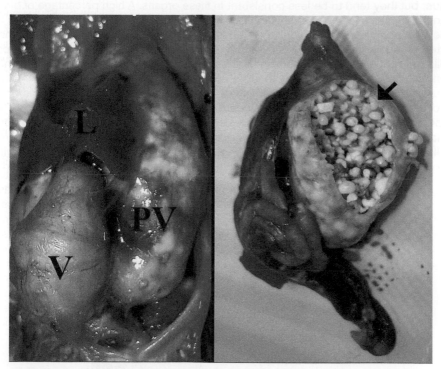

Fig. 1. Markedly dilated and thin-walled proventriculus (PV) in a cockatiel (*N hollandicus*) with experimentally induced PDD. On the right is the PV of the same bird after being removed from the carcass and cut open. Severe impaction with millet seeds is present (*arrow*). Undigested seeds can also be seen through the wall of the intestine. L, liver; V, ventriculus.

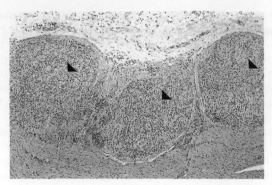

Fig. 2. Myenteric ganglioneuritis in an African gray parrot (*P erithacus*). Three adjacent sections of a large nerve on the serosal surface of the ventriculus are shown (*arrowheads*). Heavy lymphoplasmacytic infiltration can be seen. This lesion is characteristic for PDD (hematoxylin and eosin staining, original magnification ×100).

proventriculus, there is attenuation of glands and fibrosis of the mucosa. In many cases, there is infiltration of lymphocytes mixed with a few plasma cells in and around the nerves of the muscular tunics most prominent in the gizzard. Similar lesions can also be seen in the serosal and subserosal ganglia and nerves of the crop and esophagus, but they tend to be less consistent in these organs. A high percentage of birds can have lesions in the adrenal glands. These lesions can range from the infiltration of a few lymphocytes in the medullary regions to infiltration of a large number of lymphocytes mixed with few plasma cells and heterophils (**Fig. 3**). Often, the adrenocortical cells are vacuolated and hypertrophied. The ganglia, subjacent to the adrenal gland, can also have infiltration of few to large numbers of lymphocytes. In the heart, there is usually infiltration of similar cells either in the epicardial ganglia and nerves or in and around the subendocardial, myocardial, and subepicardial Purkinje fibers. The brain and spinal cord can have similar lesions characterized by mild to severe perivascular cuffing by lymphocytes scattered throughout the cerebral cortex and cerebellum, brain stem, and spinal cord (**Fig. 4**). Vestibulocochlear ganglia along with nerves and spinal ganglia can also have lymphoplasmacytic infiltration. Similarly,

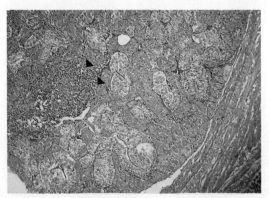

Fig. 3. Lymphoplasmacytic infiltration (*arrowheads*) of medullary areas within the adrenal gland of a cockatiel (*N hollandicus*) with experimentally induced PDD (hematoxylin and eosin staining, original magnification ×40).

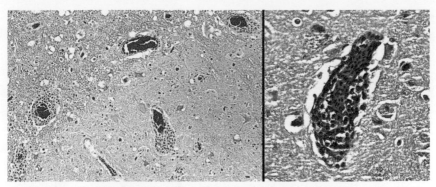

Fig. 4. Lymphoplasmacytic perivascular cuffing in the brain of a Blue-and-gold Macaw (*Ara ararauna*) with PDD (hematoxylin and eosin staining, original magnification for *left* ×100 and ×400 for *right* image).

perivascular cuffing by lymphocytes in the peripheral nerves, such as sciatic, brachial, vagus, and other nerves can be seen.[49] Lesions in the eye, when present, are characterized by moderate to severe perivascular cuffing in the optic nerves and in the choroid, ciliary body, and occasionally in the iris and pecten. Severe retinal lesions and blindness have been reported in a psittacine diagnosed with PDD.[50] Lesions in the skin include perivascular infiltration by lymphocytes and plasma cells, and occasional necrosis and infiltration of lymphocytes in the erector pili muscles.

Immunohistochemistry

IHC has been performed by investigators recently to study the tissue distribution and localization of ABV in psittacines[42–44,46] and canaries[20] Antibodies directed against recombinant ABV nucleoprotein, as well as cross-reacting antibodies against the BDV P protein, have been used as reagents for IHC. ABV nucleoprotein was demonstrated primarily in the nuclei, but was also demonstrated in the cytoplasm of neurons including Purkinje cells and glial cells (astrocytes) throughout the brain.[43,44] Studies performed using anti-BDV polyclonal antibodies have demonstrated ABV antigen in the nucleus and the cytoplasm not only of neural tissues (neurons, glial cells, dendrites, axons of brain, myenteric plexus of proventriculus, conduction fibers of the heart, and interstitial nerves in the lung) but also in other cell types including cardiomyocytes, hepatocytes, GI epithelium, and cells in the lamina propria of the intestine.[42,44] Similarly, ABV antigen has also been demonstrated in both neural and extraneural tissues, including tubular epithelia of the kidney in a canary.[20] In all studies, ABV antigen was found to be widely distributed among host cells and was not limited only to areas with microscopic lesions (**Fig. 5**).

ANTEMORTEM DIAGNOSIS
Clinical Signs

The incubation period of PDD seems to be extremely variable. Under experimental conditions, a minimum of 11 days has been reported in one study,[31] whereas in others it was approximately 1 month[43] or more.[47] The maximum time is certainly in the months range, and possibly even years in some cases.[31,43] Birds clinically affected by PDD may show symptoms related to malfunction of the digestive tract, neurologic signs, or a combination of both.[6] Sudden death with no preceding clinical symptoms occurs in some cases.

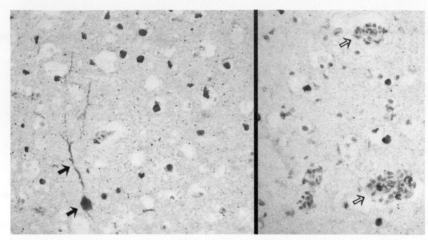

Fig. 5. IHC staining directed against avian Bornavirus nucleoprotein in the cerebrum of an African gray parrot (*P erithacus*) with PDD. The nuclei and cytoplasm of numerous neurons have stained positively (red-brown color), as has the dendritic tree of a large neuron (*solid arrows*). Viral antigen is widely distributed and can be seen within perivascular cuffs (*open arrows*) but also in areas without microscopic lesions (original magnification ×400).

Birds showing the GI form of PDD often present for marked weight loss, vomiting/regurgitation, and the presence of undigested food (eg, whole seeds, **Fig. 6**) in their feces.[6] Any of the symptoms mentioned earlier, and particularly their coexistence, should alert the clinician to a possible diagnosis of PDD; however, none of them should be considered pathognomonic. Furthermore, the severity of these symptoms varies among patients, and the symptoms may not all be noticeable at the time of presentation. Due to the feather coverage, weight loss often goes unnoticed by the bird's owner, and passing of undigested food is difficult to detect in birds that are on a pelleted diet.

The range of clinical symptoms possible with the central nervous system (CNS) form of PDD is even greater than that seen in the GI form. The signs may be subtle, ranging from a slightly dim attitude to profound neurologic deficits and/or seizures. Birds may

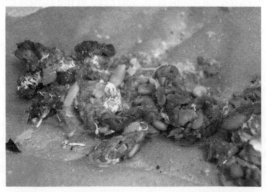

Fig. 6. Large amount of undigested seeds in the feces of an African gray parrot (*P erithacus*) with PDD.

present mildly to severely ataxic, sometimes with only one limb noticeably affected. Paraparesis is also common, and birds may be sternal at presentation with their legs either rigidly flexed or extended. Torticollis and/or abnormal head movements may be present, and central blindness has recently been described in an African gray parrot with PDD.[50] The most severe cases are presented in status epilepticus. As with the GI signs, none of these signs are specific for PDD, and other differential diagnoses should always be considered. It should be noted that mixed GI or neurologic PDD cases are common and that most birds have both GI and CNS lesions at necropsy, regardless of the clinical form observed antemortem.[14]

Hematology and Clinical Chemistry

Birds with PDD often show little or no changes in their blood work.[6,51,52] Nonregenerative anemia is the most common hematological change seen with PDD. This finding is similar to what is seen in starving birds and is likely related to GI malabsorption. Leukocytosis and heterophilia are present in some patients with PDD, but are not a consistent finding and seem to be related to stress and/or to the existence of secondary infections. Likewise, the biochemistry changes seen in birds with PDD are mainly those associated with their catabolic state. Total protein and albumin levels are often decreased,[52] and mild to moderate plasma elevations of enzymes of muscle origin (lactate dehydrogenase, creatine kinase, and aspartate aminotransferase) may be seen. Other changes are possible, but are not consistent; nevertheless, performing a chemistry panel is important for ruling out other disease conditions and for assessing the patient's general health. It is also advisable to test all birds suspected of having PDD for blood lead and zinc levels, because the symptoms of heavy metal toxicosis may mimic those of PDD.[51,53]

Fecal and Crop Cytology

There are no fecal or crop cytologic findings that are specific for PDD. However, these simple tests should always be performed as part of the diagnostic workup of birds suspected of having PDD, because they may help rule in or rule out other differential diagnoses or provide important information on changes that are secondary to PDD. It is of particular importance to rule out the presence of avian gastric yeasts (*Macrorhabdus ornithogaster*) and helminth, because these can cause GI signs similar to those seen with PDD. Changes in normal GI flora (eg, increase in gram-negative bacteria, *Clostridium* sp, and/or *Candida* yeasts) should be interpreted with caution, because they may represent a primary or a secondary process; both cases require appropriate therapy.

Diagnostic Imaging

Diagnostic imaging techniques, such as survey radiography, contrast radiography, contrast fluoroscopy, and ultrasonography, are useful aides in the diagnosis of PDD, but cannot be used to confirm or rule it out.[51,53] The most consistent finding in birds with PDD is a moderately to markedly distended proventriculus that contains mainly ingesta and variable amounts of gas. Distention of the proventriculus by gas alone is not typical of PDD. Proventricular diameter has been shown to increase over time in Spix macaws with PDD and has been suggested to be a useful indicator for performing crop biopsy.[12] Other GI compartments that may be distended include the crop, ventriculus, and small intestine; however, none of these findings are specific for PDD. The degree of distention of the various GI parts varies among birds with PDD, some showing changes only in the intestine or crop. A relatively large proventriculus may be seen in some healthy eclectus parrots, while distention of the proventriculus and crop can be physiologic in neonate birds.[51,54]

For most PDD cases, survey radiographs are the most cost-effective diagnostic imaging procedure and provide sufficient information for the assessment of the size of the relevant GI compartments (**Fig. 7**). In cases where the findings are equivocal or when the overall clinical picture does not fit well with PDD, positive contrast studies may be indicated (**Fig. 8**). The technique for performing GI contrast studies in psittacine birds has been previously described.[55,56] After the birds have been fasted for 4 hours, contrast material is introduced into the crop by gavage. Some investigators recommend dosing the patient at 25 to 50 mL/kg; however, the use of 10 to 15 mL/kg is often sufficient and reduces the risk of regurgitation and aspiration. Either barium sulfate or iodine-based contrast media may be used. Barium sulfate generally provides better and longer-lasting positive contrast compared with iodine-based products, but can cause airway irritation if accidentally aspirated and should be avoided if GI perforation is suspected. The use of barium also necessitates any GI surgery (eg, for collecting a crop biopsy) to be delayed until its complete clearance. Contrast studies may be performed with the patient anesthetized or awake. Although the disadvantages of anesthetizing the patient multiple times are obvious (increased anesthetic risk, risk of aspiration, altering GI motility), images obtained from an awake bird (eg, placed in a cardboard box or on a perch) may not always be sufficiently diagnostic. In many cases, a combination of both options may prove most practical, that is, most of the images are obtained with the bird awake, and the bird is anesthetized for a short period of time to achieve correct positioning, only once or twice, at well-chosen time points.

Contrast studies provide information not only on the size and relative positioning of the GI compartments but also on the GI transit time. In healthy psittacine birds, barium sulfate should reach the cloaca within 3 hours of administration,[55,56] often taking only 90 minutes to do so. The transit time for iodine-based products has not been well documented but appears to be significantly shorter. In some patients with PDD, transit

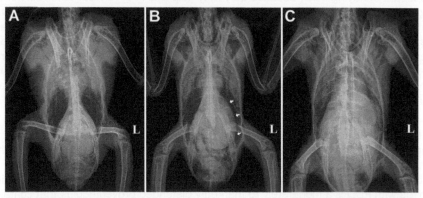

Fig. 7. Ventrodorsal survey radiographs. (*A*) A normal African gray parrot (*P erithacus*). Note the hourglass appearance of the cardiohepatic waist with abundant and symmetric airsac space on either side of it. (*B*) Moderate dilation of the proventriculus (*arrows*) in an African gray parrot with PDD. The proventriculus extends laterally beyond the liver edge at the expense of airsac space on the left. (*C*) Severe dilation of the proventriculus and ventriculus in a yellow-crested cockatoo (*Cacatua sulphurea*) with PDD. There is complete loss of the cardiohepatic waist and airsac space is markedly diminished bilaterally. Due to the general loss of peritoneal detail in this bird, a contrast study is indicated.

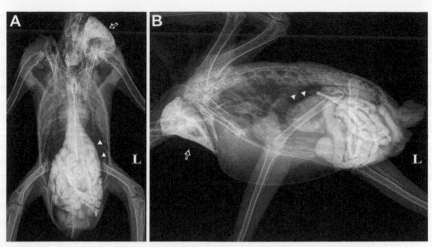

Fig. 8. (*A*) Ventrodorsal and (*B*) lateral radiographs of the African gray parrot (*P erithacus*) in **Fig. 7**B, 50 minutes after administration of 15 mL/kg iodine-based contrast medium (Ultravist 300; Schering AG, Berlin, Germany) by gavage. Although some contrast material is still present in the crop (*open arrow*), most of it has moved down the GI tract and has already reached the cloaca. It is not unusual for patients with PDD to have normal or even faster than normal GI transition time despite showing advanced clinical signs of PDD (this is the same bird that had passed the feces shown in **Fig. 6**). The proventriculus of this bird (*arrowheads*) is moderately dilated and contains mainly ingesta but also some gas. The small intestine of this bird is also mildly to moderately dilated.

time may be markedly prolonged,[6,51] whereas in others it is normal or even shortened (see **Fig. 8**). GI transit time may be altered by many pathologic and physiologic conditions; therefore, GI transit time cannot be considered a sensitive or specific indicator of PDD.

Contrast fluoroscopy can also aid the diagnosis of PDD.[52] The procedure is similar to that described earlier. After administration by gavage of 5 to 10 mL/kg barium sulfate mixed 1:1 with commercial hand-feeding formula, the awake bird is placed in a cardboard box or on a perch and observed intermittently with the fluoroscope until the barium reaches its cloaca. The main advantage of fluoroscopy compared with standard contrast studies is that it provides real-time views of the GI motility. Knowing the normal motility patterns is obviously necessary for the detection of changes. In the normal psittacine bird, boluses of ingesta can be clearly seen leaving the crop and traveling along the thoracic esophagus to the proventriculus. These boluses usually occur at an approximate rate of 1 bolus per minute, and should be unidirectional with no significant amount of barium remaining in the esophagus between boluses. The motility of the proventriculus is less pronounced than that of other GI parts, but every few minutes a large contraction followed by partial emptying into the ventriculus should be seen. Little or no proventricular motility may be present in patients with PDD with a grossly distended proventriculus. Most striking of all are the changes in normal ventricular motility seen with PDD. Because of the sequenced contraction of the thick and thin muscle pairs of its wall, a constant washing machine-like turning effect is produced and should be clearly visible in the lateral view of a healthy bird. In patients with PDD this pattern may be completely missing, often being replaced by a shallow and irregular flutter of the ventricular wall. The latter finding is the likely cause of failure of the mechanical food grinding action of the ventriculus, leading to the passing of whole seeds in the feces of patients with PDD. Peristalsis of the small intestine is bidirectional in psittacine species, with waves traveling down to the cecal remnants and back up to the pylorus. Some patients with PDD may show very fast and erratic peristaltic activity and an increase in duodenal diameter, whereas in others motility may be slower than usual. As with other imaging techniques, fluoroscopy findings should be regarded suggestive, but not confirmative, for PDD. Unfortunately, this useful technique requires costly equipment; therefore, it is not readily available to many private practitioners.

Crop Biopsy

The gold standard for diagnosing PDD has been and will likely remain histologic examination. In a live bird, this means that at least one appropriately sized biopsy from a relevant anatomic site must be obtained. Ideally, a biopsy of the serosal surface of the proventriculus and/or ventriculus should be taken because these sites are the most commonly affected by PDD.[14,15,57] However, these procedures are technically challenging and highly invasive compared with the much simpler and less invasive approach to the crop.[57]

The sensitivity of crop biopsies for detecting PDD has been a matter of controversy, with the reported prevalence of ganglioneuritis in crops of patients with PDD ranging from 22% to 76%.[14,15,49,57,58] Proper selection of the biopsy site and preparing multiple biopsy sections have been suggested to increase the sensitivity of crop biopsies.[54] The surgical approach to the crop has been previously described.[59] In brief, under general anesthesia, the bird is placed in dorsal recumbency and the skin above the crop (ie, the ventral area of the lower neck) is aseptically prepared. The skin is then incised along the ventral midline or slightly to the left of it, and the crop wall is exposed by undermining and retracting the skin laterally. The ventral portion of the crop is freed from its fascial attachments and lifted gently. Some investigators suggest that the cranial portion of the left lateral sac of the crop be preferred as the surgical site, because this area is less subject to stress and iatrogenic injury by feeding tubes.[57,59] The biopsy should include a prominent blood vessel (**Fig. 9**), because this increases the chances of obtaining nerve sections.[54,57] Stay sutures may be placed cranially and caudally to the biopsy site, which should measure no less than 12 mm at its long axis (ie, along the blood vessel). It is advisable to obtain an elliptical rather than a round biopsy (eg, 12 × 8 mm), because this enables later identification of the biopsy's original orientation. A second, smaller piece of about 2 × 2 mm should be collected in a sterile container and kept frozen for RT-PCR testing (see later discussion). The crop incision is closed in a continuous inverted (eg, Cushing's) pattern, using synthetic absorbable suture material, and the skin is closed routinely.

Following fixation for at least 2 hours in 10% buffered formalin, practitioners are encouraged to either section the biopsy themselves or provide the laboratory with specific modulation instructions. The biopsy should be cut perpendicular to its long axis, using a sharp scalpel or razor blade. Special care should be taken not to drag or compress the adventitial side because it contains most ganglia. At least 5 thin slices should be prepared and placed on edge in a histologic cassette. Under most circumstances this ensures that at least 10 medium to large nerve sections are represented, while a good biopsy includes more than 20 medium to large nerve sections (**Fig. 10**). IHC and RT-PCR for ABV are already offered by some commercial laboratories and can complement the standard histologic examination of crop tissue.

Molecular Diagnosis and Serology

The recent discovery of ABV and the development of specific molecular and serologic assays for its detection offer new diagnostic tools to avian veterinarians and

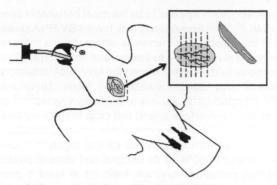

Fig. 9. Crop biopsies of about 12 × 8 mm should be collected along a prominent blood vessel. Following fixation in formalin, the biopsy should be carefully sliced perpendicular to its long axis. At least 5 thin slices should be prepared and placed on edge in a histologic cassette. An additional small piece should be frozen (fresh, without fixation) for potential RT-PCR testing.

aviculturists wishing to clear their flocks of this pathogen. However, these tools should be used cautiously, keeping in mind our limited knowledge of this novel virus and the inherent limitations of the techniques.

RT-PCR primers for conserved areas of the L, M, and N genes have been designed, and they successfully detect at least 40 ABV isolates of 5 distinct genotypes.[11,22,42,43] Quantitative real-time PCR, based on primers and probes within the P gene, has also been successfully applied to detect and quantify the presence of ABV in various tissues.[34,45] The RT-PCR assays for the highly expressed M and N genes seem to have a similar sensitivity that is somewhat higher than that of the L gene RT-PCR. Based on the limited information available to date, brain, crop, proventriculus,

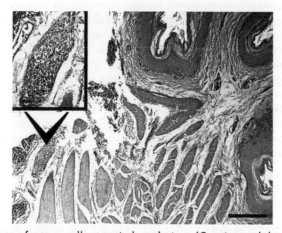

Fig. 10. Crop biopsy from a yellow-crested cockatoo (*Cacatua sulphurea*) with PDD. A ganglion with severe lymphoplasmacytic infiltration (*inset*) is present on the adventitial surface of the crop (hematoxylin and eosin staining). The biopsy of this bird included 36 sections of nerves and ganglia, of which 22 were diagnostic for PDD. All 6 slices prepared from this biopsy had at least one diagnostic lesion. However, this is not always the case with crop biopsies (original magnification for inset image ×100 and ×40 for actual image).

ventriculus, and adrenal glands appear to be the most consistent sites for postmortem detection of ABV RNA.[34,42–45] Some birds may have ABV RNA present in most major organs, as well as in the plasma,[43,45] whereas others show a more restricted distribution pattern. Therefore, it is important to test several tissue types (brain and stomachs at the least). Specimens that may be tested for ABV RNA antemortem include crop tissue, blood, choanal and cloacal swabs, and feces. Unfortunately, preliminary data show that ABV-infected birds are not consistently viremic[43,45] and shed the virus only intermittently in their saliva/feces, and that crop tissue may test ABV-negative in some patients with PDD.[43,45] Furthermore, some naturally infected birds have been reported to shed the virus without obvious clinical signs.[43,45] One such cockatiel has had ABV RNA present in 90% of its choanal and cloacal swabs during a period of 110 days[43] and has remained asymptomatic for at least 1 year thereafter (A.Y. Gancz, unpublished data, 2005–2010). These findings suggest that false-negative and false-positive results may occur when attempting to determine a bird's PDD status based on RT-PCR.

Serum from patients with PDD has been shown by Western blot analysis to contain antibodies against an unidentified ABV protein in the bird's brain. This protein was later identified to be nucleoprotein, 1 of the 2 major immunogenic proteins of Bornaviruses (the second one being P). The protein from the bird's brain was extracted and used to test other sera from birds with PDD and from control birds, with promising results.[60] Similarly, Lierz and colleagues[45] have used Western blot to test sera from symptomatic and asymptomatic ABV-positive birds. Recombinant ABV N and P proteins, as well as BDV N and P proteins, were used rather than brain extracts, and similar antibody responses were detected, regardless of the birds' clinical status. The strongest reaction was to the recombinant ABV N protein, showing minimal cross-reactivity with BDV N. Responses to both P proteins were relatively weak and variable. It was concluded that serology could not differentiate between patients with PDD and asymptomatic ABV carriers. This conclusion is also supported by the findings of another study that used Western blot and enzyme-linked immunosorbent assay to detect anti-ABV antibodies in asymptomatic ABV-positive macaws.[48]

Even with the limited data available to date on molecular and serologic assays for ABV detection, the advantages and shortcomings of these tests are already apparent. When used for the diagnosis of PDD, false-positive as well as false-negative results are possible. The tests may detect the ABV status of a bird correctly, but cannot be directly correlated to the patient's clinical status. Therefore, the definitive diagnosis of PDD in the single patient continues to be based on histology, with PCR, serology, and IHC results as supporting evidence (**Fig. 11**). The advantage of these tests is that they offer for the first time practical tools for screening birds for the causative agent of PDD. The optimal screening protocol (eg, serology vs PCR of several swabs collected serially) is yet to be determined. However, it is hoped that these tests greatly improve our ability to clear flocks from ABV and by that significantly reducing the incidence of PDD.

CLINICAL MANAGEMENT OF PDD

PDD is a devastating disease for affected birds, but it is equally devastating for their owners or caretakers. Furthermore, the disease often becomes a flock management problem, because many owners of psittacine birds have multiple birds. Transmission between birds in the home environment can be problematic and may lead to sequential illnesses and potential deaths, which may occur over a period of years. The social implications of a PDD diagnosis can also be devastating. Owners may be shunned

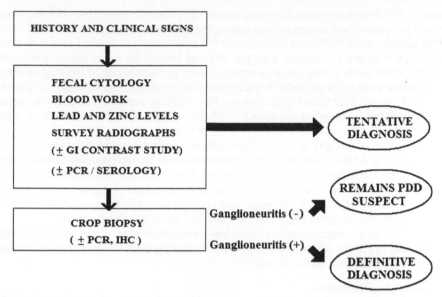

Fig. 11. A proposed diagnostic approach to PDD.

from bird club functions or social interaction with other bird owners. Pet sitters often refuse to provide care while the owner is away.

Likewise, the diagnosis of PDD in an avicultural collection can have severe financial and emotional effects on aviculturists. Counseling the owner and establishing a long-term management plan are important aspects of veterinary care. The first step in management, therefore, is client counseling, and planning not only for the affected bird but also other birds in the flock or home.

Initially the owner may be faced with difficult decisions, choosing between euthanasia and long-term management of affected birds that may remain infectious. Euthanasia may be the best decision if the bird is critically ill; however, many owners may be reluctant to choose this option. A potential compromise that may allow the client to make a more calculated decision is to treat for 3 to 4 weeks and reevaluate for treatment response.

Living with a bird that has a chronic infectious disease, which is a risk to other birds, requires a commitment of time as well as limiting birds coming and going from the home. Long-term care can entail a significant investment of time and money. The bird could be placed in a rescue center that handles birds with PDD, but rescue centers typically request monetary support for long-term treatment of the bird. Placement of the bird in a home without other birds for long-term management is another option if such a home can be found.

Although many birds with clinical PDD can be returned to being clinically normal, effective treatment typically requires months and even years. More research is needed to determine the risk to other birds from birds that have been treated but may still be latently infected.

Counseling for owners needs to include the fact that even using current therapeutic methods, the long-term consequences of treatment and risks associated with the affected bird after treatment are still unknown. It is also important to understand that the disease can take many forms and can have a long incubation period. Clinically healthy birds can be infected with ABV and pose a risk of transmission to others.[43,45,48] A clinician who only diagnoses PDD in classic emaciated vomiting birds that are passing whole seeds is only seeing the tip of the iceberg.

The second step in clinical management is assessing the disease status of their other birds that are in contact with the affected bird(s). To be in denial and avoid checking other birds in the home or aviary is placing them at risk. If the PDD is diagnosed before the bird is critically ill, most birds can be helped. Conversely, many birds that are diagnosed by either crop biopsy, ABV-PCR, or antibody to ABV may never develop naturally occurring disease.[43,45,48] ABV diagnostics are currently in their infancy. Extensive, long-term research is needed to provide the client with a reasonable prognosis, especially when multiple birds or flocks are subject to exposure.

In developing a treatment and control plan, each bird should be considered individually. To determine the extent of the problem, it is important to evaluate all birds in contact with an affected bird. Ideally all contact birds should be screened, preferably by a combination of Ag and AB tests, and possibly crop biopsy as well. In this way, asymptomatically infected birds can be identified, isolated, and treated.

Clients should be encouraged to make the commitment not to bring more birds into their homes, placing them at risk. Likewise, transferring birds to other owners without disclosure places other birds at risk.

Treatment Considerations

As an infectious disease that causes inflammation of the central and peripheral nervous system as well as the digestive system, when managing PDD thought must be given to prevention of transmission of the disease to uninfected individuals, reducing inflammation, aiding digestion, and controlling secondary infections. In many cases this must be done for a long time. With prolonged therapy and control of secondary infections, birds that are diagnosed early can return to good physical condition. However, their life expectancy cannot be predicted.

Nonsteroidal Anti-Inflammatory Drugs

Initial reports of treatment using the anti-inflammatory drug celicoxib presented the first real hope for birds with PDD.[61] Nonsteroidal anti-inflammatory drugs (NSAIDs) are a group of structurally diverse compounds used clinically for the treatment of pain and/or inflammation. NSAIDs are believed to exert their analgesic and anti-inflammatory effects through inhibition of the cyclooxygenase (COX) enzymes, which catalyze the conversion of arachidonic acid to the various prostaglandins.[62]

Two isoforms of the COX enzyme have been identified in eukaryotic cells, cyclooxygenase-1 (COX-1) and cyclooxygenase-2 (COX-2). The COX-1 protein is constitutively expressed (ie, it is present under normal conditions and does not need to be induced) and is involved in the maintenance of homeostatic conditions. For example, COX-1 plays a role in blood clotting and elicits a protective role in organs such as the GI tract. The COX-2 protein, on the other hand, is inducible and is involved in the immediate early gene response to various stimuli such as cytokines, growth factors, and ultraviolet light. Older NSAIDs such as aspirin, ibuprofen, and flurbiprofen, inhibit both forms of COX and are referred to as nonselective NSAIDs. Newer NSAIDs, such as celecoxib and rofexocib, are selective for COX-2 and are referred to as selective COX-2 inhibitors.[61–64]

In addition to their anti-inflammatory properties, NSAID therapy may have other unexpected effects. Chen and colleagues[65] found that NSAID treatment can suppress the propagation of vesicular stomatitis virus (VSV) in mice. The inhibition of COX antagonized VSV propagation using in vitro and in vivo experiments. In addition, aspirin and celecoxib prevented the disruption of the blood-brain barrier in

VSV-infected mice. In vitro experiments showed that the effect of COX inhibition was at least partially mediated by increased production of nitric oxide, a molecule that is known to inhibit VSV replication. In another study, Zhu and colleagues[66] demonstrated that COX-2 inhibitors could inhibit the production of human cytomegalovirus in human fibroblast cultures. These studies indicate that NSAIDs may have direct antiviral effects.

Celecoxib has been used successfully in treating PDD at the rate of 20 mg/kg body weight (BW) once daily if given directly orally.[67] However, unless a bird is extremely tame, stress associated with therapeutic protocols must be considered, especially because of the long-term nature of therapy. Long-term treatment success has been achieved when adding celecoxib to the bird's food at 40 mg/kg BW once daily.[67] A 200-mg capsule of celecoxib may be dissolved in 10 mL of water and used at 0.2 mL/100 g BW. The drug should be provided on a small amount of food so that the chance of consuming adequate amounts improves. The stability of this suspension has not been studied. Empirically, it is recommended that a new stock be prepared fresh at least once a week, and that it is stored under refrigeration. Many practitioners prefer to have the drug compounded. In most birds clinical response is slow and gradual, and many birds do not show much benefit for at least 2 weeks.[67]

Other NSAIDs have also been used to treat PDD. Tepoxalin (Zubrin; Schering Plough, Union, NJ, USA), a combined COX-1, COX-2, and 5-lipoxygenase (LOX) inhibitor, was used successfully in the treatment of a group of crop biopsy positive birds.[67] Through its inhibition of the LOX enzymes, this drug potentially reduces the production of leukotrienes, including leukotriene B4, that may contribute to increased GI tract inflammation. Inhibition of LOX may also reduce the GI effects routinely seen in dogs (and possibly in birds) with COX-1 inhibitors.[63]

In a pilot study comparing the effectiveness of celecoxib and tepoxalin,[67] 3 treatment groups were compared: (1) Celecoxib 40 mg/kg BW on seed mix (n = 9); (2) tepoxalin 40 mg/kg BW on seed mix (n = 8); and (3) tepoxalin 40 mg/kg BW on an extruded rice-based hypoallergenic diet (n = 14). All birds were positive on crop biopsy before treatment and underwent a second crop biopsy after at least 9 months of therapy. In group 1, 2 birds still had positive crop biopsies after 9 months' treatment, whereas in group 2, 6 birds still had positive crop repeated biopsies. The best results were found in group 3, in which lesions typical of PDD were not found in any of the 14 birds. These results may be attributable to the extruded diet readily absorbing the medication, attributable to its hypoallergenic nature and an enhanced efficacy of tepoxalin on this diet, or possibly because the species in group 3 were easier to treat effectively compared with the species in groups 1 and 2. Palm cockatoos (*Probosciger aterrimus*) were found to be particularly difficult to treat effectively, accounting for 7 out of 8 cases of treatment failure. Palm cockatoos and hyacinth macaws (*Anodorhyncus hyacinthinus*) consume much of their calories through nuts and seeds, making consistent dosing difficult.[67] In these species, some sort of soft or fresh food, such as fruits and vegetables, should be used as a vehicle for administration of the medication.

Meloxicam is another NSAID that is widely used by avian practitioners. Meloxicam is considered COX-2 preferential (not specific), and at higher dosages its COX-2 specificity is diminished.[63] However, in the authors' empiric opinion, the clinical response seen with meloxicam is inferior to that observed with celecoxib therapy.

The most common side effect of celecoxib and other COX-2 inhibitors is bleeding in the gastrointestinal tract. The risk may be higher in the first few weeks of therapy. An adult female hybrid macaw with PDD died within 7 days of initiation of celecoxib therapy, exhibiting acute proventricular bleeding.[67] The feces of birds treated with NSAIDs should be monitored daily. Treatment should be discontinued immediately if melena or fresh blood is detected, and the bird should be evaluated. Fecal cytology, including a Gram stain, should be performed to detect *Clostridium* sp and/or other potential bacterial pathogens.

Some birds seem to develop hypersensitivity to celecoxib. A mature female hyacinth macaw developed severe pruritus locally on the sides of its face while being treated with celecoxib, which subsided in severity when celecoxib therapy was discontinued.[67]

Most NSAIDs are eliminated by renal clearance and should be used with caution in birds with renal disease. In addition, NSAID-induced renal disease has been documented in birds.[68] Therefore, it is recommended that birds on long-term NSAID therapy be monitored on a regular basis for changes in their chemistry panel.

Although the inflammatory lesions in nerves are often reversed in response to NSAID therapy, these drugs are not considered a cure or a prophylactic agent for PDD.

Amantadine Hydrochloride

The prognosis of PDD is especially guarded in patients showing severe CNS disorders. Such cases have been poorly responsive to NSAID therapy alone. In the experience of one of the authors (S.C.), the addition of amantadine hydrochloride (10 mg/kg by mouth once a day or 20 mg/kg once a day on food) to the therapeutic protocol resulted in a vast improvement in outcome.

Amantadine was initially used as an antiviral against influenza viruses.[63] Its antiviral mechanism of action involves interference with a viral ion channel. Later, it was also found to have an effect in reducing the severity of symptoms of Parkinson disease, by antagonizing the *N*-methyl-D-aspartate receptor and other mechanisms that are not yet fully understood.[69] Amantadine has many effects on the brain, including release of dopamine and norepinephrine. Because of increased viral resistance, amantadine is no longer recommended for influenza treatment or prophylaxis,[70,71] but is still being used to treat various psychological disorders in humans. Common side effects in humans include appetite loss, diarrhea, nausea, lethargy, and allergic reactions. Amantadine has been used in combination with celecoxib to treat a large number of PDD patients with only rare adverse reactions, which resolved after cessation of therapy (S. Clubb, unpublished data, 2005–2010).

Other Drugs Used to Treat PDD Patients

Because of their impaired GI motility, birds with PDD often develop secondary bacterial and fungal GI infections. These should be diagnosed and treated appropriately. *Clostridium* infections are more common in birds with PDD than in birds with normal intestinal motility, and can result in bulky, black, foul-smelling feces. Vaccination for *Clostridium* should be considered. A bovine multivalent *Clostridium chauvoei/septicum/haemolyticum/novyisordellii/perfringens* types C and D bacterin-toxoid vaccine (Vision 8; Intervet Inc, Millisboro, DE, USA), administered at 0.25 to 1 mL intramuscularly or subcutaneously, has been used with empiric success. Initially, 2 doses are given 2 weeks apart with an annual booster.[67]

Gas formation and retention in the GI tract is a common finding in birds affected with PDD and can cause discomfort. Gas may be evident radiographically and/or gas bubbles may present in the feces or vomitus. Surfactants (eg, Infant's Mylicon; Johnson & Johnson, Merck Consumer Pharmaceuticals, Ft. Washington, PA, USA) provide some symptomatic relief. Many birds exhibiting GI gas or vomiting respond clinically to combination drug therapy (eg, clarithromycin, metronidazole, and sucralfate) as if they are infected with *Helicobacter* species; however, the presence of *Helicobacter* has not been confirmed in these patients.

Metoclopramide (0.5 mg/kg every 12 h by mouth or intramuscularly) is an important adjunct therapy to management of severe PDD cases.[67] It is beneficial in cases of reduced intestinal motility or intestinal stasis. Treatment is initiated by injection and later continued orally. An adverse reaction to metoclopramide has been reported in a macaw being treated for PDD.[70,71]

Birds with PDD often become anemic and hypoproteinemic. Supplement of vitamins, especially B complex vitamins, is helpful.

Husbandry Considerations

If possible, birds should be kept outside where sunlight and fresh air help in diluting and inactivating the virus; it also enhances the bird's well-being. The birds should be spread out as much as possible to reduce the concentration of virus in the environment. Stress should be kept to a minimum. The diet should be easily digestible, because ventricular and proventricular function is adversely affected by PDD. Liquid diets and pelleted diets have been developed specifically for birds with PDD, and juvenile hand-feeding formulas can also be used for initial nutritional therapy. Formulated diets are ideal because they are easier to digest than seeds; however, extreme caution should be used in converting an ill bird from a seed-based diet to a formulated diet. Extruded diets also absorb medication well, enabling long-term, stress-free therapy.

Supplementing the diet with vegetables that are high in fiber might be beneficial with early cases of PDD by stimulating intestinal motility. Birds affected by PDD often ingest foreign bodies, especially pieces of wood. These materials may then be passed through vomitus or feces. The bird may be ingesting these materials in an attempt to provide relief from intestinal discomfort. These birds may need toys and cage accessories that cannot be chewed or ingested, and may benefit from high-fiber vegetables to fill this need.

Cruciferous vegetables are beneficial sources of raffinose sugars (rich in oligofructosaccharides), which enhance viability of autochthonous flora (species of *Lactobacillus* and *Bifidobacterium*), thereby inhibiting gram-negative bacteria and *Clostridium*. However, in advanced cases these foods may linger in the intestines and ferment. Periodic supplementation with probiotics may be beneficial.

Because of the inflammatory nature of PDD, supplements that enhance nutrition and provide anti-inflammatory effects may augment conventional therapy. Antioxidants including oils, specific amino acids, and minerals, and some natural herbal anti-inflammatory agents may be beneficial. A balance of omega-3 and omega-6 fatty acids has proved to be beneficial in many inflammatory diseases. Salmon oil, flax seed oil, and safflower oil are used as sources of omega-3 and omega-6 fatty acids. Fatty acid supplementation is provided at 50 to 250 mg/kg BW of omega-3 fatty acids with an omega-3:omega-6 ratio of 1:2 to 1:6. If the bird is primarily on a seed diet, which is naturally high in omega-6 fatty acids, supplementation with salmon oil and flax seed oil helps to correct the omega-3:omega-6 ratio. Nutritional adjuncts to therapy that may be beneficial in cases with CNS signs include Ginkgo biloba, vitamin E, alpha-lipoic acid, acetyl-L-carnitine, and B-complex vitamins. There are no studies in the literature on the effect of various diets and/or nutraceuticals on birds with PDD; therefore, all recommendations made earlier are empiric.

Monitoring Progress of Therapy

Response to therapy can be monitored by periodic physical examination, monitoring body condition and weight, repeated radiographs and hematology, and plasma biochemistry analysis. Increases in body weight can be misleading, because weight gain may be associated with dilation of the proventriculus and intestinal stasis.

Monitoring by serial crop biopsies is useful. On repeated biopsy, the site of previous biopsy should be avoided because the presence of old suture material can result in nonspecific inflammatory lesions.

If monitored by radiography, the composition of the diet must be considered in evaluation, especially if the bird is primarily on a seed diet at the time of diagnosis and is converted to a more bulky extruded diet. Birds eating a primarily formulated or extruded diet tend to have a dilated GI tract as evident radiographically, which can complicate radiographic evaluation (S. Clubb, unpublished data, 2005–2010).

PREVENTION

Early epidemiologic data on PDD as well as recent studies on ABV[45] suggest that the disease and its causative agents are not equally distributed among flocks. Although in some aviaries PDD cases occur on a regular basis, the disease appears to be completely absent from other facilities (A.Y. Gancz, unpublished data). With this observation in mind, the obvious goals of PDD prevention are: (a) to avoid introducing the pathogen into new flocks and (b) to clear it from flocks where it is already present. However, until recently these goals were nearly impossible to achieve due to the disease's long incubation period and because its cause was unknown. Even facilities that quarantined all new arrivals for extended periods of time and facilities that performed crop biopsies on all of their birds were not completely safe from PDD. Now, with the discovery of ABV and the development of molecular and serologic assays for its detection, it is hoped that this situation will change.

Regular monitoring of the bird's body condition and feces (ie, looking for undigested seeds) are simple ways for detecting clinical PDD cases in flocks where the disease already exists. While still valid, these simple measures do not detect birds in early stages of PDD or birds that are asymptomatic ABV carriers.

ABV RT-PCR and serology are already offered by some commercial laboratories, and are expected to become widely available in the near future. At this point, precise recommendations as to the preferred screening protocol cannot be made, but when possible both tests should be used. Because of intermittent shedding of ABV, it is advisable to submit several serially collected oral or cloacal swabs for RT-PCR. If crop biopsies are collected, they too can be submitted for RT-PCR.

As with other infectious diseases, practicing good hygiene and following strict biosafety rules are essential for fighting PDD. Diagnostic necropsies and histopathology should be performed on all birds that die of unknown causes. Overcrowding of aviaries facilitates the spreading of PDD and should be avoided. All new additions should be quarantined and tested (see earlier) as should be any bird suspected to have clinical signs of the disease. Birds that test ABV-positive must not be allowed into existing flocks and should be removed from flocks where they already exist. These birds should be placed in a situation where they cannot infect other birds. Similar principles may be applied to smaller collections such as multiple-bird households.

SUMMARY

PDD is a fatal inflammatory disease that affects mainly psittacine birds (order: Psittaciformes). The disease was first recognized in the 1970s, but it was not until 2008 that the causative agent of PDD, a novel Bornavirus, ABV, was discovered. Since its discovery the number of publications on ABV has been increasing rapidly, with new information becoming available on an almost monthly basis. RT-PCR and serologic and immunohistochemical assays for ABV detection are already commercially available, but the knowledge regarding their optimal application is still lagging behind.

For years, PDD has posed one of the greatest diagnostic and therapeutic challenges to the avian veterinarian. It is hoped that the exciting recent progress in PDD research greatly improves our ability to diagnose, manage, and prevent this disease.

ACKNOWLEDGMENTS

The authors thank Juliet Mandelzweig for her assistance with language editing of this article.

REFERENCES

1. Woerpel RW. Clinical and pathologic features of Macaw wasting disease (proventricular dilatation syndrome). Proc West Poultry Dis Confer 1984;89–90.
2. Clark D. Proventricular dilation syndrome in large psittacine birds. Avian Dis 1984;28(3):813–5.
3. Graham DL. An update on selected pet bird virus infections. Proc Annu Conf Assoc Avian Vet 1984;267–80.
4. Turner R. Macaw fading or wasting syndrome. Proc West Poultry Dis Confer 1984;87–8.
5. Gerlach S. Macaw wasting disease—a 4-year study on clinical case history, epizootology, analysis of species, diagnosis and differential diagnosis, microbiological and virological results. Proc Conf Euro Assoc Avian Vet 1991;273–81.
6. Gregory CR, Latimer KS, Niagro F, et al. A review of proventricular dilatation syndrome. J Assoc Avian Vet 1994;8(2):69–75.
7. Gregory CR, Ritchie BW, Latimer KS, et al. Progress in understanding proventricular dilatation disease. Proc Annu Conf Assoc Avian Vet 2000;269–75.
8. Sullivan ND, Mackie JT, Miller RI, et al. First case of psittacine proventricular dilatation syndrome (macaw wasting disease) in Australia. Aust Vet J 1997;75(9):674.
9. Donelely RJ, Miller RI, Fanning TE. Proventricular dilatation disease: an emerging exotic disease of parrots in Australia. Aust Vet J 2007;85(3):119–23.
10. Lublin A, Mechani S, Farnoushi I, et al. An outbreak of proventricular dilation disease in psittacine breeding farm in Israel. Isr J Vet Med 2006;61(1):16–9.
11. Kistler AL, Gancz A, Clubb S, et al. Recovery of divergent avian bornaviruses from cases of proventricular dilatation disease: identification of a candidate etiologic agent. Virol J 2008;5:88.
12. Wyss F, Deb A, Watson R, et al. Radiographic measurements for PDD diagnosis in Spix's macaws (*Cyanospitta spixii*) at Al Wabra Wildlife Preservation (AWWP), Qatar. Proc Intern Conf Dis Zoo Wild Anim 2009;349–54.
13. Marietto-Goncalves GA, Troncarelli MZ, Sequeira JL, et al. Proventricular dilatation disease (PDD) and megaesophagus in a blue-fronted Amazon parrot (*Amazona aestiva*)—case report. Vet e Zootec 2009;16(1):69–73.
14. Shivaprasad HL, Barr BC, Woods LW, et al. Spectrum of lesions (pathology) of proventricular dilatation syndrome. Proc Annu Conf Assoc Avian Vet 1995;505–6.
15. Graham DL. "Wasting/proventricular dilation disease" a pathologists view. Proc Annu Conf Assoc Avian Vet 1991;43–4.
16. Reavill D, Schmidt R. Lesions of the proventriculus/ventriculus of pet birds: 1640 cases. Proc Annu Conf Assoc Avian Vet 2007;89–93.
17. Daoust PY, Julian RJ, Yason CV, et al. Proventricular impaction associated with nonsuppurative encephalomyelitis and ganglioneuritis in two Canada geese. J Wildl Dis 1991;27(3):513–7.
18. Shivaprasad H. Proventricular dilation disease in peregrine falcon (*Falco peregrinus*). Proc Annu Conf Assoc Avian Vet 2005;107–8.

19. Perpinan D, Fernandez-Bellon H, Lopez C, et al. Lymphoplasmacytic myenteric, subepicardial, and pulmonary ganglioneuritis in four nonpsittacine birds. J Avian Med Surg 2007;21(3):210–4.

20. Weissenböck H, Sekulin K, Bakonyi T, et al. Novel avian bornavirus in a nonpsittacine species (Canary; *Serinus canaria*) with enteric ganglioneuritis and encephalitis. J Virol 2009;83(21):11367–71.

21. Phalen D. An outbreak of psittacine proventricular dilation syndrome (PPDS) in a private collection of birds and an atypical form of PDS in a nanday conure. Proc Annu Conf Assoc Avian Vet 1986;27–34.

22. Kistler AL, Smith JM, Greninger AL, et al. Analysis of naturally occurring avian bornavirus infection and transmission during an outbreak of proventricular dilatation disease among captive psittacine birds. J Virol 2009;84(4):2176–9.

23. Gaskin JM, Homer BL, Eskeland KH. Preliminary findings in avian viral serositis: a newly recognized syndrome in psittacine birds. J Avian Med Surg 1991;5(1): 27–34.

24. Gaskin JM, Homer BL, Eskeland KH. Some unofficial thoughts on avian viral serositis. Proc Annu Conf Assoc Avian Vet 1991;38–42.

25. Mannl A, Gerlach H, Leipold R. Neuropathic gastric dilatation in psittaciformes. Avian Dis 1987;31(1):214–21.

26. Grund CH, Werner O, Gelderblom HR, et al. Avian paramyxovirus serotype I isolates from the spinal cord of parrots display a very low virulence. J Vet Med B Infect Dis Vet Public Health 2002;49(9):445–51.

27. Grund CH, Mohn U, Korbel R. Relevance of low virulent avian paramyxovirus serotype 1 for psittacine birds. Proc Annu Conf Assoc Avian Vet 2005;283–6.

28. Gough RE, Drury SE, Culver F, et al. Isolation of a coronavirus from a green-cheeked Amazon parrot (*Amazona viridigenalis* Cassin). Avian Pathol 2006; 35(2):122–6.

29. Gough RE, Drury SE, Harcourt-Brown NH, et al. Virus-like particles associated with macaw wasting disease. Vet Rec 1996;139(1):24.

30. Hartcourt-Brown NH, Gough RE. Isolation of virus-like particles associated with proventricular dilatation syndrome in macaws. Proc Euro Conf Avian Med Surg 1997;111–5.

31. Gregory CR, Ritchie BW, Latimer KS, et al. Proventricular dilatation disease: a viral epornitic. Proc Annu Conf Assoc Avian Vet 1997;43–52.

32. Gregory CR, Latimer KS, Niagro FD, et al. Investigation of eastern equine encephalomyelitis virus as the causative agent of psittacine proventricular dilatation syndrome. J Avian Med Surg 1997;11(3):187–93.

33. Rossi G, Crosta L, Pesaro S. Parrot proventricular dilation disease. Vet Rec 2008; 163(10):310.

34. Honkavuori KS, Shivaprasad HL, Williams BL, et al. Novel borna virus in psittacine birds with proventricular dilatation disease. Emerg Infect Dis 2008;14(12): 1883–6.

35. Cubitt B, Ly C, de la Torre JC. Identification and characterization of a new intron in Borna disease virus. J Gen Virol 2001;82(3):641–6.

36. Jordan I, Lipkin WI. Borna disease virus. Rev Med Virol 2001;11(1):37–57.

37. Rott R, Becht H. Natural and experimental Borna disease in animals. Curr Top Microbiol Immunol 1995;190:17–30.

38. Stitz L, Bilzer T, Planz O. The immunopathogenesis of Borna disease virus infection. Front Biosci 2002;7:d541–55.

39. Kohno T, Goto T, Takasaki T, et al. Fine structure and morphogenesis of Borna disease virus. J Virol 1999;73(1):760–6.

40. De la Torre JC. Reverse-genetic approaches to the study of Borna disease virus. Nat Rev Microbiol 2006;4(10):777–83.
41. Berg M, Johansson M, Montell H, et al. Wild birds as a possible natural reservoir of Borna disease virus. Epidemiol Infect 2001;127(1):173–8.
42. Rinder M, Ackermann A, Kempf H, et al. Broad tissue and cell tropism of avian bornavirus in parrots with proventricular dilatation disease. J Virol 2009;83(11): 5401–7.
43. Gancz AY, Kistler AL, Greninger AL, et al. Experimental induction of proventricular dilatation disease in cockatiels (*Nymphicus hollandicus*) inoculated with brain homogenates containing avian bornavirus 4. Virol J 2009;6:100.
44. Weissenböck H, Bakonyi T, Sekulin K, et al. Avian bornaviruses in psittacine birds from Europe and Australia with proventricular dilatation disease. Emerg Infect Dis 2009;15(9):1453–9.
45. Lierz M, Hafez HM, Honkavuori KS, et al. Anatomical distribution of avian bornavirus in parrots, its occurrence in clinically healthy birds and ABV-antibody detection. Avian Pathol 2009;38(6):491–6.
46. Ouyang N, Storts R, Tian Y, et al. Histopathology and the detection of avian bornavirus in the nervous system of birds diagnosed with proventricular dilatation disease. Avian Pathol 2009;38(5):393–401.
47. Gray P, Hoppes S, Suchodolski P, et al. Use of avian bornavirus isolates to induce proventricular dilatation disease in conures. Emerg Infect Dis 2010;16(3):473–9.
48. De Kloet SR, Dorrestein GM. Presence of avian bornavirus RNA and anti-avian bornavirus antibodies in apparently healthy macaws. Avian Dis 2009;53(5): 568–73.
49. Berhane Y, Smith DA, Newman S, et al. Peripheral neuritis in psittacine birds with proventricular dilatation disease. Avian Pathol 2001;30(5):563–70.
50. Steinmetz A, Pees M, Schmidt V, et al. Blindness as a sign of proventricular dilatation disease in a grey parrot (*Psittacus erithacus erithacus*). J Small Anim Pract 2008;49(12):660–2.
51. Hoefer HL. Diseases of the gastrointestinal tract. In: Altman RB, Clubb SL, Dorrestein GM, Quesenberry K, editors. Avian medicine and surgery. Philadelphia: WB Saunders; 1997. p. 419–53.
52. Boutette JB, Taylor M. Proventricular dilatation disease: a review of research, literature, species differences, diagnostics, prognosis and treatment. Proc Annu Conf Assoc Avian Vet 2004;175–81.
53. Lumeij JT. Gastroenterology. In: Ritchie BW, Harrison GJ, Harrison LR, editors. Avian medicine: principles and application. Delray Beach (FL): HBD International Inc; 1999. p. 482–521.
54. Ritchie BW, Gregory CR, Latimer KS, et al. Epizootiology of proventricular dilatation disease in breeding cockatiels. Proc Annu Conf Assoc Avian Vet 2004;41–5.
55. Smith BJ, Smith SA. Radiology. In: Altman RB, Clubb SL, Dorrestein GM, et al, editors. Avian medicine and surgery. Philadelphia: WB Saunders; 1997. p. 170–99.
56. McMillan MC. Imaging techniques. In: Ritchie BW, Harrison GJ, Harrison LR, editors. Avian medicine: principles and application. Delray Beach (FL): HBD International Inc; 1999. p. 246–61.
57. Gregory CR, Latimer KS, Campagnoli RP, et al. Histologic evaluation of the crop for diagnosis of proventricular dilatation syndrome in psittacine birds. J Vet Diagn Invest 1996;8(1):76–80.
58. Doolen M. Crop biopsy—a low risk diagnosis for neuropathic gastric dilation. Proc Annu Conf Assoc Avian Vet 1994;193–6.

59. Bennett RA, Harrison GJ. Soft tissue surgery. In: Ritchie BW, Harrison GJ, Harrison LR, editors. Avian medicine: principles and application. Delray Beach (FL): HBD International Inc; 1999. p. 1096–136.

60. Hoppes S, Gray P. An update on proventricular dilatation disease. Proc Conf Euro Assoc Avian Vet 2009;141–6.

61. Dalhausen B, Aldred S, Colaizzi E. Resolution of clinical proventricular dilation disease by cyclooxygenase 2 inhibition. Proc Annu Conf Assoc Avian Vet 2002;9–12.

62. Rao P, Knaus EE. Evolution of nonsteroidal anti-inflammatory drugs (NSAIDs): cyclooxygenase (COX) inhibition and beyond. J Pharm Pharm Sci 2008;11(2): 81s–110.

63. Plumb DC. Plumb's veterinary drug handbook. 5th edition. Available at: http://www.vin.com/Members/Drug/VDH.plx. Accessed January, 2010.

64. Clement D, Goa KL. Celecoxib: a review of its use in osteoarthritis, rheumatoid arthritis, and acute pain. Drugs 2000;59:957–80.

65. Chen N, Warner JL, Reiss CS. NSAID treatment suppresses VSV propagation in mouse CNS. Virology 2000;276(1):44–51.

66. Zhu H, Cong JP, Yu D, et al. Inhibition of cyclooxygenase 2 blocks human cytomegalovirus replication. Proc Natl Acad Sci U S A 2002;99(6):3932–7.

67. Clubb SL. Clinical management of psittacine birds affected with proventricular dilation disease. Proc Annu Conf Assoc Avian Vet 2006;85–90.

68. Echols S. Treatment and management of avian renal disease. Proc Annu Conf Assoc Avian Vet 2004;77–85.

69. Danielczyk W. Twenty-five years of amantadine therapy in Parkinson's disease. J Neural Transm Suppl 1995;46:399–405.

70. CDC. High levels of adamantane resistance among influenza A (H3N2) viruses and interim guidelines for use of antiviral agents—United States, 2005-06 influenza season. MMWR Morb Mortal Wkly Rep 2006. Available at: http://www.cdc.gov/mmwr/preview/mmwrhtml/mm5502a7.htm. Accessed January, 2010.

71. Massey JG. Adverse drug reaction to metoclopramide hydrochloride in a macaw with proventricular dilation syndrome. J Am Vet Med Assoc 1993;203(4):542–4.

The Isolation, Pathogenesis, Diagnosis, Transmission, and Control of Avian Bornavirus and Proventricular Dilatation Disease

Sharman Hoppes, DVM, DABVP-Avian[a],*, Patricia L. Gray, DVM, MS[a],
Susan Payne, PhD[b], H.L. Shivaprasad, BVSc, MS, PhD, DACPV[c],
Ian Tizard, BVMS, PhD, ACVM[d]

KEYWORDS

• Bornavirus • Parrot • Proventriculus • Encephalitis

Proventricular dilatation disease (PDD) is a common infectious neurologic disease of birds, affecting more than 50 species of psittacines, and has been reported in toucans, honey creepers, weaver finches, water fowl, raptors, and passerines.[1–9] PDD is also known as Macaw wasting disease, after the first birds observed to be affected, and neuropathic ganglioneuritis or lymphoplasmacytic ganglioneuritis, after the lesions that it causes.[1,10,11] The name PDD is derived from the predominant feature of the disease in parrots, a dilatation of the proventriculus by ingested food as a result of defects in intestinal motility. This intestinal dysfunction results from virus-induced damage to the enteric nervous system. As a result of this damage to the gastrointestinal tract, birds are unable to empty their digestive tract or digest their food, and this

[a] Small Animal Clinical Sciences, Texas A&M University, 4474 TAMU, College Station, TX 77843, USA
[b] Associate Professor, Veterinary Pathobiology Department, Texas A&M University, 4467 TAMU College Station, TX 77843, USA
[c] Professor, Avian Pathology, University of California, Davis, CAHFS-Tulare, 18830 Road 112, Tulare, CA, USA
[d] Professor and Director, The Schubot Exotic Bird Health Center, Veterinary Pathobiology Department, Texas A&M University, 4467 TAMU, College Station, TX, USA
* Corresponding author.
E-mail address: shoppes@cvm.tamu.edu

Vet Clin Exot Anim 13 (2010) 495–508
doi:10.1016/j.cvex.2010.05.014
1094-9194/10/$ – see front matter © 2010 Elsevier Inc. All rights reserved.

leads to weight loss, crop stasis, proventricular and intestinal dilatation, regurgitation, maldigestion (passing of whole seeds), and eventually starvation and death.[12] The disease is also associated with significant central nervous system damage, which may include the development of encephalitis and myelitis resulting in depression, seizures, ataxia, blindness, and tremors.[13] Affected birds may show both neurologic and gastrointestinal signs. Definitive diagnosis has been based historically on crop biopsy or necropsy findings, the pathognomonic lesions being the presence of a lymphoplasmacytic infiltration in the ganglia and myenteric plexus of the gastrointestinal tract or central nervous system.[14] Definitive diagnosis of PDD has been problematic due to the inconsistent distribution of lesions. Berhane and colleagues[1] found lesions in the crop in 43% of cases, proventriculus 36%, ventriculus 93%, duodenum 21%, heart 79%, adrenal gland 50%, spinal cord 69%, brain 46%, sciatic nerve 58%, brachial nerve 46%, and vagus nerve 46%. Similar results have been reported by Shivaprasad and colleagues.[15] Whereas necropsy has provided a clear and concise diagnosis, premortem diagnosis has proven to be more difficult (**Fig. 1**).

PDD has long been considered an infectious disease, and multiple viruses have been suggested as its cause. For example, adenovirus-like particles were demonstrated within intranuclear inclusion bodies in the cells lining the kidneys of one affected bird,[16] and a coronavirus was isolated from a bird with PDD by Gough and colleagues[17] and was suggested to be the etiologic agent. A paramyxovirus related to Newcastle disease has also been considered a likely cause, because it was reported that this virus could be isolated in up to 60% of PDD cases.[18] None of these agents, however, have been consistently present in affected birds.

In 2008, major advances were made in determining the etiology of PDD. Pyrosequencing of cDNA from the brains of parrots with PDD identified 2 strains of a novel bornavirus.[19] Using real-time polymerase chain reaction (PCR), Honkavuori and colleagues[19] confirmed the presence of this virus in brain, proventriculus, and adrenal gland in 3 birds with PDD but not in 4 unaffected birds. Kistler and colleagues[20] used a microarray approach to identify a bornavirus hybridization signature in 5 of 8 PDD cases and none of 8 controls. Using high-throughput pyrosequencing in combination with conventional PCR cloning and sequencing, a complete viral genome sequence was recovered and named avian bornavirus (ABV). During this same time, Gray and colleagues[21] succeeded in culturing ABV from the brains of 7 psittacines diagnosed

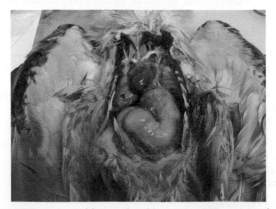

Fig. 1. Dilated proventriculus in a blue and gold macaw, PCR-positive for ABV, with histopathological lesions of PDD.

with PDD, providing a source of antigen for serologic assays and nucleic acid for molecular assays.

Bornaviruses are negative-strand RNA viruses belonging to the family Bornaviridae. Their most unique characteristic is that they undergo transcription inside the nucleus. These viruses also undergo alternative splicing, and use different initiation and termination signals than other viruses.[22] Two members of the family are known: Borna disease virus (BDV) and ABV. BDV causes neurologic disease in horses, cats, and sheep, and appears to be restricted to central Europe. While predominantly a disease of mammals, BDV has also been detected in the feces of wild mallards and corvids in Scandinavia. However, the significance of avian BDV infections and their epidemiologic significance are unclear.[23] An outbreak of neurologic disease attributed to BDV has been reported in ostriches in Israel. This diagnosis was based on serology, and unfortunately the virus isolates were lost, so the significance and etiology of this outbreak remain unclear.[24]

Experimentally, BDV has been shown to cause infections in chickens and quail. The clinical signs of BDV infection can range from a fatal meningoencephalitis to minor behavioral problems and persistent asymptomatic infection.[25] BDV appears to be only distantly related to ABV, although it is likely that one evolved from the other.

In this review the authors provide evidence that ABV is the etiologic agent of PDD. Recent findings on the transmission, epidemiology, pathogenesis, diagnosis, and control of ABV infection and PDD are also reviewed.

THE ISOLATION OF AVIAN BORNAVIRUS

Gray and colleagues[21] inoculated primary mallard embryo fibroblasts with a fresh brain suspension from a PDD infected yellow-collared macaw (*Primolius auricollis*) and African gray parrot (*Psittacus erithracus*), and succeeded in growing viruses from each. These viruses caused no detectable cytopathic effect in the duck cells. However, serum from a PDD-affected green-winged macaw (*Ara chloroptera*) that had been shown to recognize ABV N-protein was available. By performing a Western blot on infected duck cell lysates, these investigators demonstrated a progressive increase in the quantity of this viral antigen when cultured over 5 days. Indirect immunofluorescence assays on these infected cells using this same antiserum showed foci of antigen-positive cells demonstrating characteristic speckled intranuclear fluorescence (see **Fig. 1**). This speckled pattern is similar to that considered diagnostic of mammalian bornavirus infection: the stained particles are called Joest-Degen bodies and are believed to be complexes of the viral N and P proteins.[26,27] PCR assays conducted on this and other infected tissue cultures confirmed the presence of ABV. Subsequently the authors have isolated ABV by culture in duck embryo fibroblasts using material from the brains of 5 additional birds with necropsy-confirmed PDD (**Fig. 2**).

When Kistler and colleagues[20] first reported on the detection of ABV in PDD cases, they also reported several different genotypes. These genotypes differed by about 5% to 15% in their gene sequences. Given the huge diversity of species affected by PDD, the presence of diverse genotypes was unsurprising. However, Kistler's data show that specific genotypes do not favor certain avian species and appear to be of roughly equivalent pathogenicity. To date 7 different genotypes have been identified.[28,29] There is also significant genetic variation within these genotypes. Of the authors' 7 isolates, one is genotype 1 (ABV1) while the remainder belong to genotype 4 (ABV4). This predominance of genotype 4 has been observed by other groups.[28,29] This genotype could be an artifact resulting from increased pathogenicity of ABV4

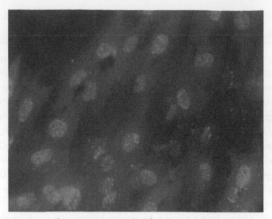

Fig. 2. Immunofluorescence photomicrograph of cultured duck embryo fibroblasts infected with an ABV isolate from a yellow-collared macaw 3 days previously. The lack of apparent cytotoxicity and presence of speckled nuclear fluorescence is typical of bornavirus infection. (Immunoflorescense stain at 10X.)

and the fact that tissue from lethal PDD cases is being selectively cultured. It is more likely, however, that it is indeed the predominant circulating genotype. The authors have also found that ABV4 is the predominant genotype in isolates from subclinical carriers of ABV (see later discussion). It is noteworthy that BDV, in contrast to ABV, shows a remarkable lack of genotypic variation. Only 2 genotypes of this virus have been identified. The reasons for this major difference between the 2 bornaviruses are unknown.

THE PATHOGENESIS OF AVIAN BORNAVIRUS INFECTION

Initial studies using immunoblots on tissues from 15 PDD-affected birds demonstrated that serum from PDD-affected birds consistently detected an antigen of 38 to 40 kDa present in their central nervous system.[30] This antigen, now known to be ABV N-protein, could also be detected in myocardium but not in other organs. Ouyang and colleagues[31] subsequently examined 24 stored avian brain samples, processed for histopathology and retained following their submission for necropsy or histopathology to the Schubot Exotic Bird Center diagnostic laboratory in 1992—a year selected at random. Thirteen of these samples were from PDD-infected birds. The remaining 11 were diagnosed with diseases other than PDD. Immunohistochemistry was performed using the macaw anti–N-protein serum and developed with a peroxidase-labeled anti-macaw serum. Cells containing ABV N-protein were found in the brain and spinal cord of all 13 PDD cases.[31] One bird not previously diagnosed with PDD also had ABV N-protein–positive cells in its cerebrum. A review of this bird's necropsy report indicated that it was most probably also suffering from PDD. ABV antigen was located in the cerebrum, cerebellum, and spinal cord. In the cerebrum it was usually found in scattered neurons and glial cells. In the cerebellum viral antigen was expressed in the Purkinje layer of the cerebellum, although Purkinje cells were never observed to contain the antigen. The cells containing the viral antigen were located adjacent to the Purkinje cells. Similar lesions have been observed in mammalian bornavirus infections.[32] All levels of affected spinal cord contained the ABV antigen in neurons and glia. Krähenbühl and colleagues[33] have also detected ABV in tissues of birds with PDD using in situ hybridization. Ten birds submitted for necropsy after dying for reasons other than PDD had no detectable N-protein in their brains.

Lierz and colleagues[34] have studied the distribution of ABV in infected cockatoos using real-time PCR on laser dissected tissues. These investigators found the virus in all organs of one bird with clinical PDD, implying viremia. In a second, apparently healthy bird, the virus was restricted to nerve ganglia. Rinder and colleagues,[29] using immunohistochemistry employing reagents developed for BDV, also found the virus to be present in multiple avian organs of affected birds. By contrast, Western blot studies by Villanueva and colleagues,[35] and the immunohistochemical studies reported by Gancz and colleagues,[36] suggested that the virus was restricted to nervous tissue.

AVIAN BORNAVIRUS IN THE EYE

Ouyang and colleagues[31] noted that ABV was detectable in the optic lobe of many PDD cases. In a single separate case of PDD in an Eclectus parrot (*Eclectus roratus*), eye fluid (vitreous and aqueous fluid) was collected on necropsy. This fluid contained so much virus that the ABV N-protein band was visible on stained electrophoresis gels. This protein band was excised and sequenced by mass spectroscopy and was confirmed to be the ABV N-protein (see **Fig. 2**). In addition, particles with a morphology consistent with that of a bornavirus were observed by immunotransmission electron microscopy (**Fig. 3**). Subsequent analysis of multiple additional eye fluid samples from PDD cases, while demonstrating the presence of occasional virus-like particles on electron microscopy, did not show the numbers of particles observed in the first bird and some contained no detectable virus-like particles, so the phenomenon is inconsistent. It is pertinent that eye lesions are a feature of some cases of PDD; choroiditis and optic neuritis predominate. The single article describing blindness in a psittacine as a result of bilateral retinal degeneration suggests that the lesions in the optic lobe may well lead to local retinal destruction or degeneration (see **Fig. 3; Fig. 4**).[13]

AUTOIMMUNITY

During the course of developing the Western blot assay, Villanueva and colleagues[30] originally used an extract of brain tissue from PDD-affected birds as their antigen source. For control purposes they used an extract of brain tissue from a bird that had died of causes other than PDD and which was both

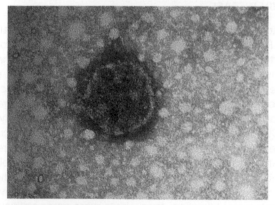

Fig. 3. Negatively stained (with phosphotungstic acid [PTA]), virus-like particle (83 nm in diameter) from the eye fluid of an Eclectus parrot with confirmed PDD and ABV infection. The image was recorded with an FEI Morgagni 268 transmission electron microscope at a magnification setting of 180,000X. (*Courtesy of* Dr Ross Payne.)

MPPKRQRSPNDQDEEMDSGEPAASRSHFPSLTGAFL
QYTQGGVDPHPGIGNEKDIHKNAVALLDQSRRELYHS
VTPSLVFLCLLIPGLHSALLFAGVQRESYLTTPVKQGE
RLITKTANFFGEKTMDQELTELQISSIFNHCCSLLIGVVI
GSSAKIKAGAEQIKKRFKTLMASINRPGHGETANLLS
VFNPHEAIDWINAQPWVGSFVLALLTTDFESPGKEFM
DQIKLVAGFAQMTTYTTIKEYLNECMDATLTIPAVALEI
KEFLDTTAKLKAEHGDMFKYLGAIRHSDAIKLAPRNF
PNLASAAFYWSKKENPTMAGYRASTIQPGSIVKEAQL
ARFRRREITRGDDGTTMPPEIAEVMKLIGVTGFAN

Fig. 4. The amino acid sequence of a 438 kDa protein isolated from the eye fluid of an Eclectus parrot. The colored sequences are the peptides shown to be identical to ABV N-protein.

seronegative and PCR-negative for ABV. During these studies, occasionally the serum of a seropositive bird would also react with antigens present in the normal bird brain. In one such case, serum from a "healthy" golden conure (*Guarouba guarouba*) was shown to react very strongly with a brain protein migrating in the 18- to 20-kDa region. Because this is the approximate molecular weight of myelin, this was investigated. This serum was also found to react with a similar-sized protein in normal chicken brain and with purified myelin basic protein (MBP) derived from that chicken brain. This ABV seropositive bird remains clinically healthy after 1 year. Serum evaluated 7 months later reacted weakly with MBP. It is proposed that the bird mounted a transient autoimmune response to myelin. Villanueva and colleagues[30] also surveyed 12 ABV-positive parrot sera for reactions with normal macaw brain and found that 3 reacted with an uncharacterized 40-kDa protein. These findings are of significance because it has been suggested that PDD results from an autoimmune response to brain gangliosides following viral infection in a manner similar to the induction of Guillain-Barré syndrome.[37] The authors do not believe that PDD is an autoimmune disease per se. However, the results described indicate that transient autoimmune responses do indeed occur in some PDD cases. The results are probably not clinically significant but may contribute to the complex pathogenesis of this disease.

EXPERIMENTAL ABV DISEASE

There is now abundant evidence proving that infection with ABV is causally associated with clinical PDD. For example, Gancz and colleagues[36] were able to induce PDD in 2 of 3 cockatiels after inoculation with ABV-infected brain homogenates. But Koch's postulates remains the standard by which an infectious agent is proven to cause a specific disease.[38] When Gray and colleagues[39] succeeded in culturing ABV4 in duck embryo fibroblasts, they also undertook a series of challenge experiments to establish Koch's postulates in 3 species of bird; mallards (*Anas platyrhynchos*), Patagonian conures (*Cyanoliseus patagonus*),[21] and cockatiels (*Nymphicus hollandicus*).[40]

Mallards. Three groups of 5, 4-day-old, SPF mallard chicks were infected by the oral, intraocular, and intramuscular routes.[39] Over a period of 6 weeks, no consistent clinical signs attributable to ABV infection occurred. However, the mallards were shown to be infected with ABV4 because their feces were positive by PCR when tested at weekly intervals. Likewise, these birds were seropositive for antibodies to ABV N-protein after 3 weeks. The mallards were euthanized at 3 to 8 months. On necropsy, no lesions compatible with PDD were observed. Histopathology of relevant organs showed no evidence of viral infection.

Patagonian conures. Three Patagonian conures, at least 15 years old, shedding psittacine herpesvirus but otherwise healthy, were used in a second challenge experiment.[21] Two were placed in isolation and administered passage 6 cultured ABV4 by both the oral and intramuscular routes. The third, uninfected conure was housed in a separate aviary and inoculated with uninfected duck embryo fibroblasts (DEFs). The 2 infected birds became seropositive at 21 days and became fecal shedders by 35 days. Aviary workers reported that they were eating but losing weight. On day 64, one of these birds was found dead in its cage. Necropsy showed an emaciated bird with gross lesions typical of PDD. The next day, the second infected bird was examined; it too was very thin and was euthanized. Necropsy again revealed gross changes consistent with PDD. Tissues were examined histologically, revealing typical PDD lesions—lymphocytic ganglioneuritis throughout the intestine as well as a lymphoplasmacytic encephalitis and myocarditis. PCR assays on the brains of these birds were strongly positive for ABV. The RNA from these brains was sequenced and shown to be identical to the ABV4 challenge strain. The control bird was euthanized 77 days after receiving uninfected tissue culture. Necropsy and histopathological examination of this bird showed no evidence of PDD. PCR of 4 separate brain samples from the control bird was negative for ABV.

Cockatiels. Payne and colleagues[40] have also challenged cockatiels with cultured ABV4 that had been passaged 6 times in DEFs. Four cockatiels were inoculated with ABV-M24 using the same routes and doses as the Patagonian conures described above. Two additional birds were inoculated with uninfected tissue culture and retained as negative controls. The inoculated birds remained in apparent good health until day 92 post infection. On that day, one bird was found dead in its cage. Necropsy revealed gross lesions typical of PDD. The remaining 3 infected birds were apparently healthy but their daily feed intake and activity levels declined. On day 110, 2 birds began showing neurologic signs, ataxia, and inability to walk. All 3 infected birds were euthanized humanely. Histopathology showed that 2 of these birds were suffering from PDD with lesions of unusual severity. The lesions were especially severe in the gastrointestinal tract and adrenal gland. The brain and spinal cord had mild to severe multifocal perivascular cuffing and gliosis randomly scattered throughout. The nerves had mild to moderate multifocal perivascular cuffing. The adrenal gland had a severe infiltration of lymphocytes and plasma cells in the medullary regions. The crop, proventriculus, ventriculus, and intestine had a severe infiltration of lymphocytes and a few plasma cells in the serosal and subserosal nerves and ganglia that also extended between muscle fibers. The bird with mild neurologic signs, but no gastrointestinal signs, had mild lesions compatible with PDD. The control, sham-infected birds remained healthy until euthanized on day 120. Their gross necropsy was unremarkable but on histopathology, they showed the presence of scattered lymphoid nodules throughout the spleen, kidney, and liver. It is important that in this study, the cockatiels were shown to be subclinical carriers of ABV4 prior to challenge. Their susceptibility indicates that they were not immune to the challenge virus despite prior exposure. This finding will be of significance in seeking to vaccinate against this virus and is discussed further below (**Fig. 5**).

DIAGNOSIS OF AVIAN BORNAVIRUS INFECTION

Animals mount a detectable antibody response to bornavirus infection. In mammals, immunofluorescence, enzyme-linked immunosorbent assay (ELISA), and Western blotting have been widely employed. In birds, Western blotting has been employed successfully to detect antibodies to ABV. For example, Villanueva

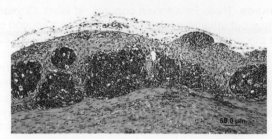

Fig. 5. Severe PDD lesions in the ventriculus of experimentally infected cockatiels. (*Courtesy of* H.L. Shivaprasad.)

and colleagues[35] used a Western blot assay to test for antibodies to ABV in the serum of 117 psittacine birds. A lysate from ABV-infected DEFs served as the source of antigen. The predominant antigen recognized by these birds was the 38-kDa N-protein. Thirty of these birds were confirmed positive for PDD by biopsy or necropsy, whereas the remaining 87 birds were apparently healthy or were suffering from non-PDD related disease. Sera from 27 of the 30 PDD cases (90%) contained antibodies to ABV N-protein. Seventy-three (84%) of the 87 apparently "healthy" birds were seronegative. In addition, sera from 7 wild macaws and one mealy Amazon parrot trapped in the Peruvian Amazon rainforest were negative. Most of the positive sera recognized only the N-protein in infected DEF cells. These positive sera also reacted strongly with 2 different preparations of recombinant N-protein. One clone was generated in an *Escherichia coli* vector, the other was generated in Chinese hamster ovary (CHO-K1) cells. A small proportion of the positive sera could also recognize cloned bornaviral P-protein generated in an *E coli* vector, a finding also reported by Lierz and colleagues.[34]

Although the development of antibodies to ABV largely corresponded with the development of clinical PDD and provides a much superior diagnostic procedure than, for example, crop biopsy, it must be pointed out that 14 apparently healthy normal birds possessed detectable antibodies to ABV. It is believed that these birds are infected by ABV but have yet to develop clinical disease. As discussed later in this article, "healthy" or subclinical carriers of ABV are apparently common so the presence of seropositive healthy birds is not unexpected. It is unclear at this time whether these seropositive birds will eventually, inevitably, develop clinical PDD. Villanueva and colleagues[35] also demonstrated that many seronegative birds were infected with ABV as detected by fecal PCR. Thus positive serology will be of limited usefulness in any disease eradication programs. The Western blot assay is also a slow and expensive test. A more practical and economic test would be an ELISA that employs purified, cloned ABV N-protein as the test antigen. Such a test is under development.

THE TRANSMISSION OF AVIAN BORNAVIRUS

Given the apparent sporadic nature of PDD cases and the apparent lack of explosive disease outbreaks, it has long been believed that the causal agent was slowly or inefficiently transmitted. New evidence indicates that this is by no means the case. The infection is indeed common and widespread among captive psittacines, at least in North America. That said, infection does not appear to inevitably or immediately cause PDD. Healthy or subclinical carriers of several species have been documented.

Fecal-Oral Route

The PCR using sequences from the N-gene as a primer readily detects ABV in fecal samples from infected birds. The authors have examined multiple samples from both feces, and cloacal swabs of large numbers of normal and PDD-affected birds. Any PCR products detected were confirmed by sequencing. For example, in the experimentally infected groups of birds, mallards began to shed virus in feces at week 14, yet showed no clinical disease.

A group of 15 "healthy" cockatiels from a single aviary, with no history of PDD or exposure to other birds, was screened for ABV by fecal PCR. Six were positive on first testing, 4 more on testing a week later, and 2 more on a third test. Thus, 12 of these birds were eventually ABV positive; only 2 were also positive by Western blot. The presence of so many PCR-positive birds in a "healthy" colony of cockatiels prompted the authors to screen other cockatiel colonies. A second colony of about 50 birds that practices no biosecurity and purchases birds at random from dealers was tested, and 2 of 10 fecal samples were PCR positive. The owner claimed that he had no significant health problems having lost only 5 birds in the last year (2009). The authors consider a 10% loss of some significance. A third cockatiel colony tested practiced fairly rigorous biosecurity and purchased very few birds from outside. From this colony, none of 15 fecal samples were PCR positive. This study is ongoing, but it is clear that there are "healthy" cockatiels shedding ABV. Lierz and colleagues[34] have also shown that apparently healthy birds within an aviary where clinical cases were occurring were also shedding ABV as detected by fecal swabs.

In an unintentional study on the transmission of ABV, the 15 cockatiels were housed on arrival with the control, uninfected mallards. The cockatiels were in suspended cages while the mallards were housed on the floor of the isolation building. Within days, mallards were observed to be eating cockatiel droppings. The cockatiels were tested and found to be shedding ABV4 in their feces. Fourteen days later, fecal samples from the mallards were also positive for the presence of ABV4 by PCR.

Respiratory Route

A dry-filter unit (DFR 1000) was used to test air for the presence of ABV in the authors' infected aviary. A very high volume of air (700 L/min) was drawn through a filter for 24 hours. The filter was subsequently washed and the washings tested by PCR for the presence of ABV. The air was sampled at 4 separate sites ranging from 11 in (28 cm) to 150 in (381 cm) from a cage containing a known ABV-infected bird. Each site was tested 3 times. All filters within the aviary were PCR-positive, indicating the presence of ABV in the air. Three samples were taken from a room adjacent to the aviary where birds were handled, and 2 of these samples were positive. Of 3 samples taken within 4 ft (122 cm) of an external aviary door, 1 was weakly positive. Of 3 samples taken 15 ft (457 cm) from this door, none were positive. Thus ABV was present both in the aviary itself and in a nearby workroom. It is possible that this disease can be transmitted by the respiratory route. It is of interest that pulmonary lesions have been described in cases of PDD with lymphocytoplasmic infiltrates observed in nerve ganglia associated with the large pulmonary blood vessels.[41]

ABV Shedding

While the authors have chosen to focus on the presence of ABV in the feces of affected birds, the shedding of this virus from other sites has also been examined. For this purpose the authors have had available 3 healthy African gray parrots known to be persistent shedders of ABV. These birds were swabbed at weekly intervals for 7 weeks and at longer intervals thereafter. The virus was detected by PCR not only in feces and cloacal swabs but also in swabs from the nares, the choana, and from the feathers in the axilla. This shedding was variable both between individuals and locations. One bird (**Table 1**) shed virus from all test sites on every sampling. Another bird shed virus intermittently and at times only choanal swabs were positive. The third bird was also a frequent shedder but not as consistent as the first.

ABV IN OTHER AVIAN SPECIES

PDD has largely been restricted to captive psittacines. However, there have been reports of a similar disease in Canadian geese (*Branta canadensis*),[42] and several passerine and piciform species.[41] Using fecal PCR the authors have tested feces from 102 ducks (*Anatidae* sp), a toco toucan (*Ramphastos toco*), 6 rock doves (*Columba livia*), 2 mourning doves (*Zenaida macroura*), 1 Carolina wren (*Thryothorus ludovicianus*), 2 eastern screech owls (*Megascops asio*), 2 barred owls (*Strix varia*), 2 barn owls (*Tyto alba*), 1 peregrine falcon (*Falco peregrinus*), 2 red-shouldered hawks (*Buteo lineatus*), and 1 red-tailed hawk (*Buteo jamaicensis*). All except the toucan were negative. The toco toucan was housed in a flight cage together with multiple macaws, some of which were shedding ABV4. The toucan was known to eat macaw droppings. The ABV detected in its feces was of genotype 4 and the bird was healthy at the time of sampling. Weissenböck and colleagues[43] recently published an article describing PDD and ABV in a canary (*Serinus canaria*) in Hungary. The genotype of this virus was found to be intermediate between other ABV genotypes and BDV. The significance of this is unclear but it is entirely plausible, given the presence of BDV in European ducks,[23] that ABV may have evolved from BDV. As described earlier, the authors succeeded in infecting mallards with ABV4 but no disease resulted within 8 months. The authors have tested serum from a domestic Muscovy duck (*Cairina moschata*) submitted to a veterinary clinic because of a tumor, whose serum was positive for antibodies to ABV N-protein by Western blotting. However, given the issues regarding the specificity and significance of Western blotting in humans, the significance of this single positive result is unclear at this time.

CONTROL AND PREVENTION OF ABV INFECTION

The control of viral infections in many cases depends on appropriate management practices and infection control. No data are available to the authors regarding the survival of ABV in the environment. However, it is an enveloped RNA virus of similar size and structure to Newcastle disease virus (NDV); both are enveloped Mononegavirales. ABV would be expected therefore to show a sensitivity profile similar to that observed in NDV. The authors therefore suggest that NDV can be used as a surrogate and that disinfectants and cleansing agents that are effective for NDV will likely be effective for ABV. Control would include isolation, traffic control, sanitation and thorough cleaning, and the use of disinfectants such as phenols, formaldehyde, or hypochlorites such as bleach. With the availability of a fecal PCR, it should also be possible to control the admittance of ABV-infected birds to aviaries. It must be pointed out, however, that not all birds are constant ABV shedders. Thus, as with psittacine herpesviruses, repeated testing may be required to exclude any specific bird as an ABV carrier.

The authors have treated a group of clinically healthy, seropositive, ABV-shedding African gray parrots (*Psittacus erithacus*) with the antiviral drug amantadine for 6 weeks, with no apparent effect on fecal viral shedding. Amantidine was tested because there have been anecdotal reports of its therapeutic affect in parrots with PDD.[44] The authors are currently looking at other antiviral compounds and are using

Table 1
Avian bornavirus PCR shedding over a 5-month period

		19-May-09	21-Jul-09	08-Sep-09	15-Sep-09	22-Sep-09	29-Sep-09	01-Oct-09
AG1 = African gray "Juniper"	Nares	POS	POS	POS	POS	POS	POS	POS
	Choana	POS	POS	POS	POS	POS	POS	POS
	Skin	POS	POS	POS	POS	POS	POS	POS
	Cloaca	POS	POS	POS	POS	POS	POS	POS
AG2 = African gray "Quincy"	Nares	NEG	NEG	NEG	NEG	NEG	NEG	NEG
	Choana	POS	POS	POS	POS	POS	POS	POS
	Skin	NEG	NEG	NEG	NEG	NEG	NEG	NEG
	Cloaca	POS	POS	POS	POS	POS	NEG	NEG
AG3 = African gray "George"	Nares	POS	POS	NEG	POS	NEG	POS	POS
	Choana	POS	POS	POS	POS	POS	POS	POS
	Skin	POS	POS	POS	POS	POS	POS	POS
	Cloaca	POS	POS	POS	POS	POS	POS	POS
AG8 = African gray "Zelda"	Nares	NEG	NEG	NEG	NEG	NEG	NEG	NEG
	Choana	NEG	NEG	NEG	NEG	NEG	NEG	NEG
	Skin	NEG	NEG	NEG	NEG	NEG	NEG	NEG
	Cloaca	NEG	NEG	NEG	NEG	NEG	NEG	NEG

Juniper, Quincy, and George were all crop biopsy positive and serologically positive for ABV. Zelda has been consistently negative on PCR, serology, and crop biopsy.

virus shedding as a marker of efficacy. Treatment protocols will have to be developed, although experience with mammalian encephalitides suggests that it may be difficult to identify an effective antiviral therapy.

It is generally believed that Borna disease in mammals is in large part immunologically mediated.[45–47] Immunosuppressive or anti-inflammatory treatments appear to reduce the severity of disease while immune stimulation may in some cases increase its severity. Thus Borna disease is believed to belong to that group of infections whereby immune responses increase severity and vaccination may be contraindicated.

It is certainly true that most birds suffering from PDD are strongly seropositive, implying that antibodies to the immunodominant N-protein are not protective. The authors' cockatiel study described herein also provided clear evidence that prior exposure to ABV is not protective. In addition, there are obvious economic issues involved in the commercial production of a vaccine for use in a small, specialized market.

SUMMARY

Multiple investigators have now demonstrated that ABV is consistently present in cases of PDD. Likewise, Koch's postulates have been fulfilled in 2 species, cockatiels and Patagonian conures. ABV has been demonstrated in the lesions of PDD cases. All available evidence supports the contention that ABV is the etiologic agent of PDD. Diagnostic tests such as Western blots or fecal PCR can identify many, but not all ABV-infected birds, and should be employed to control the spread of this disease. Such tests may be very useful for diagnosis and in epidemiologic studies.

ACKNOWLEDGMENTS

We would like to thank Dr Ross Payne who undertook the transmission electron microscopy of the virus.

REFERENCES

1. Berhane Y, Binnington B, Hunter B, et al. Peripheral neuritis in psittacine birds with proventricular dilation disease. Avian Pathol 2001;73:563–70.
2. Gregory C, Ritchie B. Advances in understanding of proventricular dilation disease (PDD): detection of virus and viral nucleic acid in infected birds. Proc Annu Conf Assoc Avian Vet 1999;41–3.
3. Ritchie B. Epizootiology of proventricular dilatation disease in breeding cockatiels. Proc Annu Conf Assoc Avian Vet 2004;41–5.
4. Boutette JB, Taylor M. Proventricular dilation disease: a review of research, literature, species differences, diagnostics, prognosis, and treatment. Proc Annu Conf Assoc Avian Vet 2004;175–81.
5. Shivaprasad HL. Proventricular dilatation disease in a peregrine falcon. Proc Annu Conf Assoc Avian Vet 2005;107–8.
6. Hadley T. Atypical presentation of proventricular dilatation disease in a yellow-headed Amazon. Proc Annu Conf Assoc Avian Vet 2005;353–5.
7. Clark D. Proventricular dilation syndrome in large psittacine birds. Avian Dis 1984;28:813–5.
8. Phalen D. An outbreak of psittacine proventricular dilation syndrome (PPDS) in a private collection of birds and an atypical form in a Nanday conure. Proc Annu Conf Assoc Avian Vet 1989;27–34.

9. Gregory CR, Ritchie BW, Latimer KS, et al. Progress in understanding proventricular dilatation disease. Proceedings of the International Aviculture Society. Orlando (FL); 1998. p. 1–6.

10. Turner R. Macaw fading or wasting syndrome. Proc 33rd West Poult Dis Conf 1984;87–8.

11. Suedmeyer W. Diagnosis and clinical progression of three cases of proventricular dilation syndrome. J Assoc Avian Vet 1992;6:159–63.

12. Gregory CR, Latimer KS, Niagro FD, et al. A review of proventricular dilatation syndrome. J Assoc Avian Vet 1994;8:69–75.

13. Steinmetz A, Pees M, Schmidt V, et al. Blindness as a sign of proventricular dilatation disease in a grey parrot (Psittacus erithracus erithracus). J Small Anim Pract 2008;49:660–2.

14. Schmidt RE, Reavill DR, Phalen DN. Pathology of pet and aviary birds. Iowa: Iowa State Press; 2003. p. 47–55.

15. Shivaprasad HL, Barr BC, Woods LW, et al. Spectrum of lesions (pathology) of proventricular dilation syndrome. Proceedings of the Association of Avian Veterinarians. Philadelphia; 1995. p. 507–08.

16. Heldstab A, Morgenstern D, Ruedi A, et al. Pathologie einer endemieartig verlaufenden neuritis im magen/darmberich bei groBpapageien. Int Symp Zoo Animal 1985;317–24 [in German].

17. Gough RE, Drury SE, Culver F, et al. Isolation of a coronavirus from a green-cheeked Amazon parrot (Amazona viridigenalis Cassin). Avian Pathol 2006;35:122–6.

18. Grund CH, Werner O, Gelderblom HR, et al. Avian paramyxovirus serotype I isolates from the spinal cord of parrots display a very low virulence. J Vet Med 2002;49:445–51.

19. Honkavuori KS, Shivaprasad HL, Williams BL, et al. Novel bornavirus in psittacine birds with proventricular dilatation disease. Emerg Infect Dis 2008;14:1883–6.

20. Kistler AL, Gancz A, Clubb S, et al. Recovery of divergent avian bornaviruses from cases of proventricular dilatation disease: identification of a candidate etiologic agent. Virol J 2008;5:88.

21. Gray P, Hoppes S, Suchodolski P, et al. Use of avian bornavirus isolates to induce proventricular dilatation disease in conures. Emerg Infec Dis 2010; 16(3):473–9.

22. Briese T, de la Torre JC, Lewis A, et al. Borna disease virus, a negative-strand RNA virus, transcribes in the nucleus of infected cells. Proc Natl Acad Sci U S A 1992;89:11486–9.

23. Berg M, Johansson M, Montell H, et al. Wild birds as a possible natural reservoir of Borna disease virus. Epidemiol Infect 2001;127:173–8.

24. Malkinson M, Weismann Y, Ashash E, et al. Borna disease in ostriches. Vet Rec 1993;133:304.

25. Ludwig H, Kraft W, Kao M, et al. Bornavirus infection (Borna disease) in naturally and experimentally infected animals: its significance for research and practice. Tierarztl Prax 1985;13:421–53.

26. Joest E, Degen K. Über eigentümliche Kerneinschlüsse der Ganglienzellen bei der enzootischen Gehirn-Rückenmarksentzündung der Pferde. Z Infkrankh Haustiere 1909;6:348–56 [in German].

27. Herzog S, Rott R. Replication of borna disease virus in cell cultures. Med Microbiol Immunol 1980;168:153–8.

28. Weissenböck H, Bakonyi T, Sekulin K, et al. Avian bornaviruses in psittacine birds from Europe and Australia with proventricular dilatation disease. Emerg Infect Dis 2009;15:1453–9.

29. Rinder M, Ackermann A, Kempf H, et al. Broad tissue tropism of avian bornavirus in parrots with proventricular dilatation disease. J Virol 2009;83:5401–7.
30. Villanueva I, Gray P, Tizard I. Detection of an antigen specific for proventricular dilation disease in psittacine birds. Vet Rec 2008;163:426.
31. Ouyang N, Storts R, Tian Y, et al. Detection of avian bornavirus in the nervous system of birds diagnosed with proventricular dilatation disease. Avian Pathol 2009;38:393–401.
32. Eisenman LM, Brothers R, Tran MH, et al. Neonatal borna disease virus infection in the rat causes a loss of Purkinje cells in the cerebellum. J Neurovirol 1999;5: 181–9.
33. Krähenbühl I, Lehner A, Hilbe M, et al. Detection of avian bornavirus in parrots with proventricular dilatation disease (PDD) by in-situ hybridization. J Comp Path 2009;141:294.
34. Lierz M, Hafez HM, Honkavuori KS, et al. Anatomical distribution of avian bornavirus in parrots, its occurrence in clinically healthy birds and ABV-antibody detection. Avian Pathol 2009;38:491–6.
35. Villanueva I, Gray P, Mirhosseini N, et al. The diagnosis of proventricular dilatation disease: use of a western blot assay to detect antibodies against avian borna virus. Vet Micro 2010;143:196–201.
36. Gancz AY, Kistler AL, Greninger AL, et al. Experimental induction of proventricular dilatation disease in cockatiels (Nymphicus hollandicus) inoculated with brain homogenates containing avian bornavirus 4. Virol J 2009;6:11.
37. Rossi G, Crosta L, Pesaro S. Parrot proventricular dilatation disease. Vet Rec 2008;163:310.
38. Koch R (1890). Ueber bakteriologische Forschung, Verhandl, des X. Internatl Med Congr, Berlin. August Hirschwald, Berlin: 1891. p. 35.
39. Gray P, Villaneuva I, Mirhosseini N, et al. Experimental infection of birds with avian bornavirus. Proceeding of the Association of Avian Veterinarians. Milwaukee; 2009. p. 7.
40. Payne S, Shivaprasad HL, Mirhosseini N, et al. Unususal and severe lesions of proventricular dilatation disease in Cockatiels (Nymphicus hollandicus) as healthy carriers of avian bornavirus and subsequently infected with a virulent strain of the same ABV genotype. Vet Micro, in press.
41. Perpiñán D, Fernández-Bellon H, López C, et al. Lymphocytic myenteric, subepicardial, and pulmonary ganglioneuritis in four nonpsittacine birds. J Avian Med Surg 2007;21:210–4.
42. Daoust PY, Julian RJ, Yason CV, et al. Proventricular impaction associated with nonsuppurative encephalomyelitis and ganglioneuritis in two Canada geese. J Wildl Dis 1991;27:513–7.
43. Weissenböck H, Sekulin K, Bakonyi T, et al. Novel avian bornavirus in a nonpsittacine species (canary; Serinus canaria) with enteric ganglioneuritis and encephalitis. J Virol 2009;83:11367–71.
44. Clubb SL, Meyer MJ. Clinical management of psittacine birds affected with proventricular dilatation disease. Proc Annu Conf Assoc Avian Vet 2006;85–90.
45. Stitz L, Dietzschold B, Carbone KM. Immunopathogenesis of Borna disease. Curr topics Microbiol Immunol 1995;190:75–92.
46. Morimoto K, Hooper DC, Bornhorst A, et al. Intrinsic responses to Borna disease virus infection of the central nervous system. Proc Natl Acad Sci U S A 1996;93: 13345–50.
47. Schwemmie M, Lipkin WI. Models and mechanisms of Bornavirus pathogenesis. Drug Discov Today 2004;1:211–6.

Advanced Diagnostic Approaches and Current Management of Thyroid Pathologies in Guinea Pigs

Jörg Mayer, DMV, MSc, DABVP (ECM)[a],*, Robert Wagner, DVM, PhD, DECVDI[b],
Olivier Taeymans, VMD, DABVP-Exotics[a]

KEYWORDS

- Thyroid pathologies • Hyperthyroidism
- Hypothyroidism • Guinea pig

Primary pathology of the thyroid in the guinea pig was described in the literature more than 40 years ago.[1,2] Recently, a relatively high incidence of thyroid pathology in guinea pigs has been reported.[3] The relative prevalence was reported to be 4.6% at one pathology facility, making thyroid pathology the second most commonly reported after lymphoma (Garner, personal communication, 2006); however, there is no scientific report that describes the clinical case of a confirmed hyperthyroid state of a guinea pig in the English literature. Contrary to this observation, the German literature states that hyperthyroidism is a relatively commonly observed clinical presentation in guinea pigs.[4] This might be attributable to several factors. One observation is that hyperthyroidism is not currently listed as a disease in the major clinical textbooks dealing with exotic companion mammals and clinicians might not include the condition in the differential diagnosis list when confronted with an animal that displays typical signs. Until very recently, there was no good clinical resource that provided validated reference values for thyroid hormone levels in the guinea pig and clinicians had problems interpreting the results of a hormone profile if it was run. In addition, surgery to remove the affected gland or to take a biopsy of the affected tissue is relatively difficult; therefore, there is no fast or easy diagnostic process.

The authors have encountered multiple clinical cases of clinical hyperthyroidism in the guinea pig, which responded positively to clinical treatment. Hyperactive thyroids

[a] Department of Clinical Sciences, Tufts University Cummings School of Veterinary Medicine, 200 Westboro Road North Grafton, MA 01536, USA
[b] Division of Laboratory Animal Resources, University of Pittsburgh, S 1049 Biomedical Science Tower, 200 Lothrop Street, Pittsburgh, PA 15261, USA
* Corresponding author.
E-mail address: joerg.mayer@tufts.edu

in the guinea pig appear to exist causing typical clinical signs. An early accurate diagnosis of this pathologic state is important in the clinical setting. One of the authors (R.W.) has encountered a few clinical cases of hypothyroidism in guinea pigs. Hypothyroidism appears to be a rare condition and has been described anecdotally in the German literature.[4] Because of the rarity of hypothyroidism, the text focuses mainly on the guinea pig as a hyperthyroid case. A short description of the clinical presentation of the hypothyroid animal is included at the end of the text.

THE TYPICAL CLINICAL PRESENTATION

It appears that hyperthyroidism can affect guinea pigs of all ages. Most reported cases are in guinea pigs older than 3 years. It has been reported that the prevalence of thyroid pathology can reach up to 30% in some groups of guinea pigs after 3 years of age.[5] Thyroid hyperplasia, adenoma, and carcinoma all have been responsible for clinical problems; unfortunately, the exact numbers of the distribution of malignant versus benign lesions are not known and further research is needed to link the pathologic and clinical findings. In the authors' experiences, there may be a slight predilection for females but statistical confirmation of any gender predilection is lacking. In the dog it is common that clinically detectable thyroid neoplasias represent mostly carcinomas and less frequently adenomas.[6] A relatively high incidence for carcinomas in the guinea pig was also observed in a recent review of thyroid pathology in the guinea pig. It was found that approximately 55% of thyroid neoplasms of the guinea pig were adenocarcinomas.[7] Further studies are needed to determine if the hyperthyroid guinea pig patient behaves more like the cat or the dog in regard to the distribution of carcinoma versus adenoma and functional pathology versus nonfunctional enlargement of the thyroid gland.

TYPICAL CLINICAL SIGNS

In reviewing multiple cases, clinical signs vary significantly; however, some changes are consistently found and can be considered key clinical signs. These include hyperactivity and hyperesthesia combined with the observation that the animals often are polyphagic but appear thin or are losing weight. Other common but inconsistent clinical findings include diarrhea or soft stool, polyuria/polydipsia, and a palpable mass in the neck. Progressive alopecia has also been reported (**Fig. 1**).[4] Occasionally, the

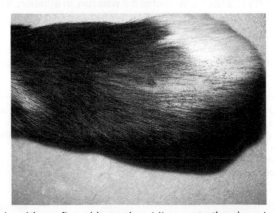

Fig. 1. A guinea pig with confirmed hyperthyroidism, note the alopecia over the dorsum.

patient has tachycardia and should be examined for cardiovascular abnormalities. In a recent review of the pathology of the thyroid gland in guinea pigs, the most common co-condition was pulmonary congestion, followed by atrophy of fat.[7]

DIAGNOSIS

The diagnosis of this condition can be difficult, as results from various diagnostic tests can often be inconclusive. In guinea pigs, the T4 and T3 blood concentrations can be unreliable for both disease diagnosis and treatment monitoring. It is possible to encounter an animal with severe clinical signs without significant elevations in T4/T3 levels. As a baseline for normal values, recently published material on serum thyroxine concentrations in clinically healthy pet guinea pigs is now available,[8] making the diagnosis a bit easier. The investigators concluded that normal thyroxine concentrations in the healthy guinea pig ranged from 14.2 to 66.9 nmol/L (1.1–5.2 mg/dL) with a median value of 27.0 nmol/L (2.1 mg/dL) (**Tables 1** and **2**). If a swelling of the neck is noted during the physical examination, a fine-needle aspirate with cytologic evaluation can aid in the diagnosis of thyroid tumor but it cannot assess endocrine activity. One author (R.W.) found that fluid aspirated from the neck mass often reveals extremely high T4 concentrations and correlates well with systemic T4 elevation (**Fig. 2**). In rare cases in which T4/T3 levels fall below expected normal values, keep in mind that advanced stages of hypothyroidism can mimic hyperthyroidism as mentioned later in the text.

DIAGNOSTIC IMAGING

In human medicine the thyroid imaging approach is based on the preliminary clinical evaluation. If lesions are smaller than 2 cm it is recommended that lesions are evaluated by ultrasound (US), if possible in combination with a US-guided fine-needle aspirate for cytology (**Fig. 3**). More advanced imaging, such as computed tomography (CT) and magnetic resonance imaging (MRI), is not routine and is more restricted to specific indications such as the evaluation of the extent of substernal goiters, characterization of large neck masses, estimation of local invasiveness of thyroid carcinomas, and detection of local and distant metastases.[6]

In cats, nuclear medicine is considered the imaging modality of choice in the diagnosis and treatment of hyperthyroidism. A benefit of this technique in cases of neoplasia is the potential to detect local and distant metastases. Most thyroid tumors in dogs, however, are not hypersecreting thyroid hormones and therefore do not result in increased radiopharmaceutical uptake of the radioisotope as compared with cats.[9–11] The use of nuclear medicine in cases of canine primary hypothyroidism remains controversial, as false negative results and variation in normal uptake have been reported.[6,11–14] A benefit of this technique in cases of neoplasia is the potential

Table 1 Gender-specific values for thyroid hormone in the guinea pig (n = 6)[28]	
T4 male: 2.9 ± 0.6 μg/dL	T3 male: 39 ± 17 ng/dL
T4 female: 3.2 ± 0.7 μg/dL	T3 female: 44 ± 10 ng/dL
Free T4 male: 1.26 ± 0.41 ng/dL	Free T3 male: 257 ± 35 pg/dL
Free T4 female: 1.33 ± 0.25 ng/dL	Free T3 female: 260 ± 59 pg/dL

Data from Castro MI, Alex S, Young RA, et al. Total and free serum thyroid hormone concentrations in fetal and adult pregnant and nonpregnant guinea pigs. Endocrinology 1986;118(2):533–7.

Table 2
Gender-specific values for thyroid hormone in the guinea pig according to Müller
and colleagues

Sex	N	Thyroxine (μg/dL)		
		Median	Minimum	Maximum
Females	16	2	1.1	5
Males	16	2.2	1.1	4.5
Castrated male	8	2.7	1.5	5.2
All animals	40	2.1	1.1	5.2

Data from Müller K, Müller E, Klein R, et al. Serum thyroxine concentrations in clinically healthy pet guinea pigs (Cavia porcellus). Vet Clin Pathol 2009; 38:507–10.

to detect local and distant metastases. Although the availability of testing equipment and of this diagnostic test are not widespread, the interested clinician should try to locate a local veterinary or human medical facility that is equipped with a gamma camera.

Hyperactive thyroid tissue and potential metastatic tissue were demonstrated in a guinea pig using nuclear scintigraphy. In this case, diagnostic images were obtained 60 to 80 minutes after injection (**Fig. 4**).[15] The role of thyroid scintigraphy as a specific tool for the identification of hyperthyroidism in guinea pigs still has to be determined; however, it appears that it is one of the most precise diagnostic tools to document the function of a potentially abnormal thyroid gland.

As an alternative choice of imaging, an ultrasound examination of the thyroid can be performed to detect any anatomic changes in the gland. Because of its very superficial location, high-frequency transducers of at least 10 MHz should be used to examine the thyroid gland (see **Fig. 4**). The location of the thyroid gland in the guinea pig has been reported to be at a significantly different location than in the dog or cat. According to the anatomic drawings by Popesko and Rajtova,[16] the gland is located between the rami mandibulae and is therefore located significantly more cranially than when compared with other species (**Fig. 5**A). In the clinical setting, however, a nodule in the neck is often palpated where one would expect the thyroid in other species.

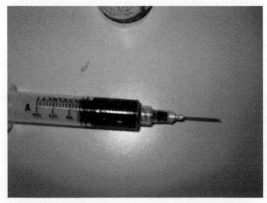

Fig. 2. Fluid aspirated from a swelling on the ventral neck in a guinea pig with typical clinical signs of hyperthyroidism.

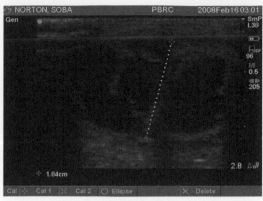

Fig. 3. An ultrasound examination of the thyroid gland in the guinea pig, note the cystic compartment.

A thorough anatomic review with histologic analysis will be required to confirm anatomic location of the gland. Please refer to **Fig. 5**, B and C, as examples of the anatomic location of a confirmed thyroid tumor in a guinea pig.

Analogous to dogs, carcinoma in the guinea pig may potentially benefit from an MRI study. This imaging technique has the potential to better define local tissue invasion, as it has a higher contrast resolution than US. This technique is also not hampered by gas when trying to visualize tissue invasion dorsal to the trachea and is less operator dependant than US.[17]

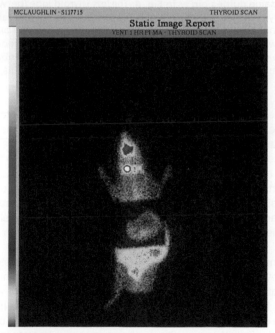

Fig. 4. A ventral color scintigram of the abnormal guinea pig taken 60 minutes after administration of the radiopharmaceutical illustrates a subjectively increased pattern of uptake of the right thyroid.

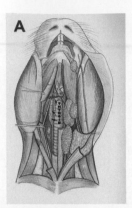

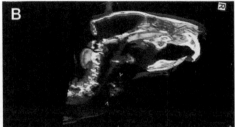
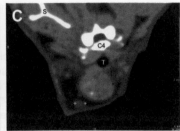

Fig. 5. (*A*) An anatomic sketch of the location of the thyroid in the guinea pig, note the rostral location of the gland when compared with other species. (*B*) Three-dimensional maximum intensity projection (3D-MIP) reconstructed CT image showing the enlarged left thyroid lobe of the same guinea pig as in **Fig. 4**. The left thyroid lobe (between white arrowheads) is moderately enlarged and shows multiple central areas of mineralization. (*C*) Transverse CT image of the thyroid gland of the same guinea pig as in **Figs. 4** and **5B** displayed in a soft tissue window. The left thyroid lobe (between black asterisks) is moderately enlarged and shows multiple central areas of mineralization. The right thyroid lobe (between white plus signs), is unremarkable. C4, fourth cervical vertebra; S, right scapula; T, trachea.

CT could also have a potential benefit, as thyroid tissue is expected to be hyperattenuating because of the presence of iodine (high atomic number) and therefore should result in easy detection of normal thyroid tissue. CT also has the advantage to be simultaneously able to look for pulmonary metastatic disease[17] (**Fig. 5**B, C).

However, if no access to specialized imaging is available or the owner declines imaging, the tentative diagnosis can be made by the combination of history, clinical presentation, physical examination, and blood work. In suspect cases, a trial therapy of methimazole can be started, as the response to medical treatment is usually very fast and obvious (ie, weight gain or behavior change within 48 hours after start of trial therapy).

During the diagnostic process, it is important to avoid a "thyroid storm," which can be triggered by any stressful event such as excessive handling or the mechanical (ie, surgical) manipulation of the gland. Keeping the animal in a calm environment and handling it gently is the best way to prevent an adverse event. It is important to remember that the condition is chronic and urgent acute treatment is often not needed. If secondary pathologic problems exist, such as congestive heart failure, it is important to address these issues immediately to prevent complications during the thyroid therapy (for a list of potential complications see the Medical Treatment).

THERAPY

Once the clinical diagnosis has been established, multiple treatment therapies exist for hyperthyroidism. Each treatment has distinct advantages and disadvantages. The owner should be made aware of all these factors when deciding which treatment option to choose. The goal of treatment is to return thyroid hormone levels to normal with a subsequent resolution of the clinical signs. Optimally, the owner should be informed about all different treatment options and should be educated about the positive and negative attributes of each treatment option. A significant factor in the decision-making process is often the cost involved with the treatment along with the potential risks associated with the treatment. To provide the owner with accurate information about treatment options, it is important to locate certain specialty clinics (eg, specialty surgery service, I-131 treatment facility). Exact costs associated with each procedure should be detailed so as to provide a realistic estimate and avoid disappointment later on.

As outlined in the following section, treatment can range from oral medication to invasive surgery to remove the pathologic tissue.

Medical Treatment

The medical treatment of choice in the guinea pig is extrapolated from clinical feline medicine. To the authors' knowledge, no pharmacologic study has been published on the therapeutic use of antithyroid drug in the guinea pig; however, some data are available on the use of propylthiouracil (PTU) in guinea pigs. PTU is a thioamide drug used to treat hyperthyroidism and pharmacologically is similar to methimazole. Studies have shown that pharmacokinetic behavior of PTU in the guinea pig is similar to that in humans. Plasma levels are reached after 2 hours in guinea pigs and within 1 to 2 hours in humans.[18] Therefore, extrapolation of the pharmacokinetic data of methimazole from humans to guinea pigs appears adequate.

The drugs of choice are methimazole or carbimazole, as these drugs are used in cats with the same problem. These antithyroid drugs directly suppress thyroid hormone production. Drug dosages for methimazole have been extrapolated from cat dosages and successful anecdotal use ranges from 0.5 to 2.0 mg/kg orally once to twice a day. Carbimazole is now also available in the United States and drug dosages for guinea pigs are reported at 1 to 2 mg/kg orally once a day.[4] The appropriate dose would be determined by repeated assays of serum thyroid hormone levels. Because methimazole is available only in 5- and 10-mg tablets, it is often prepared by a compounding pharmacy. One author (J.M.) suggests compounding it into a liquid of 10 mg/kg to avoid large or small dosing volumes and also to accomplish good drug distribution in compounded liquids. The use of transdermal methimazole in premium lecithin organogel gel has been reported to have therapeutic success in cats that do not tolerate oral dosing. One author (R.W.) has had clinical success with transdermal methimazole in guinea pigs; however, transdermal application has been shown to cause depigmentation of brown guinea pig skin.[19] The depigmentation effect is also observed in humans, where the dermal application of methimazole can be used in hyperpigmentation disorders.[20] Caution should be used with this delivery method in any animal other than cats because of this side effect.

Advantage

Oral medical treatment is considered the least invasive option to treat patients. The clinical response is usually seen very fast, ie, within 48 hours, and the drugs are not very expensive. The drug is usually given orally once daily, which aids medication and owner compliance significantly. A few refractory cases require twice-daily dosing. Because of the ease of treatment with minimal side effects, the drug can be used as a trial therapy in suspect cases, where appropriate diagnostics are not an option. If clinical signs improve significantly on the drug and return once medication is stopped, there is a strong clinical suspicion for hyperthyroidism and a tentative diagnosis can be made.

Disadvantage

The main drawback of the oral treatment is that the medication needs to be given for life, as the discontinuation of the medication will result in return of clinical signs very fast (ie, 24–48 hours). As mentioned previously, it can be difficult to monitor the effect of the medication based on hormone levels; the efficacy of the treatment often needs to be guided by the clinical response. In dogs and cats, the drug has been reported to cause some minor side effects such as vomiting, anorexia, and depression. Eosinophilia, leukopenia, and lymphocytosis may be seen with drug administration. When observed in cats, these clinical pathology changes are usually transient and do not require cessation of therapy.[21] Cases of toxicity because of an accidental overdose, agranulocytosis, hepatopathy, and thrombocytopenia are deleterious side effects reported in other domestic species.[21]

It is unclear to what extent these potential side effects affect guinea pigs. To date, no side effects during the therapeutic use of methimazole have been reported in the guinea pig.

Surgical Excision

Surgery to excise the affected gland is possible and a technical paper on the procedure was published more than 30 years ago.[22] Multiple articles exist in the scientific literature where a complete thyroidectomy in guinea pigs was performed experimentally.[23] Before surgery is attempted, the authors strongly suggest having diagnostic imaging performed to evaluate if the disease is uni- or bilateral. The 2 imaging techniques of choice are US examination or scintigraphy. Although the US examination will reveal morphologic abnormalities and vascular involvement, scintigraphy will locate functional, ectopic tissue if present.

Advantage

Surgical removal of all pathologic tissue can be curative. After a successful surgery there is no need to medicate the animal long term; however, frequent rechecks of the hormone levels are still recommended as the disease has the potential to recur. It is advisable to submit the removed tissue to a pathologist for histopathologic evaluation.

Disadvantage

Surgical excision can be complicated because of the anatomic location of the thyroid gland. Possible complications include recurrent laryngeal nerve damage and the stimulation of aberrant thyroid tissue. The surgery should be performed by a specialist with access to microsurgical instruments. One of the authors (R.W.) encountered several thyroid carcinomas that could not be surgically excised because of the extensive vascular nature and other vital tissue involvement. Surgery should ideally not be attempted before the animal is medically stabilized so as to avoid postsurgical complications, such as a thyroid storm (C. Orcutt, personal communication, 2008).[24] It is interesting to note that human patients with hyperthyroidism (and those receiving exogenous thyroid replacement) may be susceptible to developing severe hypertension and tachycardia when given ketamine. However, the veterinary significance of this potential complication is unknown.[21]

The total removal of all thyroid gland in a guinea pig involves also removing the parathyroid glands, as they are embedded throughout the thyroid tissue. To prevent postoperative hypocalcemia, which would be fatal immediately after surgery, it is important to provide a source of calcium, such as 1.0% calcium lactate or calcium gluconate orally once a day. Calcium should be provided at least for 7 to 10 days post-operatively before a weaning trial of the calcium can be started.

Percutaneous Ethanol Injection

In cats, the destruction of abnormal tissue by the direct injection with alcohol has been published.[24] The injected alcohol will necrotize the glandular tissue and leave it nonfunctional. Alcohol ablation was attempted 2 times on the same guinea pig with only transient improvement; eventually the guinea pig died 1 month after the last alcohol injection (R.W.). The authors do not recommend the percutaneous use of ethanol to treat this disease.

Radioactive Treatment with I-131

Two authors (R.W., J.M.) have each treated one patient with I-131 and the patients had a good quality of life after radiation treatment. Both animals weighed approximately 700 g at the time of diagnosis and received 1 miC of I-131 subcutaneously once. One patient lived for 14 months after the treatment and then died of chronic renal failure. The second guinea pig is doing well 6 months after treatment. Both patients rapidly regained weight after the treatment with the radioactive iodine. Hyperactive behavior ceased and hormone levels returned to normal.

There was no indication of azotemia in the affected guinea pigs before the treatment; neither of the guinea pigs diagnosed had elevated blood urea nitrogen (BUN) at the time of diagnosis. Renal problems might not be a common clinical finding in hyperthyroid guinea pigs.

Advantage

In one author's (J.M.) opinion this can be considered the best treatment option for different reasons (**Figs. 6–8**). First, the treatment can achieve long-term control of the disease and, second, it has the potential to be curative. The treatment with I-131 renders all hyperfunctional thyroid tissue, including ectopic tissue, nonfunctional. This treatment is less invasive than surgery, has a higher success rate, and can be given intravenously or subcutaneously. It appears that the dose of 1 miC achieved good clinical results in 2 guinea pigs.

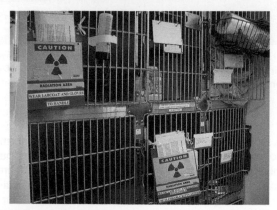

Fig. 6. Cages with signs of radiation after the animal has been injected with radioactive material for either a diagnostic scintigraphy or for treatment with I-131.

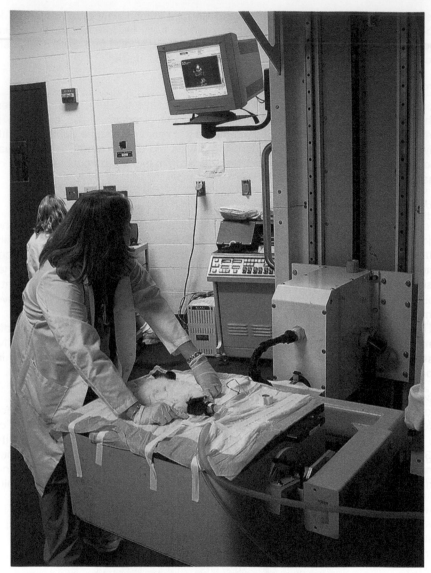

Fig. 7. The anesthetized guinea pig rests on top of the gamma camera for the scintigraphy procedure. Even minimal motion will result in an inaccurate capture of the image details obtained by the gamma camera.

Disadvantage

The patient needs to be brought to a special clinic that can perform this procedure. The clinic needs to be an approved specialty facility with state department of health and Nuclear Regulatory Commission permits for use of I-131. There are few clinics that are allowed to use radioactive materials; in addition, no clinical data on the use of this treatment in guinea pigs are available. Often state approval for individual cases has to be obtained if species other than dogs or cats are being treated. Relapse of the hyperthyroid status is possible. Isolation at the treatment facility for 1 to 7 days after

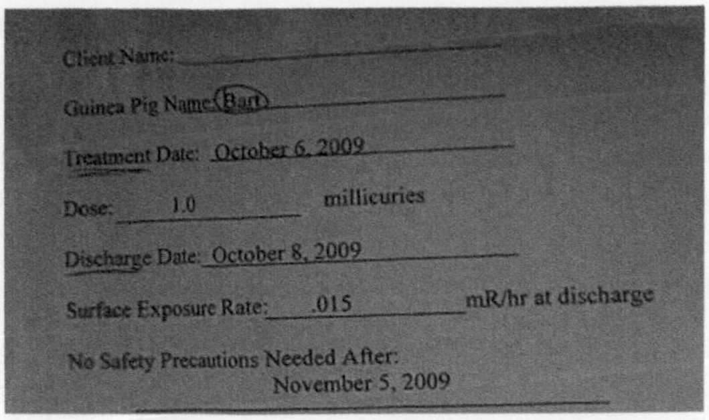

Client Name: _____

Guinea Pig Name: Bart

Treatment Date: October 6, 2009

Dose: _____ 1.0 _____ millicuries

Discharge Date: October 8, 2009

Surface Exposure Rate: ____.015_____ mR/hr at discharge

No Safety Precautions Needed After:
                November 5, 2009

Fig. 8. Treatment sheet of a guinea pig receiving radioactive iodine treatment (I-131). As you can see, the animal was discharged within 48 hours after the treatment but the owner had to collect all waste products of the animal and store it for about 30 days before they can be discharged in the normal trash.

therapy is required, as treated animals will be radioactive. Proper radiation doses for guinea pigs still need to be determined. If the administered dose is too high, there is a risk of causing iatrogenic hypothyroidism in the animal.

RECOMMENDED MONITORING

The monitoring intensity for the treated animal depends on the method of treatment. The least critical side effects are expected with radioactive and medical treatment. The highest risks for complications are associated with surgical treatment. Monitoring the animal after treatment is important to judge and gauge the success of the therapy and to recognize potential complications early on to avoid a fatal outcome. The evaluation of the ionized calcium of postsurgical patients is of utmost importance to ensure that the parathyroid glands were not completely removed during the thyroidectomy.

Medical Therapy

Monitoring for side effects of medication is indicated but the authors have not noticed any significant side effects when using recommend doses. As a general routine for recheck examination, the following parameters should be monitored after medical treatment is started: complete physical examination, blood work, and T4/T3 blood levels at 2 weeks posttreatment. If the patient is normal, reassess the patient 6 months after treatment or earlier if adverse effects or recurrent signs of hyperthyroidism are noted.

Thyroidectomy

In addition to the monitoring mentioned previously for medical management, in a surgical case the blood work should include ionized calcium if a bilateral thyroidectomy was performed. Oral calcium supplementation is needed to avoid an immediate fatal hypocalcaemia. The ionized calcium would need to be checked immediately after surgery and then at 2 weeks after surgery.

Radioactive Iodine Therapy

The recheck should include what is done with medical therapy. Again, the physical examination and patient history are very important. Descriptions of changes in behavior or eating habits should be discussed in great detail.

PROGNOSIS

The prognosis can be good in cases where the problem was diagnosed early and response to treatment is good. In severe cases and in cases where the animal is debilitated, the prognosis is less favorable. Sometimes secondary complications can occur such as secondary pneumonia, or aspiration of food with a ravenous appetite.

HYPOTHYROIDISM IN THE GUINEA PIG

Hypothyroid conditions of the guinea pig appear much less frequently in the clinical setting than hyperthyroidism. The low end of the normal thyroxine level is reported to be 1 µg/dL.[8] If the value falls significantly below this level and the animal shows typical signs of hypothyroidism, a thyroid-stimulating hormone (TSH) stimulation test is indicated.

Typical clinical signs that have been reported are a decrease in activity and increase in body weight. Often these changes are subtle and the gradual onset often goes

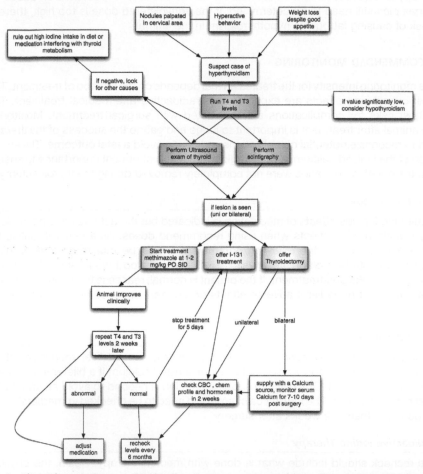

Fig. 9. Algorithm used as a guide for the diagnosis and treatment of hyperthyroidism in an exotic small mammal patient.

unnoticed by the owner. A detailed anamnesis with questions about a change in activity over a longer time period is important. In chronic cases, the clinical presentation can mimic the signs of hyperthyroidism; animals have been reported to lose weight and even lose hair. The alopecic areas are often observed in the dorsal area and the inner thighs. Sometimes bradycardia can also be ausculted.[4]

Diagnosis

One of the authors (R.W.) uses the following routine to diagnose hypothyroidism in the guinea pig: 100 μg of thyrogen, a recombinant human TSH (rhTSH) is given intramuscularly and plasma T4 concentrations are determined before and 4 hours after TSH injection. An increase of at least 1.5 times prestimulation T4 concentrations at 4 hours poststimulation is considered a normal response.

Therapy

If the animal is not presented in the late stage of the disease, medical management can be successful in controlling the condition. Oral L-thyroxine at a dosage of 10 μg/kg once a day can be given.[4] Blood thyroxine levels should be rechecked 2 weeks and then 2 months after the initiation of the therapy.

SUMMARY

Diagnosing hyperthyroidism in nontraditional species is challenging because of multiple factors (**Fig. 9**). Interpretation of thyroid values can be considered to be difficult even in species for which tests have been validated (eg, dog and cats). In cats with early or mild forms of hyperthyroidism, the serum thyroid levels might fall well within described normal reference values. In addition, the presence of a concurrent secondary problem might lower the T4 value back into the reference value in a true hyperthyroid patient.[25] Because of these common problems, it has been suggested to perform a "free" T4 test or a TSH stimulation test, as these assays are considered more sensitive for the diagnosis of early stages of hyperthyroidism.[26] Another more reliable method to diagnose functional pathologies of the thyroid gland is nuclear medicine. For a more detailed discussion on how to perform and evaluate scintigraphy of suspect cases please see Mayer and colleagues.[15]

It appears that functional (clinical) hyperthyroidism truly exists in the guinea pig population. Although no clear pattern about the sex predilection can be seen in the examined cases here, it is interesting to note that in human medicine it is known that differences exist between the activity of the thyroid gland of males and females. A greater tendency to thyroid hypertrophy exists in the female.[27,28] It has been discovered that a parallelism exists between the anatomic characteristics of the thyroid gland and the intensity of its metabolic activities and production of hormone. In the female guinea pig during the sexual cycle, the number of mitoses in the thyroid gland is therefore about 3 times higher than in the male. In human medicine, this would correspond to the predilection of hyperthyroidism in females.[27] In addition, it is mentioned that there is a female sex-linkage of mixed thyroid tumors in humans and canines.[2] It is speculative if this also applies to the guinea pig.

REFERENCES

1. Mosinger M. Sur la carcinoresistance du cobaye. Premiere partie. Les tumeurs spontanees du cobaye. Bulletin de l'Association Francaise pour l'etude du Cancer 1961;48:217 [in French].

2. Zarrin K. Thyroid carcinoma of a guinea pig: a case report. Lab Anim 1974;8(2): 145–8.

3. Gibbons P, Garner M. Pathological aspects of thyroid tumors in guinea pigs. Proceedings of the AEMV Milwaukee (WI): 2009. Page 81.

4. Ewringmann A, Glöckner B. Leitsymptome bei Meerschweinchen, Chinchilla und Degu. Diagnostischer Leitfaden und Therapie. 1st edition. Stuttgart/Germany: Enke publishing; 2005. October 2005.

5. Percy DH, Barthold SW. Pathology of laboratory rodents and rabbits. 3rd edition. Ames (IA): Blackwell Publishing Professional; 2007.

6. Taeymans O, Peremans K, Saunders JH. Thyroid imaging in the dog: current status and future directions. J Vet Intern Med 2007;21:673–84.

7. Gibbons P, Garner M. Tumors of the thyroid gland in guinea pigs (Cavia porcellus). Manuscript in preparation 2009.

8. Müller K, Müller E, Klein R, et al. Serum thyroxine concentrations in clinically healthy pet guinea pigs (*Cavia porcellus*). Vet Clin Pathol 2009;38(4):507–10.

9. Kintzer PP, Peterson ME. Nuclear medicine of the thyroid gland. Scintigraphy and radioiodine therapy. Vet Clin North Am Small Anim Pract 1994;24:587–605.

10. Marks SL, Koblik PD, Hornof WJ, et al. 99mTc-pertechnetate imaging of thyroid tumors in dogs: 29 cases (1980–1992). J Am Vet Med Assoc 1994;204:756–60.

11. Daniel GB, Brawner WR. Thyroid scintigraphy. In: Daniel GB, Berry CR, editors. Textbook of veterinary nuclear medicine. North Carolina (NC): American College of Veterinary Radiology; 2006. p. 181–98.

12. Adams WH, Daniel GB, Petersen MG, et al. Quantitative ^{99m}Tc-pertechnetate thyroid scintigraphy in normal beagles. Vet Radiol Ultrasound 1997;38:323–8.

13. Ferguson DC. Update on diagnosis of canine hypothyroidism. Vet Clin North Am Small Anim Pract 1994;24:515–39.

14. Catherine J, Scott-Moncrieff R, Guptill-Yoran L. Endocrine disorders. Hypothyroidism. In: Ettinger SJ, Feldman EC, editors. Textbook of veterinary internal medicine. St. Louis (MO): Elsevier-Saunders; 2005. p. 1535–43.

15. Mayer J, Hunt K, Eshar D, et al. Thyroid scintigraphy in a guinea pig with suspected hyperthyroidism. Exotic DVM 2009;11(1).

16. Popesko P, Rajtova V. A colour atlas of anatomy small laboratory animals: 2. Bratislava, Mosby: Elsevier; July 1, 1992.

17. Taeymans O, Schwarz T, Duchateau L, et al. Computed tomographic features of the normal canine thyroid gland. Vet Radiol Ultrasound 2008;49:13–9.

18. Benker G, Reinwein D. Pharmacokinetics of antithyroid drugs. Klin Wochenschr 1982;60:531–9.

19. Kasraee B. Depigmentation of brown guinea pig skin by topical application of methimazole. J Invest Dermatol 2002;118(1):205–7.

20. Kasraee B, Handjani F, Parhizgar A, et al. Topical methimazole as a new treatment for postinflammatory hyperpigmentation: report of the first case. Dermatology 2005;211(4):360–2.

21. Plumb DC. Plumb's veterinary drug handbook. 5th edition. Ames (IA): Wiley-Blackwell; 2005.

22. Kromka MC, Hoar RM. An improved technique for thyroidectomy in guinea pigs. Lab Anim Sci 1975;25(1):82–4.

23. Moltke E, Lorenzen I. Effect of thyroidectomy and thyroxine on the mucopolysaccharides of wounds and skin. Acta Endocrinol 1960;34:407–10.

24. Goldstein RE, Long C, Swift NC, et al. Percutaneous ethanol injection for treatment of unilateral hyperplastic thyroid nodules in cats. J Am Vet Med Assoc 2001;218(8):1298–302.

25. Peterson ME, Gamble DA. Effect of nonthyroidal illness on serum thyroxine concentrations in cats: 494 cases. J Am Vet Med Assoc 1990;197(9):1203–8.
26. Peterson ME, Melian C, Nichols R. Measurement of serum concentrations of free thyroxine, total thyroxine, and total triiodothyronine in cats with hyperthyroidism and cats with nonthyroidal disease. J Am Vet Med Assoc 2001;218(4):529–36.
27. Chouke KS, Friedman H, Loeb L. Proliferative activity of the thyroid gland of the female guinea pig during the sexual cycle. The Anatomical Record 2005;63(2):131–7.
28. Castro MI, Alex S, Young RA, et al. Total and free serum thyroid hormone concentrations in fetal and adult pregnant and nonpregnant guinea pigs. Endocrinology 1986;118(2):533–7.

Updates and Advanced Therapies for Gastrointestinal Stasis in Rabbits

Marla Lichtenberger, DVM, DACVECC[a],*,
Angela Lennox, DVM, DABVP (Avian)[b]

KEYWORDS

- Rabbit • Gastric stasis • Fluid therapy

UNDERSTANDING GASTROINTESTINAL STASIS IN RABBITS

Gastrointestinal stasis is currently a vaguely defined term for decreased gastrointestinal motility. The term gastric stasis syndrome was previously proposed,[1] but falls short of an accurate description, as in many cases portions of the gastrointestinal tract other than the stomach are affected. Capello has recently proposed the term rabbit gastrointestinal syndrome (RGIS) to define a complex of clinical signs, symptoms, and concurrent pathologic conditions affecting the digestive apparatus of the rabbit. The following pathologic conditions can be included, and often occur in combination:

Gastric impaction
Gastric gas accumulation
Intestinal impaction
Intestinal gas accumulation
Intestinal obstruction
Primary gastroenteritis
Adhesions
Neoplasia
Pancreatitis
Liver disease (hepatic lipidosis, torsion, cholangiohepatitis).

In many cases, underlying cause of RGIS is uncertain. Symptoms may be secondary to any disease producing alterations in fluid balance (dehydration/shock) and/or alterations in gastrointestinal motility. Lichtenberger has recognized RGIS associated with nonspecific hepatitis and pancreatitis confirmed histopathologically,

---

[a] Milwaukee Emergency Clinic for Animals, 4670 South 108th Street, Greenfield, WI 53228, USA
[b] Avian and Exotic Animal Clinic, 9330 Waldemar Road, Indianapolis, IN 46268, USA
* Corresponding author.
E-mail address: MarlaL@erforanimals.com

Vet Clin Exot Anim 13 (2010) 525–541
doi:10.1016/j.cvex.2010.05.008
1094-9194/10/$ – see front matter © 2010 Elsevier Inc. All rights reserved.

and in some cases suspected at ultrasound. It should also be noted that psychogenic stress is well defined in terms of negative impact on gastrointestinal motility.[2]

Impaction can be produced by overaccumulation of normal gastrointestinal contents due to alterations in motility, or desiccation of normal contents due to dehydration. Impaction of various portions of the gastrointestinal tract with foreign material has also been reported.[3]

In terms of gastrointestinal obstruction, it is noteworthy that true gastric (pyloric) obstruction is uncommonly reported in clinical practice. However, a 2006 study of postmortem findings in Angora rabbits reported a death rate of 28.6% over a 5-year period, which the investigators attributed to the presence of a large, firm trichobezoar in the pyloric region of the stomach.[4] Most cases of true obstruction in pet rabbits are reported to occur in the proximal duodenum, or the ileocecolic junction.[5] Other sites of lower gastrointestinal obstruction have been described as well, including cases of multiple obstructions (Capello, personal communication, December 2009) The most commonly reported cause of obstruction is tightly packed hair; other less commonly mentioned objects include carpet fibers and locust bean seeds.[5] Harcourt-Brown[5] has also described intestinal obstruction secondary to herniation, and tapeworm cysts. In all cases, obstruction can be complete or partial; in many cases absolute diagnosis is difficult.

Malnutrition and alterations in diet are often implicated in cases of RGIS and include low-fiber diets, excess carbohydrates, and rapid diet change.[1] The fiber requirements of rabbits are well described. Increased carbohydrate consumption can produce disruption of motility, leading to alterations in the cecal pH and disruption of the complex bacterial flora of the hindgut.[1]

Primary gastroenteritis (bacterial, viral, parasitic) is uncommon, and full discussion is beyond the scope of this article.

Clinical symptoms of RGIS vary in severity and can include depression, reluctance to move, teeth grinding, abnormal posture suggestive of abdominal discomfort, reduced food intake to anorexia, reduced to absent stool production or abnormal stool character, and presence of excessive or uneaten cecotrophs.

Physical examination findings in cases of RGIS can be unremarkable but also can include fluid imbalances (dehydration, shock), abdominal distention, including gastric and intestinal distension, and gastric tympany. Other symptoms may be related to ongoing underlying conditions. Severely ill rabbits in hypovolemic shock are often hypothermic, with pale mucus membranes and decreased capillary refill time, and altered mentation (depressed to comatose). Indirect blood pressure is low or unobtainable.[6]

When ill rabbits present for examination it is important to determine if RGIS is present and if so, begin treatment and a diagnostic workup to determine underlying contributing factors. Identification of underlying cause is often difficult; the authors and others have encountered many rabbits presenting with evidence of RGIS whereby attempts to identify an underlying cause are unfruitful. In many cases, these patients respond positively to supportive therapy including fluids, hand feeding, and motility-enhancing drugs.

INITIAL PRESENTATION AND EVALUATION: DECISION-MAKING

All ill rabbits are evaluated as quickly as possible.

Decision 1

Can this rabbit tolerate manual restraint, evaluation, and treatment?
Most pet rabbits tolerate handling well. However, in some severely ill or stressed patients, handling and treatment may worsen clinical condition. Delay of treatment

carries risk as well. For these cases, the authors highly recommend sedation.[7] Sedation is an underutilized option for ill rabbits. Benefits are multiple and include reduction of anxiety and stress, as well as relief of pain. Relief of pain is of particular benefit, as many diseases of rabbits produce discomfort to at least some degree. The authors recommend midazolam (Baxter Healthcare Corp, Deerfield, IL, USA) in combination with an opioid analgesic.

Midazolam At sedation doses, this drug has a wide margin of safety in humans and many species, and clinical experience has revealed the same in rabbits. Dosages are reduced further when combined with an opioid, and when used in ill or debilitated patients.[8] Dosages are listed in **Table 1**.

Opioids At lower doses, these drugs are generally safe in many species, and are reversible. Butorphanol (Dolorex; Intervet, Millboro, DE, USA), buprenorphine (Buprenex; Reckitt Benckiser, Richmond, VA, USA), and others are commonly used by the authors and others as analgesics for rabbits.[9] For ill rabbits, select shorter-acting drugs with a lower dose range and combine with midazolam.

There is considerable debate over the use of opioids in rabbits with decreased gastrointestinal motility, as these drugs can produce dose-dependent reduction of motility in humans and other species.[10] As most gastrointestinal disease is painful, and pain and distress are potent depressors of gastrointestinal motility, the authors and others believe that the use of opioids are fully justified when used with appropriate measures to support the gastrointestinal tract (eg, fluids and motility-enhancing drugs).

Table 1
Drugs mentioned in this article for use in treatment of rabbits with suspected gastrointestinal disease

Drug	Dosage	Comments
Midazolam	0.25–0.25 mg/kg IV, IM, SC	For sedation; use lower dosages in ill rabbits; synergistic when combined with an opioid
Butorphanol	0.20–0.4 mg/kg IM	For analgesia, and sedation when combined with midazolam
Hydromorphone	0.10 mg/kg IM	For more severe pain; use in combination with midazolam for added sedation
Cisapride	0.5 mg/kg every 8 h PO	Oral solution available through compounding pharmacies
Ranitidine	0.5 mg/kg every 24 h IV or SC	May be synergistic with cisapride
Trimebutine		Motility regulator Not available in the USA but may be legally imported by veterinarians for personal use
Fentanyl/ketamine constant rate infusion	Fentanyl = 5–10 µg/kg/min + ketamine = 1–2 mg/kg/h	Added to crystalloid fluids at rates appropriate for correction of fluid deficits and/or maintenance. Drugs are added to fluids or placed in a syringe pump to provide hourly dosage

Dosages/rates for fluid support are given in the text.

Thorough physical examination should proceed carefully, with attention to changes in condition.

Decision 2

What type of fluid support is indicated?

As gastrointestinal motility is affected by patient hydration, and RGIS negatively impacts hydration, all patients with signs or symptoms suggestive of RGIS should receive fluids.[11]

Guidelines for fluid type and rate determination are presented in the section on fluid administration. In general, subcutaneous fluids are only appropriate for those stable patients with normal hydration to mild dehydration.[6] Oral fluid replacement is only appropriate when obstruction is unlikely and the gastrointestinal tract is judged to be functional. Replacement needs are calculated as described below, and administered in subcutaneous boluses, or per os as applicable. Moderately dehydrated rabbits, or those showing evidence of shock require direct vascular support.[6] Options include intravenous (cephalic, lateral saphenous, auricular vessels) or intraosseous access (femur, tibia).[12] Although intraosseous access is not technically considered direct vascular access, functionally it is equivalent to intravenous access.[13]

Placement of an intravenous catheter is straightforward and is greatly facilitated by sedation, as described above, with topical anesthesia of the venipuncture site. Topical anesthesia helps to reduce sudden pullback of the limb at the moment of skin penetration. The site is prepared and lidocaine gel applied to the skin. After 5 to 10 minutes roll the skin away from the vein and inject lidocaine into the dermis and subcutis. It is important to wait an additional 5 to 10 minutes to allow the drug to take effect. Choose a 24- to 25-gauge catheter. Note that intact male rabbits often have particularly tough skin that complicates catheterization. For these patients, gently roll the skin away from the catheter site as described for local infusion of lidocaine, and puncture with a 22-gauge needle; allow the skin to roll back into position over the vein and introduce the catheter via the puncture site. Intraosseous catheterization is an option when intravenous access (standard or cut-down technique) is impossible. The site of entry is prepared, and the bone cavity entered with a spinal needle of larger injection gauge, 22 to 18. The catheter is secured with tape and fitted with an injection port. Placement is facilitated with sedation and local analgesia, in the form of topical lidocaine, and lidocaine injected under the skin and into the periosteum at the entry site.[13]

Decision 3

When should diagnostic workup proceed?

In the stable patient, diagnostic workup can proceed when practical. The authors have found that ill, sedated patients often tolerate diagnostic imaging and venipuncture for diagnostic sampling without additional anesthesia, which should be avoided. In many cases, workup can proceed immediately after catheterization. For those patients where clinical judgment indicates struggling and resistance to handling may carry increased risk, but speedy diagnostic workup is indicated, consider a slight increase in dosage of midazolam/opioid, or the addition of very low dose ketamine (see **Table 1**), or low concentration (2%–3%) isoflurane delivered via face mask.

Decision 4

Can this patient be managed medically or will surgical intervention be required?

Due to frequent uncertainties in exact underlying diagnoses, and complications related to complex gastrointestinal anatomy and physiology, determination of prognosis and selection of ideal therapy can be difficult. As mentioned earlier, all rabbits with evidence of gastrointestinal disease should receive fluids. Whereas some patients present strongly suggesting the presence of gastrointestinal obstruction or other condition requiring surgical intervention, many presentations are far less certain. In these cases, decision-making relies on response to medical therapy, with progress determined by changes in physical condition and as demonstrated radiographically (see later discussion).

While surgical intervention is generally reported as associated with poor overall prognosis,[11] some investigators have suggested that earlier surgical intervention may improve survival. In an article examining outcomes in 76 cases of gastric dilation and intestinal obstruction, survival rate for rabbits with evidence of intestinal obstruction (dilated stomach, suggestive radiographic findings) undergoing exploratory surgery was 40%.[5]

DIAGNOSTIC WORKUP FOR RABBITS WITH RGIS
Radiography

Radiography remains the single most important diagnostic test for evaluation of the gastrointestinal tract of the rabbit and for monitoring response to therapy.[3] Lichtenberger has found ultrasonographic evidence of hepatitis and pancreatitis in some rabbits with RGIS. In theory, ultrasound may be helpful in identification of obstructions; however, gas accumulation may reduce its value. Blood work is important to help identify underlying abnormalities (anemia, hypoproteinemia) and disease conditions (renal disease), but is nonspecific for gastrointestinal disease.

Radiographs are important for evaluation of location, size, shape and, to some extent, contents of the gastrointestinal tract.[3,5,11] Abdominal radiographs of the normal rabbit are somewhat variable and depend on the current phase of digestion. The stomach is oval-shaped and located caudal to the liver, mostly on the left quadrant. The caudal border does not extend beyond the last rib. There is always some ingesta in the partially filled stomach that is evenly mixed with fine pockets of gas. On the ventrodorsal projection the stomach shape is asymmetric, with the largest curvature on the left side. The stomach is relatively small compared with the rest of the gastrointestinal tract.[3]

The small intestine contains digesta as well, and gas is evenly dispersed. The cecum may be partially to completely filled. When full, the cecum occupies the majority of the abdomen. The distal colon may contain fecal material that takes on the characteristic shape of hard fecal pellets (**Fig. 1**).

Abnormal findings include larger pockets of gas anywhere throughout the gastrointestinal tract, from stomach to colon.[3] An abnormal stomach may begin to take on a more filled to round shape as contents accumulate. There may be impaction of the stomach with accumulation of intestinal gas, or gas accumulation in both stomach and intestine (**Figs. 2 and 3**). The cecum may be impacted, or distended with gas. Rabbits with partial to complete intestinal obstruction may demonstrate typical radiographic findings, including rounded fluid and gas-filled stomach with a gas pattern ending abruptly in the proximal duodenum, or elsewhere. The authors have observed cases of obstruction with gas present both proximal and distal to the site of obstruction, likely a result of obstructive accumulation of gas, and accumulation due to secondary functional ileus. In cases of ingestion of foreign material, radiodense material may appear anywhere along the gastrointestinal tract.

Capello and Lennox describe "gastric repletion," a potentially pathogenic condition of rabbits adapted to inappropriate, low-fiber diets. The stomach appears overfull on radiographs, but there is no abnormal gas, and rabbits in general do not present with

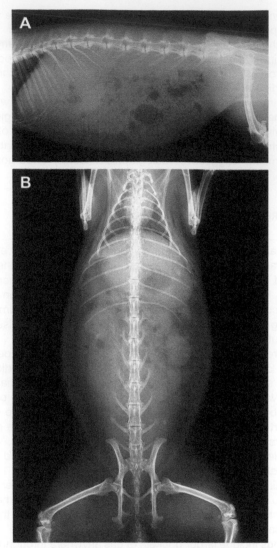

Fig. 1. Lateral (*A*) and ventrodorsal (*B*) radiographs of the abdomen of a normal 1.4-kg intact female rabbit. (*Reprinted from* Capello V, Lennox AM. Clinical radiology of exotic companion mammals. Ames (IA): Wiley-Blackwell; 2008. p. 88–9; with permission.)

symptoms of gastrointestinal disease (**Fig. 4**). The condition is likely related to inadequate dietary fiber. In cases of gastric repletion, the stomach appears overfilled, and extends caudal to the most distal rib. These rabbits are likely at risk for eventual development of gastrointestinal disease.[3]

Radiography is always interpreted along with changes in clinical condition of the patient. Serial radiography is of critical importance for helping to determine response to therapy and changes in therapy (**Boxes 1** and **2**; **Fig. 5**; **Tables 2** and **3**). Radiographs are repeated every 3 to 4 hours in critical patients with evidence of obstructive disease, to as long as every 24 hours in more stable, less severe patients.

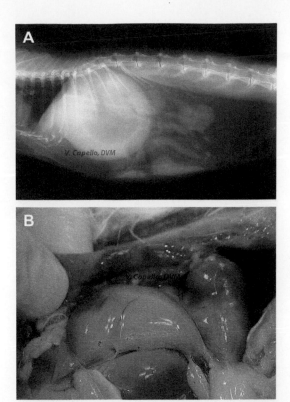

Fig. 2. Lateral radiograph (*A*) and necropsy specimen (*B*) of a rabbit with a duodenal obstruction due to a trichobezoar. Note the overfilled, round stomach with absence of gastrointestinal contents elsewhere along the tract.

Contrast radiography is not commonly described in rabbits, but may be useful, especially in cases of suspected partial or complete obstruction.

Other Diagnostic Testing

Other diagnostic tests (hematology, clinical chemistries, urinalysis) are nonspecific for RGIS or primary gastrointestinal disease, but are useful for evaluation of overall patient condition and as an aid to rule out other underlying conditions.

FLUID ADMINISTRATION FOR RABBITS WITH RGIS

A fluid therapy plan involves the type, quantity, and rate of fluid to be administered. The primary goal is to give the least amount of fluids possible to reach the desired end points of resuscitation. The general principles of fluid administration, including fluid type and rate of administration, are well established in traditional pet species; the authors and others have found these principles practical and efficacious in rabbits as well.

There are 3 phases for fluid resuscitation: correction of perfusion deficits, rehydration, and maintenance.[6,14,15] Fluids used include isotonic crystalloids, colloids, and blood products.[15–17] Isotonic crystalloids (lactated Ringer solution and others) are often used together with colloids in the resuscitation phase.[14,15] Hetastarch (Hospira Inc, Lake Forest, IL, USA) is the most commonly used colloid due to cost and

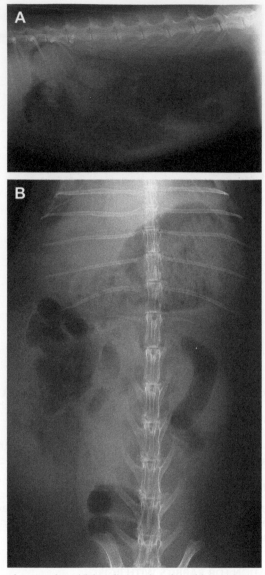

Fig. 3. Lateral (*A*) and ventrodorsal (*B*) radiographs of a rabbit with gastrointestinal stasis as evidenced by gas accumulation throughout the gastrointestinal tract. This rabbit responded well to 24 hours of supportive care, including fluids, hand feeding, analgesia, and motility-enhancing drugs.

availability. Oxyglobin (OPK Biotech, Cambridge, MA, USA) is a colloid with the added advantage of oxygen-carrying ability.

Treatment of Hypovolemic Shock in the Rabbit

Characteristics of hypovolemic shock in the rabbit

According to Lichtenberger, rabbits with hypovolemia commonly present in the decompensatory stage of shock, similar to that commonly seen in the cat

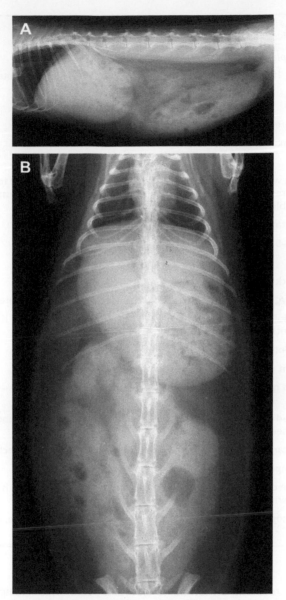

Fig. 4. Lateral (*A*) and ventrodorsal (*B*) radiographs of a rabbit with gastric repletion, or overfilling of the gastrointestinal tract without other evidence of gastrointestinal disease. This finding is common in rabbits on inappropriate diets. In most cases, rabbits are clinically normal but may be at risk for developing gastrointestinal disease in the future. *Reprinted from* Capello V, Lennox AM. Clinical radiology of exotic companion mammals. Ames (IA): Wiley-Blackwell; 2008. p. 106; with permission.

(see **Box 1**). The earlier compensatory stages of shock commonly observed in the dog and bird are generally not seen in rabbits. This difference may be partially explained by the response of rabbit baroreceptors to inadequate arterial stretch in the shock state: sympathetic fiber stimulation occurs concurrently with vagal

---

Box 1
Correction of perfusion deficits adapted for the rabbit

Decompensatory phase of shock (Bradycardia, hypotension, hypothermia)

- Slow bolus over 10 minutes of hypertonic saline 7.2%/7.5% (3 mL/kg) + Hetastarch (3 mL/kg) IV or IO

↓

- External and core body temperature warming over 1–2 h
- Crystalloids at maintenance (3–4 mL/kg/h)

↓

- When patient is warmed to 98°F (36.7°C), use slow IV/IO fluids (see below) to correct indirect systolic blood pressure to >90 mm Hg (after each bolus recheck blood pressure-repeat bolus 3–4 times until blood pressure is normal)

  Crystalloids (lactated Ringer solution, normosol, Plasmalyte) at 15 mL/kg

  Hetastarch at 3–5 mL/kg

↓

Unresponsive shock to above protocol:

- Consider oxyglobin at 2 mL/kg slow bolus, and if systolic blood pressure is >90 mm Hg:

  Start crystalloid constant rate infusion (CRI) to correct dehydration or if not dehydrated then at maintenance (3–4 mL/kg/h)

  Start oxyglobin CRI at 0.2 mL/kg/h

- If the patient continues to be unresponsive:

  Check blood glucose, blood urea nitrogen, acid base, and electrolytes—correct if abnormal

  Check packed cell volume (PCV) and total protein; consider whole blood transfusion if PCV is <20 (see blood transfusion in text)

  Check echocardiogram for abnormal heart function and correct contractility if abnormal

  Recheck temperature of patient and warm again if hypothermic

- If the patient continues to be unresponsive and systolic blood pressure is <90 mm Hg (but patient is normothermic):

  Consider vasopressors in the doses recommended for small animals (ie, norepinephrine, dopamine)

---

fiber stimulation, resulting in normal to slow heart rate. This finding contrasts with those in dogs under similar conditions whereby fiber stimulation results in tachycardia.[14,15]

Many rabbits with clinical evidence of shock demonstrate bradycardia (<180 beats/min), hypotension (systolic blood pressure <90 mm Hg), and hypothermia (temperature lower than 97°F [36.1°C]).

Treatment of hypovolemic shock

Earlier recommendations for the treatment of hypovolemic shock included rapid administration of crystalloids administered in volumes equivalent to several times the patient's blood volume. However, rapid resuscitation with crystalloids alone can result in significant pulmonary and pleural fluid accumulation. Newer

Box 2
Estimation of dehydration deficits and calculation of fluid replacement needs for the rabbit

Estimation of percentage dehydration:

>10% = dry mucous membranes, suction eyes, altered mentation, very significant skin tenting

7%–9% = dry mucous membranes, skin tenting

5%–7% = dry mucous membranes and mild skin tenting

4%–5% = dry mucous membrane

Fluid requirements of dehydration deficits calculation:

%dehydration × kg × 1000 mL/L = fluid deficit (L)

This amount is added to maintenance requirements (3–4 mL/kg/h) + any losses (ie, diarrhea)

Replacement over how many hours based on how fast the losses occurred:

Losses occurred in <24 h = acute so replace dehydration deficit over 6–8 h

Losses occurred over 24–72 h = chronic, so replace over 24 h

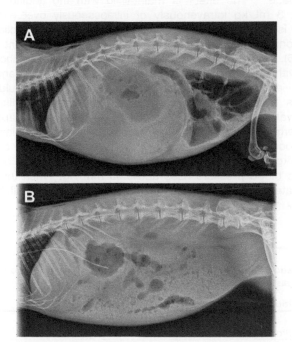

Fig. 5. Changes in clinical condition, and changes noted radiographically are used to determine response to therapy, and determine if changes in therapy are indicated. In this case, foreign body obstruction was listed in the differential diagnosis based on extreme distention of the stomach (*A*). However, radiographs taken after 12 hours of intensive supportive measures, including intravenous fluid therapy, indicated medical management was effective (*B*). This rabbit was discharged 24 hours later. Note the presence of a nasogastric tube for support feeding in (*B*).

Table 2 Radiographic findings associated with improving or declining condition in rabbits with suspected gastrointestinal disease	
Improving Condition	**Declining Condition**
Reduction of the size of individual gas accumulations	Increasing gas accumulations
Changes in gas accumulation pattern-gas has moved or appears to have "broken up"	Specific areas of gas accumulation unchanged
Presence of formed stool in the distal colon	
Decrease rounded appearance of the stomach	Stomach size increasing, shape more rounded

Findings must be interpreted in conjunction with changes in the patient's overall clinical condition.

recommendations include a combination of crystalloids, colloids, and rewarming procedures.[14,15]

Begin with a bolus infusion of 7.2%–7.5% hypertonic saline (3 mL/kg as a slow bolus over 10 minutes) to rapidly draw fluid from body compartments into the intravascular space.[16] The effect is maintained with the addition of Hetastarch administered at 3 mL/kg intravenously or intraosseously over 5 to 10 minutes. Blood pressure is monitored; once it is above 40 mm Hg systolic, maintenance volumes of isotonic crystalloids are administered, while the patient is aggressively warmed (**Fig. 6**). Warming and restoration of normothermia should ideally be accomplished within 1 to 2 hours using both external techniques and core temperature warming via administration of warm intravenous fluids. Fluids are warmed with intravenous fluid warmers or by running the intravenous fluid line through a pan of hot water. In many cases, once rectal temperature approaches 98°F (36.6°C), adrenergic receptors can begin to respond to catecholamines and fluid therapy, and blood pressure will increase. At this point, boluses of isotonic crystalloids (10 mL/kg) with Hetastarch (5 mL/kg) can be repeated over 15 minutes until the systolic blood pressure rises above 90 mm Hg. When the systolic blood pressure is greater than 90 mm Hg, the rehydration phase of fluid resuscitation begins (see **Box 1**).

Table 3 Physical examination findings associated with improving or declining condition in rabbits with suspected gastrointestinal disease	
Improving Condition	**Declining Condition**
Eating on own Taking hand feeding well	Not eating on own Refusing hand feeding
Appearance of formed stool	Decreasing to absent stool
Resolution of fluid deficits (hypovolemia, dehydration)	No resolution of fluid deficits
Normal posture, grooming activities noted	Continued abnormal, painful posture
Reduction in gas accumulation as detected via palpation or percussion	Gas accumulation as detected via palpation or percussion increasing or unchanged

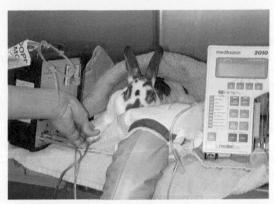

Fig. 6. Indirect Doppler blood pressure can be used to help guide fluid resuscitation for hypovolemic shock in the rabbit. The blood pressure is assessed on the forelimb. Fluids are given until the indirect systolic blood pressure is greater than 90 mm Hg.

Treatment of nonresponsive shock

If end-point parameters (normal blood pressure, heart rate, mucous membrane color, and capillary refill time) are still not obtained after 3 to 4 boluses of Hetastarch and crystalloids, the patient is evaluated and treated for causes of nonresponsive shock (ie, excessive vasodilation or vasoconstriction, anemia, hypoglycemia, electrolyte imbalances, acid-base disorder, cardiac dysfunction, hypoxemia).[14,15]

If PCV suggests marked anemia (<20%), consider whole blood transfusion. Alternatively, administer oxyglobin, at 2 mL/kg boluses over 10 to 15 minutes until restoration of normal heart rate and blood pressure (systolic blood pressure >90 mm Hg); this can be followed by a CRI of oxyglobin at 0.2 to 0.4 mL/kg/h.

Hypoglycemia is treated with an initial bolus of 50% dextrose at 0.25 mL/kg as a 1:1 dilution with saline. Parenteral use of dextrose should be conservative, as it may induce compartmental shifts in electrolytes and water, which could ultimately lead to further hypovolemia. Blood glucose is determined 1 hour later. If hypoglycemia persists, continue CRI of low-concentration dextrose, for example, 1.25% dextrose in crystalloids, while rechecking blood glucose every 2 to 3 hours.

SPECIFIC THERAPY FOR TREATMENT OF DEHYDRATION AND CALCULATION OF MAINTENANCE FLUIDS

The percentage of dehydration can be subjectively estimated based on body weight, mucous membrane dryness, decreased skin turgor, sunken eyes, and altered mentation (see **Box 2**).[6,14] As mentioned above, dehydration deficits greater than 5% ideally require intravenous fluid replacement using a constant-rate infusion of a crystalloid fluid. Fluid requirements for dehydration are calculated as:

% dehydration × kg × 1000 mL/L = fluid deficit (L)

Dehydration requirements should be added to fluids volumes for daily maintenance requirements (3–4 mL/kg/h) and ongoing losses, for example, diarrhea and polyurea. If fluid losses occurred in the last 12 to 24 hours (acute loss), then dehydration deficits are ideally replaced over 6 to 8 hours. If losses occurred over 24 to 72 hours, then dehydration deficits are replaced over 24 hours.[6,14–16]

Whereas urinary catheterization of companion mammals is often used as an objective measurement of urinary output, this is not usually practical in rabbits. Alternatively, urine output can be subjectively evaluated by periodically comparing the weight of absorbent bedding.

Another objective way to assess whether the fluid volume is adequate is to evaluate body weight regularly throughout the day, as acute weight loss is commonly associated with fluid loss.

If the patient is hypoproteinemic, administer a constant rate infusion (CRI) of Hetastarch at 0.8 mL/kg/h during the rehydration phase, combined with crystalloids at rehydration rates. The addition of Hetastarch helps maintain oncotic pressures in the intravascular space during rehydration therapy.[14–16]

Hydration status should be reevaluated frequently and rates readjusted accordingly. Maintenance fluids are provided until the patient is able to assimilate adequate fluids via eating and drinking.

Nutritional Support

Provision of nutrition should proceed as quickly as possible, and is important for prevention and/or treatment of RGIS.[11] Contraindications of enteral support include suspected partial or complete intestinal obstruction, or stasis whereby the stomach is already full. It must be kept in mind that fluid therapy plays an important role, as the gastrointestinal tract must be hydrated to facilitate motility and function.

In general, rabbits tolerate hand feeding via syringe extremely well. The feeding syringe is placed into the diastema, which is the large space between the incisors and premolars. Syringe feeding must be performed slowly with small volumes to prevent aspiration.

The most suitable enteral diets for syringe feeding in rabbits have a high percentage of nondigestable fiber, low fat, and relatively low carbohydrates. Herbivore enteral diets are commercially available from Oxbow Pet Products (www.oxbowhay.com). The Oxbow products have been specifically formulated for nutritional support of herbivorous small mammals and rodents. The kcal is given on a dry matter basis, with 2.69 kcal per gram of dry weight of the powder. When mixed as directed, Critical Care Enteral powder:water 1:1.5 v/v provides approximately 1.9 kcal/mL.

When syringe feeding is refused or inadequate, and feeding is determined to be appropriate based on patient condition, feeding via nasogastric tube should be considered. Two diets have been designed for use with a nasogastric tube: Critical Care (Oxbow Fine Grind Critical Care) and Emeraid Herbivore Elemental Diet (Lafeber, Chicago, IL, USA). These diets should be fed as recommended by the manufacturer. For placement of the nasogastric tube, use a 3.5F to 8F Argyle tube (Surgivet, Waukesha, WI, USA). Length necessary to reach the stomach is determined by measuring from the tip of the nose to the last rib (see **Fig. 7**). To decrease the risk of esophageal perforation, a stylet should never be used. A local anesthetic (2% lidocaine gel) is placed into the rabbit's nostril. The rabbit must be properly restrained while protecting its back, and the head is ventrally flexed but with the neck straight (to avoid compression of the trachea) by an assistant (see **Fig. 8**). The tube is passed ventrally and medially into the ventral nasal meatus. The end of the tube is advanced until it reaches the stomach. The tube is sutured to the nasal area and on the forehead, between the eyes. The remainder of the tube end is taped around the neck (**Fig. 9**). Verification of placement is determined with a radiograph and/or by aspiration of gastric contents

Regardless of the level of nutritional support selected, food should be available at all times for voluntary consumption. In some cases it is helpful to provide the rabbit with its customary diet served in a familiar bowl. Offering fresh grass, greens, or hay may stimulate appetite.

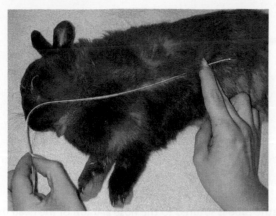

Fig. 7. Nasogastric tubes are placed in rabbits for enteral feeding. The length of tube required is determined by measuring to the last rib of the rabbit.

Promotility Medications and Analgesia

Prokinetics are used frequently, and both scientific and anecdotal reports indicate that these drugs help promote gastrointestinal motility in rabbits.[17,18] Drugs most commonly mentioned include metoclopramide (Baxter Healthcare Corp, Deerfield, IL, USA) and cisapride, or cisapride-like drugs, which are preferred by the authors.

Oral cisapride in rabbits is absorbed rapidly from the gastrointestinal tract, with a plasma half-life similar to that in dogs.[18] Other data show that cisapride may modify the contractile responses of the isolated rabbit intestine to ranitidine, having a potentiating effect up to a certain concentration. The conclusion is that coadministration of the 2 drugs may lead to enhanced motility.[18]

Timebutine is a motility-regulating drug for humans that has been anecdotally reported as extremely useful for use in rabbits with RGIS. There is limited scientific information available on the effects of trimebutine in rabbits.[19] Timebutine is not currently available in the United States, but may be legally imported by veterinarians

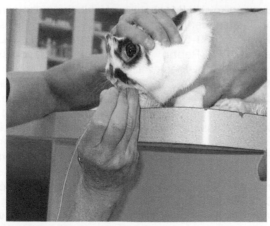

Fig. 8. The nasogastric tube is lubricated with lidocaine gel and placed into the nose of the rabbit. The head is flexed slightly, and the tube passed into the ventral nasal cavity, then advanced to the stomach.

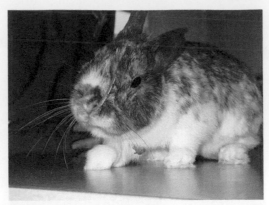

Fig. 9. The nasogastric tube is sutured to the nose and top of the head (between the eyes). The remainder of the tube can be coiled and taped around the neck.

in small quantities for personal use. Oral formulations are available in Canada and parts of Europe; an injectable form is available in Italy. Motility-enhancing drugs are contraindicated in cases of suspected gastrointestinal obstruction.[20]

Analgesia is important for rabbits with RGIS. Use of opioids is discussed earlier in the section on sedation. Analgesia can be delivered in bolus doses, or for rabbits with suspected severe gastrointestinal pain in the form of CRI. Drugs commonly used by Lichtenberger are fentanyl and ketamine combined in low doses delivered with crystalloids (see **Table 1**).

REFERENCES

1. Brooks DL. Nutrition and gastrointestinal physiology. In: Quesenberry K, Carpenter J, editors. Ferrets, rabbits, and rodents: clinical medicine and surgery. 2nd edition. St. Louis (MO): WB Saunders; 2004. p. 155–60.
2. Berezine TP, Ovsiannikov VI. [Mechanism of inhibition of the contractile activity in the jejunum and ileum under psychogenic stress in rabbits]. Ross Fiziol Zh Im I M Sechenova 2009;95(6):639–51 [in Russian].
3. Capello V, Lennox AM. Rabbit. In: Clinical radiology of exotic companion mammals. Ames (IA): Wiley-Blackwell; 2008. p. 54–167.
4. Mondal D, Risam KS, Sharma SR, et al. Prevalence of trichobezoars in Angora rabbits in sub-temperate Himalayan conditions. World Rabbit Science 2006; 14(1):33–8 [in Russian].
5. Harcourt-Brown FM. Gastric dilation and intestinal obstruction in 76 rabbits. Vet Rec 2007;161:409–14.
6. Lichtenberger ML. Fluid resuscitation and nutritional support in rabbits with gastric stasis or gastrointestinal obstruction. Exotic DVM 2005;7(2):34–8.
7. Divers S, Lennox AM. Sedation and anesthesia in exotic companion mammals. Proc Annual Conf Assoc Exotic Mam Vet 2009.
8. Midazolam injection. Drug insert online. Available at: www.drugs.com/pro/midazolam-injection.html. Accessed February 10, 2010.
9. Lichtenberger M, Ko J. Anesthesia and analgesia for small mammals and birds. Veterinary Clin North Am Exot Anim Pract 2007;10(2):293–315.

10. Miaskowski C. A review of the incidence, causes, consequences and management of gastrointestinal effects associated with postoperative opioid administration. J Perianesth Nurs 2009;24(4):222–8.

11. Jenkins J. Gastrointestinal diseases. In: Quesenberry K, Carpenter J, editors. Ferrets, rabbits, and rodents: clinical medicine and surgery. 2nd edition. St Louis (MO): WB Saunders; 2004. p. 161–71.

12. Tein Tay E, Hafeez W. Intraosseous access. EMedicine Journal 2008. Available at: http://www.emedicine.com/proc/TOPIC80431.HTM. Accessed April 11, 2008.

13. Lennox AM. Intraosseous catheterization of exotic animals. J Exotic Pet Med 2008;17(4):300–6.

14. Rudloff E. Kirby R. Colloid and crystalloid resuscitation In: Dhupa N. editor, The Veterinary Clinics of North America Small Animal Practice, critical care, Philadelphia: W.B. Saunders; 2001. p. 1207–96.

15. Haskins S. Fluid therapy. In: Kirk R, Bistner S, Ford R, editors. Handbook of veterinary procedures and emergency treatment. Philadelphia: WB Saunders; 1990. p. 574–600.

16. Velasco IT, Rocha e Silva M, Oliveira MA, et al. Hypertonic and hyperoncotic resuscitation from severe hemorrhagic shock in dogs: a comparative study. Crit Care Med 1989;17:261–4.

17. Michiels M, Monbalie J, Hendricks R, et al. Pharmacokinetics and tissue distribution of the new gastrokinetic agent cisapride in rat, rabbit, and dog [abstract]. Arzneimittelforschung 1987;37(10):59–67.

18. Langer JC, Branlett G. Effect of prokinetic agents on ileal contractility in a rabbit model of gastroschisis. J Pediatr Surg 1997;32(4):605–8.

19. Li C, Qian W, Hou X. Effect of four medications associated with gastrointestinal motility on Oddi sphincter in the rabbit. Pancreatology 2009;9(5):615–20.

20. Paul-Murphy J. Critical care of the rabbit. J Exotic Pet Med 2007;10(2):437–61.

Ferret Coronavirus-Associated Diseases

Jerry Murray, DVM[a],*, Matti Kiupel, DrMedVet, MS, PhD, DACVP[b],
Roger K. Maes, DVM, PhD[c]

KEYWORDS

- Ferret • Coronavirus • Hypergammaglobulinemia • Granuloma
- Feline infectious peritonitis • *Mustela putorius furo*

Coronaviruses are large, enveloped, positive-stranded RNA viruses classified under the genus *Coronavirus* within the family Coronaviridae, order Nidovirales.[1] Based on sequence homology, they are subdivided into three groups.[2] Group 1 coronaviruses include some important causes of enteric disease in domestic animals, including transmissible gastroenteritis virus of swine, feline coronavirus (FCoV), and canine coronavirus. Both the ferret enteric coronavirus (FRECV) and the ferret systemic coronavirus (FRSCV) were recently identified as group 1 coronaviruses.[3,4] Ferret enteric coronavirus causes an enteric disease called *epizootic catarrhal enteritis* (ECE).[3,5] More recently, a new systemic coronavirus-associated disease closely resembling the granulomatous or dry form of feline infectious peritonitis (FIP) was reported in the United States and Europe.[6,7] This article focuses on coronaviral diseases of ferrets, with emphasis on the clinical signs, pathology, pathogenesis, diagnosis, treatment, and prevention of the ferret systemic coronavirus-associated disease.

FERRET EPIZOOTIC ENTERITIS

In March of 1993 a novel enteric disease was reported in domestic ferrets along the east coast of the United States.[5] Initial clinical signs included lethargy, hyporexia or anorexia, and vomiting. These signs were quickly followed by a profuse, foul-smelling, bright green watery diarrhea with a high mucus content, and dehydration. During the more chronic stages of the disease, feces of affected ferrets commonly contained grainy material described as resembling birdseed. Based on the clinical

[a] Animal Clinic of Farmers Branch, 14021 Denton Drive, Dallas, TX 75234, USA
[b] Department of Pathobiology and Diagnostic Investigation, Diagnostic Center for Population and Animal Health, Michigan State University, 4125 Beaumont Road, Room 152A, Lansing, MI 48910, USA
[c] Department of Microbiology, Diagnostic Center for Population and Animal Health, Michigan State University, 4125 Beaumont Road, Room 161, Lansing, MI 48910, USA
* Corresponding author.
E-mail address: aferretvet@cs.com

Vet Clin Exot Anim 13 (2010) 543–560
doi:10.1016/j.cvex.2010.05.010
1094-9194/10/$ – see front matter © 2010 Elsevier Inc. All rights reserved.

presentation, the disease was commonly referred to as *green slime disease*. After a detailed review of the gross and microscopic lesions and the discovery of an enteric coronavirus within affected intestines, the name *epizootic catarrhal enteritis* was introduced.[5]

ECE is a highly contagious diarrheal disease with outbreaks usually involving 100% of the ferrets in the household, breeding facility, or rescue shelter. Even though the morbidity for ECE commonly reaches 100%, overall mortality rate is low (<5%). During the initial outbreaks, young ferrets commonly presented with milder, often subclinical disease, but older ferrets were more severely affected and had higher mortality rates. The disease quickly spread throughout the United States and to several other countries.[5]

On gross examination of ferrets with ECE, the mucosa of the affected portion of the small intestine is hyperemic, and the intestinal wall appears thin. The microscopic lesions of ECE include diffuse lymphocytic enteritis, with villus atrophy, fusion, and blunting; vacuolar degeneration and necrosis of the apical epithelium; or a combination of all these lesions.[5] Immunohistochemistry using a monoclonal antibody against group 1c coronavirus antigen detected large numbers of coronavirus-infected epithelial cells.[3,5] Transmission electron microscopy identified coronavirus-like particles, approximately 120 nm in diameter, in cytoplasmic vacuoles of apical enterocytes and at the cell surface.[5] Similar viral particles were observed electron-microscopically in fecal samples from multiple ferrets.[5]

In subsequent studies, partial sequences of the polymerase, spike, membrane protein, and nucleocapsid genes were identified using coronavirus consensus polymerase chain reaction (PCR) assays.[3] Based on analyses of these data and the complete sequence of the nucleocapsid gene, the ECE-associated coronavirus was found to be a novel coronavirus most closely related to group 1 coronaviruses. This coronavirus was identified as FRECV and shown to be more similar to feline coronavirus, porcine transmissible gastroenteritis virus, and canine coronavirus than to porcine epidemic diarrhea virus and human coronavirus 229E.[3] In situ hybridization using oligoprobes based on FRECV-specific sequences confirmed infection of villar epithelial cells with FRECV in ferrets with ECE.[3]

Based on serologic data and screening of fecal samples by PCR, FRECV seems to be widely distributed in the ferret population in the United States. However, severe clinical ECE has been reported rarely over the past couple of years.

FERRET SYSTEMIC CORONAVIRUS–ASSOCIATED DISEASE

An emerging systemic disease of ferrets characterized by pyogranulomatous perivasculitis and peritonitis was first recognized in Spain in 2004.[6] Shortly thereafter, the disease was also described in the United States.[7,8] Clinically and pathologically, the disease closely resembled FIP. FIP is a fatal, multi-systemic, immune-mediated disease of cats caused by virulent mutants of FCoV. The FIP viruses are believed to arise spontaneously from persisting low pathogenic to nonpathogenic feline enteric coronavirus strains.[9] This concept was, however, challenged in a recent publication.[10] Similar to FIP, this novel disease in ferrets was characterized by positive immunohistochemical labeling of the cytoplasm of intralesional macrophages for coronaviral antigen.[7,11]

Recent publications confirmed the detected coronavirus to be a novel group 1 coronavirus and named it *ferret systemic coronavirus*.[4,7] Partial sequence analysis showed FRSCV to be more similar to FRECV than to other group 1 coronaviruses, including FCoV.[3,4] The similarities in clinical disease and microscopic lesions between FRSCV and FIP virus suggested a similar pathogenesis for FRSCV-associated disease and FIP, but experimental proof is needed.

Clinical Signs

FRSCV-associated disease causing FIP-like lesions has been reported in mostly young ferrets, with most younger than 18 months.[7] Clinical signs in ferrets are nonspecific, similar to those described in cats with the granulomatous or dry form of FIP.[6,12,13] Common clinical signs include diarrhea, weight loss, lethargy, hyporexia or anorexia, and vomiting. These gastrointestinal signs may lead to loss of body condition and moderate to severe emaciation. Signs of central nervous system disease include hind limb paresis or paraparesis, ataxia, tremors, and seizures. Animals may present with primary neurologic disease, including head tilt and seizure activity. Less common clinical signs include sneezing, coughing, labored breathing, nasal discharge, dehydration, bruxism, systolic heart murmur, jaundice, focal areas of erythema of the skin, green colored urine, reddened rectal mucosa, and rectal prolapse.[7,14] Ocular signs have not yet been reported. On abdominal palpation, large abdominal masses, splenomegaly, and renomegaly are common findings. Peripheral lymphadenopathy has been reported in a few cases, and some ferrets also had fevers ranging from 103°F to 105.4°F.[7,14]

Pathology

Gross lesions observed in ferrets with FRSCV infection closely resemble those described in cats with the dry form of feline infectious peritonitis.[7,12,15] The most commonly observed gross lesion consists of multifocal to coalescing white to tan irregular nodules or plaques ranging from 0.5 to 2.0 cm in diameter dispersed over serosal surfaces (**Figs. 1–3**). Nodules are usually oriented along vasculature pathways. The peritoneum, particularly the intestinal serosa and the mesentery, are most commonly affected (see **Fig. 1**), with the mesentery being multifocally and irregularly thickened by pale white firm nodules and plaques.

Similar nodules can be commonly found on the surface or extending into the parenchyma of numerous other organs, with the liver (see **Fig. 2**), kidneys, spleen, and lung

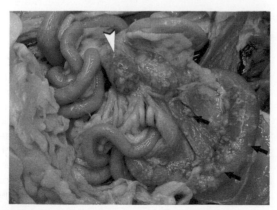

Fig. 1. FRSCV-associated granulomatous peritonitis. Multifocal to coalescing, white firm nodules (*black arrows*) of varying size are widely distributed throughout the mesentery following the vasculature. The mesenteric lymph nodes (*arrowhead*) are enlarged and contain similar nodules that replace normal parenchyma and commonly extend through the capsule. (*Courtesy of* Dodd Sledge, DVM, Lansing, MI, USA.)

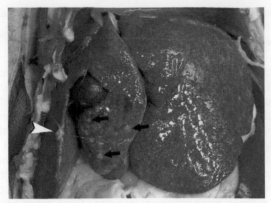

Fig. 2. FRSCV-associated granulomatous hepatitis and fibrinous peritonitis. The hepatic capsule is covered by thick strands of fibrin (*arrowhead*). Multifocal, white firm nodules are randomly distributed over the hepatic serosa and commonly extend into the parenchyma. (*Courtesy of* Dodd Sledge, DVM, Lansing, MI, USA.)

most commonly affected. The mesenteric lymph nodes are affected in most cases. They can be enlarged up to eight times their normal size, with a highly irregular capsular surface characterized by dozens of slightly raised white nodules. On cut surface, the normal parenchyma is often replaced by granulomatous inflammation (see **Fig. 3**).

Other less-specific gross lesions include the commonly observed splenomegaly, and occasional renomegaly and hepatomegaly. Based on current knowledge, ferrets with FRSCV infrequently present with serous effusions into the body cavities that are characteristic of the effusive or wet form of FIP; however, fibrinous exudate is rarely encountered (see **Fig. 2**). In animals with neurologic signs, gross lesions within the nervous system were rather limited. Some moderate meningeal opacity around the medulla and choroid plexuses of the fourth ventricle may be observed. On transverse sections, the choroid plexi can be slightly thickened and viscous exudates may be visible.

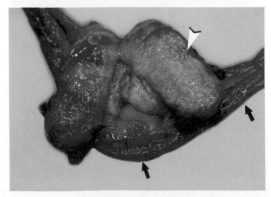

Fig. 3. FRSCV-associated granulomatous lymphadenitis. Section of jejunum (*black arrows*) and cross section of a severely enlarged mesenteric lymph node (*arrowhead*). The lymph node parenchyma is effaced by severe, diffuse granulomatous inflammation. (*Courtesy of* Dodd Sledge, DVM, Lansing, MI, USA.)

Histologic lesions are characterized by severe pyogranulomatous inflammation and are most commonly observed in the mesentery and along the peritoneal surface. Pyogranulomatous inflammation commonly encompasses the small intestine and focally expands or destroys the muscularis and serosa (**Fig. 4**). Pyogranulomas are characterized by central areas of necrosis composed of cellular debris and degenerative neutrophils surrounded by epithelioid macrophages with additional layers of lymphocytes and plasma cells (**Fig. 5**). Rare multinucleated giant cells have been described.

Necrosis is an inconsistent feature, but microgranulomas may be composed predominantly of epithelioid macrophages. Variable degrees of fibrosis surround some granulomas. Granulomatous inflammation is often localized around vessels and frequently involves the adventitia, with inflammatory cells migrating into the medial tunics of small veins and venules (**Figs. 6** and **7**). Similar areas of multifocal pyogranulomatous inflammation commonly expand and obliterate the normal architecture of the lymph nodes and other infected organs, resulting in nephritis, pancreatitis, adrenalitis, meningitis, myocarditis, and pneumonia.

In animals with neurologic signs, the primary lesions may be localized entirely within the brain and consist of a severe pyogranulomatous leptomeningitis, choroiditis, ependymitis, and encephalomyelitis. The inflammatory process is centered on vessels, particularly venules (see **Fig. 7**), along the inner and outer surfaces of the brain, with only focal extension into the underlying parenchyma. The most severe parenchymal extension of the inflammatory reaction is usually observed periventricularly.

Immunohistochemistry using a monoclonal antibody against group 1c coronavirus antigen shows strong positive intracytoplasmic staining of macrophages within the center of pyogranulomas (**Fig. 8**).[7,8,11]

Transmission electron microscopy of areas of pyogranulomatous inflammation revealed macrophages with spherical, enveloped viral particles, 70 to 140 nm in diameter, in membrane-bound cytoplasmic vacuoles and free within the cytoplasm.[7] Occasionally, circumferential spikes were observed along the outer wall of the virions.

Pathogenesis

Current knowledge of the pathogenesis of FRSCV-associated disease is rather limited. No experimental reproduction of the disease has occurred, so most of the

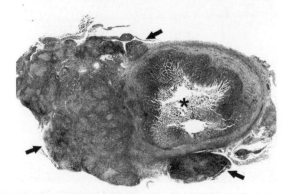

Fig. 4. FRSCV-associated granulomatous peritonitis. The asterisk indicates the lumen of a cross section of jejunum. Circumferentially encompassing the small intestine and extending into the mesentery is severe granulomatous peritonitis (*black arrows*). Hematoxylin and eosin staining (orginal magnification ×4).

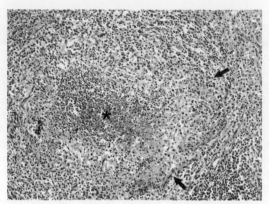

Fig. 5. FRSCV-associated pyogranulomatous peritonitis. A higher magnification of the pyogranulomatous lesions of **Fig. 4** shows the necrotic center composed of cellular debris and degenerative neutrophils (*asterisk*) surrounded by epithelioid macrophages (*black arrows*) followed by lymphocytes and plasma cells and a rim of fibroblasts. Hematoxylin and eosin staining (original magnification ×10).

current hypotheses are drawn from clinical observations, pathologic examinations, and genetic analysis of the ferret coronaviruses. The clinical signs of the systemic form, with which FRSCV has been associated, are certainly similar to those seen in cats affected with the granulomatous or dry form of FIP. Likewise, the gross and histopathologic lesions associated with the systemic form are nearly identical to those seen in the tissues of cats affected with the granulomatous form of FIP. The limited number of FRSCV strains analyzed thus far differ significantly from FRECV strains in the gene encoding for the spike protein, but additional FRECV and FRSCV strains must be analyzed to either substantiate or modify current data.[4]

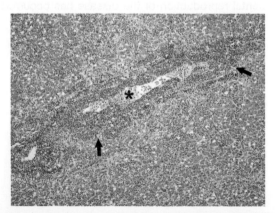

Fig. 6. FRSCV–associated granulomatous vasculitis and hepatitis. The inflammatory reaction is centered around vessels (*asterisk*) and composed of macrophages admixed with neutrophils, lymphocytes, and plasma cells that form thick perivascular cuffs (*black arrows*) that also migrate through the vascular wall and extend into the surrounding hepatic parenchyma. Hematoxylin and eosin staining (original magnification ×10).

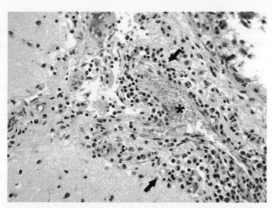

Fig. 7. Ferret systemic coronavirus–associated granulomatous vasculitis. Granulomatous vasculitis is also observed in the brain and most commonly affects the periventricular and meningeal vessels (*asterisk*). Inflammatory cells (*black arrows*), including macrophages admixed with lymphocytes, plasma cells, and a few neutrophils, surround affected vessels and infiltrate the vascular media. Hematoxylin and eosin staining (original magnification ×40).

Diagnosis

Because no pathognomonic clinical signs exist for FRSCV-associated disease, diagnostic testing is required to confirm the diagnosis. Typical hematologic signs include nonregenerative anemia, hyperglobulinemia, hypoalbuminemia, and thrombocytopenia. Serum protein electrophoretograms show a polyclonal hypergammaglobulinemia.[7,14,16,17] Differential diagnoses for hypergammaglobulinemia in domestic ferrets include Aleutian disease, lymphoma/lymphosarcoma, multiple myeloma, chronic infection (*Helicobacter*), or chronic inflammation from inflammatory bowel disease.[7,14,16,18] Counterimmunoelectrophoresis testing for anti-Aleutian disease parvovirus antibodies should be performed to exclude Aleutian disease as a differential.[7,16]

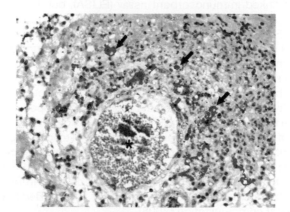

Fig. 8. Ferret systemic coronavirus-associated granulomatous vasculitis. Large numbers of macrophages within the inflammatory reaction surrounding and infiltrating into a large vessel (*asterisk*) contain abundant amounts of coronaviral antigen as indicated by the red chromogen (*black arrows*). Immunohistochemistry against coronavirus type 1 antigen using an alkaline phosphatase detection system, hematoxylin counterstaining (original magnification ×40).

Biochemical changes are variable and reflect damage to abdominal organs, such as kidneys, liver, pancreas, and the gastrointestinal tract (see **Figs. 1–3**). Serum chemistry abnormalities include elevated serum lipase, elevated blood urea nitrogen, elevated serum alanine transferase, elevated alkaline phosphatase, and elevated serum gamma glutamyl transferase.[7] Urinalysis results have only been reported for four cases of FRSCV-associated disease, but abnormal findings include green urine, proteinuria, blood, and rare bilirubin crystals.[7] The greenish color of the urine is likely caused by high levels of biliverdin. Biliverdin may be from microhemorrhage into tissues and extravascular destruction of red blood cells as part of the vasculitis and disseminated intravascular coagulation. A similar mechanism has been reported in cats with FIP.[13] Radiographs may show abdominal masses, splenomegaly, and nephromegaly. Patchy densities in the lungs have been reported in at least one ferret.[17]

The Diagnostic Center for Population and Animal Health at Michigan State University is offering PCR-based testing to detect ferret coronavirus infections. To determine whether ferrets are shedding FRECV, fecal swabs or samples are preferred. A combination of unfixed and fixed tissues containing granulomatous lesions is used to detect ferret coronavirus in ferrets affected with the systemic form.

The two reverse transcription PCR (RT-PCR) assays amplify a portion of the spike gene. Based on available data, these assays are genotype-specific. An example of the data included in a recent article is presented in **Fig. 9**.[4] The authors are currently examining whether these assays also have pathotype specificity. Ultimately clinical, pathologic, and molecular diagnostic data must be combined to determine the final diagnosis.

In addition to viral RNA detection using RT-PCR, the laboratory offers a serologic test to detect antibodies to ferret coronaviruses. The main purpose of this test is to determine whether ferrets were previously exposed to a ferret coronavirus. Thus far this test has been used exclusively to detect evidence of previous FRECV infection. As is the case for feline coronavirus, overinterpretation of titer levels can lead to erroneous conclusions, and therefore interpretation requires a good understanding of the limitations of this test.

Serum antibody tests are frequently used to help diagnose FIP in cats.[13,19] Feline serum antibody tests can include immunofluorescent antibody (IFA), virus neutralization, and enzyme-linked immunosorbent assay (ELISA), but IFA is most commonly used.[13] In general, a high antibody titer is suggestive of FIP, and a low or negative antibody titer makes FIP less likely.[13] Unfortunately, these tests are not specific for FIP. Many healthy cats will have a positive antibody titer from exposure to the feline enteric coronavirus, but most of them will not develop FIP.[13,19]

In the few ferrets that have been tested for serum antibody titers with the feline IFA or ELISA test, antibody titers have been negative.[7] In an attempt to improve the sensitivity and specificity of FIP testing, PCR tests have been developed. These tests detect viral RNA from the feline coronavirus. A RT-PCR test was developed recently to detect messenger RNA of the M gene of the feline coronavirus in macrophages/monocytes.[20] The M gene is only expressed during viral replication; therefore, detection of replicating coronavirus in the blood is thought to be more specific for FIP in cats.[20] Unfortunately, the M gene of the ferret coronavirus is very different from that of the feline coronavirus, and therefore this test will not work for ferrets. (Bernhard Kaltenboeck, DVM, PhD, personal communication, 2008).

Typical clinical signs, blood work results, and a polyclonal gammopathy on serum protein electrophoresis are suggestive of FRSCV-associated disease but are not definitive. Typical microscopic lesions are very suggestive of a diagnosis of FRSCV-associated disease; however, definitive diagnosis requires positive

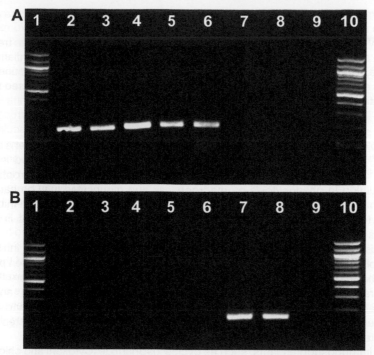

Fig. 9. S-gene genotype-specific diagnostic reverse-transcription polymerase chain reaction on clinical samples. (*A*) Genotype 1–specific assay, 157-bp–positive amplicon observed only on lanes 2 through 6. (*B*) Genotype 2–specific assay, 147-bp–positive amplicon observed only on lanes 7 and 8. Lanes 1 and 10: 100-bp DNA ladder; Lane 2: FRSCV MSU-1–positive lung; Lane 3: FRSCV MSU-1–positive kidney; Lane 4: FRSCV WADL–positive lymph node; Lane 5: FRSCV MSU-S–positive spleen; Lane 6: FRSCV MSU-S–positive intestine; Lane 7: FRECV MSU-2–positive feces; Lane 8: FRECV 1202–positive feces; Lane 9: negative control (sterile water). MSU, Michigan State University; WADL, Washington Animal Disease Diagnostic Laboratory. (*From* Wise A, Kiupel M, Garner MM, et al. Comparative sequence analysis of the distal one-third of the genomes of a systemic and an enteric ferret coronavirus. Virus Res 2010;149:42–50; with permission.)

immunohistochemistry staining of the coronavirus antigen in macrophages within areas of granulomatous inflammation. The monoclonal antibody FIPV3-70 has been used and is recommended to detect the FRSCV antigen.[7,11] However, this antibody cross-reacts with all group 1 coronaviruses and will also detect FRECV.

Further differentiation of FRSCV from FRECV remains a major challenge. Based on sequence data from a limited number of enteric and systemic strains, FRSCV and FRECV are closely related but are genetically distinct. In fact, current data indicate that FRSCV differs significantly more from FRECV than FIPV does from FCoV. Two ferret coronavirus-specific RT-PCR assays were developed as a result of these genetic findings, and these assays are the current gold standard to differentiate FRSCV from FRECV.

Treatment

Currently no cure exists for ferrets with FRSCV-associated disease; most died of the disease or were humanely euthanized because of advanced disease. Nonetheless, some ferrets have survived for several months after diagnosis, and one of the authors (JM) has a long-term survivor of more than 3 years.[7,14,16]

FRSCV-associated disease is an immune-mediated disease, and therefore treatment is aimed at suppressing the immune system, suppressing the excessive inflammatory response, and eliminating or reducing the systemic coronavirus through immune modulation. In addition, symptomatic treatment and nutritional support can be used to try to ameliorate the clinical signs and improve the ferret's quality of life.[14,16,17]

Immune suppression

Prednisolone (Pediapred) is the main medication used to suppress the ferret's immune system.[16] Prednisolone suppresses both the humoral and cell-mediated immunity (CMI).[21–26] Prednisolone decreases chemotaxis and phagocytosis by macrophages.[21] The reduction in phagocytosis by macrophages and monocytes may be caused by inhibition of Fc receptors or steroid receptor–mediated events.[23,27] The inhibition of phagocytosis may help decrease the amount of circulating coronavirus in macrophages and monocytes.

Prednisolone also has potent anti-inflammatory effects. Prednisolone inhibits the release of arachidonic acid from membrane phospholipids, and this inhibition prevents the synthesis of prostaglandins, thromboxanes, and leukotrienes, which are the main mediators of inflammation.[22] In addition to its immunosuppressive and anti-inflammatory actions, prednisolone may increase the ferret's appetite and make it feel better.[16] A high dose of prednisolone (1–2 mg/kg twice daily) is suggested initially, with a gradual tapering of the dose over time.[16]

Other immunosuppressants, such as cyclophosphamide (Cytoxan) and chlorambucil (Leukeran), have been used in the treatment of felines with FIP.[13,19,25] The goal of these two chemotherapy medications is to cause additional immunosuppression and lower the prednisolone dose; however, cyclophosphamide should not be used in ferrets because it may lower the CMI and cause the wet form of FIP to develop (John August, BVetMed, MS, MRCVS, personal communication, 2007, and Diane Addie, PhD, BVMS, MRCVS, personal communication, 2007). Azathioprine (Imuran), another immunosuppressant, has a greater effect on humoral immunity than on CMI.[22] It is very myelotoxic in cats; therefore, it is not recommended for treatment of cats with FIP.[19,22,25] However, it is used anecdotally for treating inflammatory bowel disease and Aleutian disease in ferrets; therefore, it might be worth trying azathioprine with prednisolone for additional immunosuppression, to lower the gamma globulin level, and to lower the prednisolone dose.

Immune modulation

The goal of immune modulation is to help reduce or eliminate the systemic coronavirus. Immune modulators used in feline FIP cases include a polyprenyl immunostimulant and interferon.[24–26,28–32] Polyprenyl immunostimulant is a new, investigational veterinary product composed of phosphorylated and linear polyisoprenols. It has been shown to increase T-helper lymphocytes and Th-1 cytokines, and has been used for the treatment of numerous viral diseases.[28,32] It enhances cell-mediated immunity through Toll-like receptors (Alfred Legendre, DVM, MS, personal communication, 2010).

In a recent pilot study, polyprenyl immunostimulant was used to treat three cats with the dry form of FIP. Two cats experienced long-term remission of more than 2 years when treated with a dose of 3 mg/kg orally, two to three times a week. The third cat was only treated for a few months with a twice-daily dose of 1 mg/kg subcutaneously, and survived for 14 months.[28] Polyprenyl immunostimulant does not seem to work for cases of the wet form of FIP, but it did seem to be effective in the three cats with the dry form of FIP.[28] Polyprenyl immunostimulant is available as part of a field trial through the College of Veterinary Medicine at the University of Tennessee (Tanya Kuritz, PhD, personal communication, 2009). Polyprenyl immunostimulant has a very wide margin of safety in cats, dogs, and mice, but studies are needed to assess its safety and efficacy in ferrets (Alfred Legendre, DVM, MS, personal communication, 2009).

Interferon is another immune modulator that has been studied in feline FIP.[13,24–26,29–32] Both feline interferon omega and human interferon alpha have been shown to inhibit feline coronavirus replication in vitro.[13,32] Recombinant feline interferon omega is available in some European countries and Japan and has been used to treat cats with FIP.[19,24–26] In one uncontrolled study in Japan, a recombinant feline interferon omega was used with dexamethasone or oral prednisolone to treat 12 cats with suspected FIP; 4 older cats with the wet form of FIP experienced long-term remission of greater than 2 years with this treatment.[30]

A recent placebo-controlled, double-blind study with feline interferon omega did not show any effect on survival time or quality of life. This study used either feline interferon omega or placebo along with antibiotics and glucocorticoids; however, the only long-term survivor (200 days) was in the interferon treatment group.[31] Another feline researcher anecdotally reports one third of the cats improve with feline interferon omega treatment.[26] Recombinant human interferon alpha has also been used in cats, but in one experimental study did not reduce mortality significantly.[29]

Vasculitis medications

Vasculitis is one of the common inflammatory lesions in cats with FIP and ferrets with FRSCV-associated disease.[7,11,13,17,19,26,33] Recent research has shown that tumor necrosis factor alpha (TNF-α), interleukin-1 beta (IL-1β), matrix metalloproteinase-9 (MMP-9), and major histocompatibility complex II (MHC II) are all involved in the pathogenesis of vasculitis in feline FIP.[33] Thus, medications that decrease these promoters of vasculitis may help improve the vasculitis, decrease the inflammation, and alleviate some of the clinical signs. Pentoxifylline is a methylxanthine derivative with hemorrheologic, immunomodulatory, and anti-inflammatory effects.[34–42] Pentoxifylline is a nonspecific phosphodiesterase inhibitor.[34–39] Phosphodiesterase inhibition will increase cyclic adenosine monophosphate (cAMP), which increases red blood cell deformability, decreases red blood cell destruction, and improves microcirculation and tissue oxygenation. In addition, increasing cAMP decreases platelet aggregation and blood viscosity.[34,42] Furthermore, pentoxifylline also inhibits TNF-α synthesis and lowers IL-1 levels.[34–36,39–41] Plus pentoxifylline can decrease fibrosis.[34,36] Pentoxifylline has been used to treat feline FIP by some veterinarians with anecdotal improvement, but no studies have been published yet.[19,25] A suggested dose for pentoxifylline in cats is 20 to 25 mg/kg twice daily (Alice Wolf, DVM, personal communication, 2008).

Doxycycline (Vibramycin) is a bacteriostatic antibiotic in the tetracycline family. In addition to its antibiotic properties, it also has anti-inflammatory properties, including inhibition of MMPs.[43–51] MMPs are a family of proteolytic enzymes that degrade various components of the extracellular matrix, and include collagenases, gelatinases, stromelysins, matrilysins, and membrane-type MMPs.[43] Doxycycline can also inhibit TNF-α production, decrease fibrosis, and inhibit leukocyte adhesion to endothelial cells.[44,50,51] Broad-spectrum antibiotic treatment is recommended during immunosuppressive therapy to prevent secondary bacterial infection.[16,25,26] Doxycycline can be used for this purpose, and its inhibition of MMPs and TNF-α may help decrease damage to the blood vessels. A published dose of doxycycline for ferrets is 10 mg/kg twice daily.[52]

Ozagrel (Xanbon) is a thromboxane synthetase inhibitor that has been studied in cats with FIP.[53] Thromboxane synthetase inhibitors suppress production of thromboxane A2, which is a potent platelet aggregating agent. Platelet aggregation is associated with progression of the vasculitis in FIP.[53] The reported dose for ozagrel in cats is 5 to 10 mg/kg twice daily.[53]

Aspirin (Ascriptin) or acetylsalicylic acid is a nonsteroidal anti-inflammatory drug. Its main mechanism of action is inhibition of inflammatory mediators through cyclooxygenase (COX) inhibition. Aspirin decreases platelet aggregation through inhibiting prostaglandin and preventing the formation of thromboxane A2. However, it can also cause gastric irritation and ulceration, and ferrets as a species are very prone to gastric ulcers. Therefore aspirin, especially with concurrent prednisolone, would have to be used with extreme caution, if at all, in ferrets.

Prednisolone is also used to treat vasculitis.[23] Prednisolone can prevent the formation of thromboxanes,[22] and can also inhibit TNF-α, IL-1, MHC-II, and platelet aggregation.[21-23,54,55] Combining prednisolone, pentoxifylline, and doxycycline may have a synergistic effect on decreasing inflammation and vasculitis.[34,48]

Symptomatic treatment

Symptomatic treatment can be used to help alleviate some of the clinical signs. Common clinical signs have involved the gastrointestinal tract and have included hyporexia and anorexia, weight loss, vomiting, dehydration, and diarrhea.[7,14,16,17] Gastroprotectant therapy can be used to help reduce nausea and inappetence, and prevent gastric ulcers secondary to high doses of prednisolone. Sucralfate (Carafate oral suspension) can be administered orally at a dose of 75 to 100 mg/kg, 10 to 15 minutes before each feeding and before prednisolone administration.[56,57] Antacids such as cimetidine hydrochloride (Tagamet), famotidine (Pepcid AC), ranitidine (Zantac), and omeprazole (Prilosec) can be used to reduce gastric acid. Omeprazole and famotidine have the advantage of only once-a-day administration; however, cimetidine also has some beneficial effects on the immune system.[57-62] Cimetidine is a type 2 histamine receptor blocker, and can have antiviral activity, stimulate the CMI, and increase T-lymphocyte levels.[24,58-62] Therefore, cimetidine, 10 mg/kg, administered three times daily is the suggested antacid.

Vomiting can be controlled with either maropitant citrate (Cerenia) or metoclopramide (Reglan). Dehydration can be corrected with fluid therapy. Critical ferrets and those with excessive water loss from vomiting or diarrhea may benefit from intravenous fluids, and those with severe hypoalbuminemia may benefit from administration of colloids or a blood transfusion. For noncritical ferrets, subcutaneous fluids can be used, and most owners are capable of giving subcutaneous fluids at home.[56] For ferrets that are stable, a veterinary oral electrolyte solution such as the chicken-flavored Rebound OES, or human electrolyte solutions such as grape-flavored Pedialyte or Gatorade can be used.

Diarrhea is one of the common problems and is likely caused by the pyogranulomatous inflammation in the gastrointestinal tract; however, a fecal parasite examination should be performed to rule out concurrent coccidiosis (*Eimeria* or *Isospora* species) and giardiasis.[14] Pyogranulomatous intestinal inflammation can lead to maldigestion and malabsorption of nutrients and protein-losing enteropathy. Empiric treatment for diarrhea with antibiotics, probiotics, and antidiarrheals, along with immunosuppressive therapy, may be useful in these cases.

Antiulcer antibiotics such as clarithromycin (Biaxin oral suspension) in combination with amoxicillin (Amoxi-drops) or amoxicillin with clavulanic acid (Clavamox drops) can be used to treat *Helicobacter mustelae* in the stomach and provide broad-spectrum coverage for the intestinal tact.[56,63] Additional antibiotics such as enrofloxacin (Baytril), marbofloxacin (Zeniquin), or kanamycin (Amforol oral suspension) can be used to cover gram negative bacteria. Probiotics for cats such as Proviable KP paste or Fortiflora may help restore the normal bacterial flora and improve the diarrhea. Antidiarrheals such as kaolin-pectin (Proviable KP paste), loperamide (Imodium A-D), or activated attapulgite (Amforol oral suspension) can be useful in firming up the feces.

Nutritional support

Maintaining proper protein, fat, and calorie intake is critical during treatment. Sick ferrets usually do not eat enough food to cover their nutritional needs, and therefore need nutritional support.[56,57] Ferrets will often eat a soft food when they refuse their normal dry kibble, and therefore veterinary diets designed for recovery, such as Hill's a/d, Royal Canin's recovery RS, Carnivore Care, Iams maximum calorie, or human meat-based baby foods, such as those designed for the first and second stage of solid foods, are usually accepted by inappetant ferrets.[16,56,57] Ferrets particularly like the turkey or chicken baby foods and Hill's a/d.[16,56] Another option is to make a gruel out of their regular food by grinding it up and adding warm water. Most of these soft foods can be hand-fed or syringe-fed frequently to maintain protein, fat, and caloric needs.

Supplementing vitamins and minerals may also be beneficial. Anemia is one of the common blood abnormalities, and therefore supplemental iron along with erythropoietin (Epogen, Procrit) may help increase the red blood cell production. Chronic diarrhea may be helped by cobalamin (vitamin B_{12}) supplementation. Parental administration of cobalamin at a dose of 250 µg subcutaneously once a week is an empiric recommendation.[64] Vitamin B complex at a dose of 1 to 2 mg/kg subcutaneously may be used to increase the ferret's appetite.[56] Vitamin B complex can also be added to the subcutaneous fluids or be given orally.

Antioxidants

Antioxidants may be useful to reduce the free radicals and reactive oxygen species that are produced from the inflammatory response and hyperactive immune response. Melatonin is a natural hormone that is a potent antioxidant and free radical scavenger.[65–67] Melatonin also has some anti-inflammatory effects, including decreasing TNF-α, decreasing IL-1B, and inhibiting MMPs.[68–73] Melatonin also has some immune modulation effects and antiviral effects.[74–79] Furthermore, melatonin stimulates the appetite, so it would be another way to treat the inappetence and weight loss. Melatonin is available as a liquid, a tablet, or an injectable implant for ferrets.

Another strong antioxidant is superoxide dismutase (SOD). SOD may have an additional beneficial effect on the immune system because it can increase the ratio of CD4+ to CD8+ lymphocytes in cats.[80] S-adenosylmethionine (SAMe) and silybin are other antioxidant therapies that should be beneficial. SAMe can increase glutathione levels and increase hepatic cell repair and regeneration, whereas silybin is an antioxidant. Together they are reported to help protect the liver, which may be useful during long-term prednisolone use.[81] Other antioxidants like vitamins A, C, and E may also be helpful.[26] One possible side effect from vitamin C supplementation is the formation of calcium oxalate uroliths.[82] Calcium oxalate was the third most common ferret urolith and accounted for 10.5% of all the ferret uroliths analyzed at the University of Minnesota Urolith Center, and therefore vitamin C must be used with caution.[83]

Prevention

Guidelines for prevention of FIP in cats can be modified for prevention of FRSCV-associated disease.[24,26] Prevention of FRSCV-associated disease currently is best accomplished by avoiding exposure to the ferret coronavirus. Unfortunately, FRECV is assumed to be ubiquitous in most multiple-ferret homes, shelters, and breeding farms.[5] Nonetheless, reducing fecal contamination of the environment through disinfecting the litter boxes, cages, and bowls with sodium hypochlorite (bleach) weekly, keeping litter boxes away from food and water bowls, and vacuuming up litter around litter boxes and in the ferret room at least once a week may help.[26] For breeders, isolation and early weaning of the kits may help prevent exposure.

SUMMARY

Ferret FIP-like disease is a new and almost-always fatal disease associated with the systemic ferret coronavirus; however, it is still worth treating most cases. Treatment may temporarily improve the condition and allow the ferret and owner several months of quality life. Long-term clinical remission may even be possible in some cases. The hope is that ongoing research will lead to new and more effective treatment options for this recently recognized ferret disease.

ACKNOWLEDGMENTS

Dr Murray would like to thank the pathologists (Drs Matti Kiupel, Mike Garner, Gaymen Helman, Shane Stiver, and Bruce Williams) and feline infectious peritonitis experts (Drs Diane Addie, John August, Alice Wolf, Richard Weiss, Bernhard Kaltenboeck, Al Legendre, and Niels Pedersen) who helped him understand the immunopathogenesis and treatment strategies for this new disease. He would also like to thank Dr Katrina Ramsell and the Web site www.catvirus.com.

REFERENCES

1. Lai MMC, Perlman S, Anderson LJ. Coronaviridae. In: Knipe DM, Howley PM, editors. Fields virology. 5th edition. Philadelphia: Lippincott Williams & Wilkins; 2007. p. 1305–35.
2. Gonzalez JM, Gomez-Puertas P, Cavanagh D, et al. A comparative sequence analysis to revise the current taxonomy of the family Coronaviridae. Arch Virol 2003;148(11):2207–35.
3. Wise AG, Kiupel M, Maes RK. Molecular characterization of a novel coronavirus associated with epizootic catarrhal enteritis (ECE) in ferrets. Virology 2006; 349(1):164–74.
4. Wise A, Kiupel M, Garner MM, et al. Comparative sequence analysis of the distal one-third of the genomes of a systemic and an enteric ferret coronavirus. Virus Res 2010;149(1):42–50.
5. Williams B, Kiupel M, West K, et al. Coronavirus associated epizootic catarrhal enteritis in ferrets. J Am Vet Med Assoc 2000;217(4):526–30.
6. Martinez J, Ramis AJ, Reinacher M, et al. Detection of feline infectious peritonitis virus-like antigen in ferrets. Vet Rec 2006;158(15):523.

7. Garner MM, Ramsell K, Morera N, et al. Clinicopathologic features of a systemic coronavirus-associated disease resembling feline infectious peritonitis in the domestic ferret (Mustela putorius). Vet Pathol 2008;45(2):236–46.
8. Juan-Salles C, Teifke JP, Morera N, et al. Pathology and immunohistochemistry of a disease resembling feline infectious peritonitis in ferrets (Mustela putorius furo). Vet Pathol 2006;43(5):845.
9. Rottier PJM, Nakamura K, Schellen P, et al. Acquisition of macrophage tropism during the pathogenesis of feline infectious peritonitis is determined by mutations in the feline coronavirus spike protein. J Virol 2005;79:14122–30.
10. Brown MA, Troyer JL, Pecon-Slattery J, et al. Genetics and pathogenesis of feline infectious peritonitis virus. Emerg Infect Dis 2009;15(9):1445–52.
11. Martínez J, Reinacher M, Perpiñán D, et al. Identification of group 1 coronavirus antigen in multisystemic granulomatous lesions in ferrets (Mustela putorius furo). J Comp Pathol 2008;138:54–8.
12. Hartmann K. Feline infectious peritonitis. Vet Clin North Am Small Anim Pract 2005;35:39–79.
13. Pedersen NC. A review of feline infectious peritonitis virus infection: 1963–2008. J Feline Med Surg 2009;11:225–58.
14. Perpinan D, Lopez C. Clinical aspects of systemic granulomatous inflammatory syndrome in ferrets (Mustela putorius furo). Vet Rec 2008;162(6):180–3.
15. Weiss RC, Scott FW. Pathogenesis of feline infectious peritonitis: pathologic changes and immunofluorescence. Am J Vet Res 1981;42:2036–48.
16. Murray J. Clinical management of systemic coronavirus in domestic ferrets. In: Proceedings of the 29th Annual AAV Conference & Expo with AEMV. Savannah (GA), August 11–14, 2008. p. 51–5.
17. Ramsell KD, Garner MM, Maes R, et al. A disease resembling feline infectious peritonitis in the domestic ferret. In: Proceedings of the International Ferret Symposium. Portland, June 22–24, 2007.
18. Garner MM. Focus on diseases of ferrets. Exotic DVM 2003;5(3):75–80.
19. Addie D, Belak S, Boucraut-Baralon C, et al. Feline infectious peritonitis. ABCD guidelines on prevention and management. J Feline Med Surg 2009;11:594–604.
20. Simons FA, Vennema H, Rofina JE, et al. A mRNA PCR for the diagnosis of feline infectious peritonitis. J Virol Methods 2005;124:111–6.
21. Tizard I. Drugs that affect the immune system. In: Veterinary immunology. 4th edition. Philadelphia: WB Saunders; 1992. p. 447–56.
22. Gregory CR. Immunosuppressive agents. In: Bonagura JD, editor. Kirk's current veterinary therapy XIII. Philadelphia: WB Saunders; 2000. p. 509–13.
23. Taylor HG, Samanta A. Treatment of vasculitis. Br J Clin Pharmacol 1993;35: 93–104.
24. Addie DD, Ishida T. Feline infectious peritonitis: therapy and prevention. In: Bonagura JD, Twedt DC, editors. Kirk's current veterinary therapy XIV. St Louis (MO): Saunders Elsevier; 2009. p. 1295–8.
25. Hartmann K. Diagnosis and treatment of feline infectious peritonitis. In: August JR, editor. Consultations in feline internal medicine, vol. 6. St. Louis (MO): Saunders Elsevier; 2010. p. 62–76.
26. Addie DD, Jarett O. Feline coronavirus infections. In: Greene CE, editor. Infectious diseases of the dog and cat. 3rd edition. St Louis (MO): Saunders Elsevier; 2006. p. 88–102.
27. Jones CJP, Morris KJ, Jayson MIV. Prednisolone inhibits phagocytosis by polymorphonuclear leucocytes via steroid receptor mediated events. Ann Rheum Dis 1983;42(1):56–62.

28. Legendre AM, Bartges JW. Effect of polyprenol immunostimulant on the survival times of three cats with the dry form of feline infectious peritonitis. J Feline Med Surg 2009;11(8):624–6.
29. Weiss RC, Cox NR, Oostrom-Ram T. Effect of interferon or *Propionibacterium acnes* on the course of experimentally induced feline infectious peritonitis in specific-pathogen-free and random-source cats. Am J Vet Res 1990;51(5):726–33.
30. Ishida T, Shibanai A, Tanaka S, et al. Use of recombinant feline interferon and glucocorticoid in the treatment of feline infectious peritonitis. J Feline Med Surg 2004;6(2):107–9.
31. Ritz S, Egberink H, Hartmann K. Effect of feline interferon-omega on the survival times and quality of life of cats with feline infectious peritonitis. J Vet Intern Med 2007;21(6):1193–7.
32. Kennedy MA. An update on feline infectious peritonitis. Vet Med 2009;104(8): 384–91.
33. Kipar A, May H, Menger S, et al. Morphologic features and development of granulomatous vasculitis in feline infectious peritonitis. Vet Pathol 2005;42(3):321–30.
34. Marsella R. Pentoxifylline. In: Bonagura JD, Twedt DC, editors. Kirk's current therapy XIV. St Louis (MO): Saunders Elsevier; 2009. p. 397–400.
35. Scott DW, Miller WH, Griffin CE. Dermatologic therapy. In: Muller & Kirk's small animal dermatology. 6th edition. Philadelphia: WB Saunders; 2001. p. 241.
36. Mendes JB, Campos PP, Rocha MA, et al. Cilostazol and pentoxifylline decrease angiogenesis, inflammation, and fibrosis in sponge-induced intraperitoneal adhesion in mice. Life Sci 2009;84(15–16):537–43.
37. Deree J, Lall R, Melbostad H, et al. Neutrophil degranulation and effects of phosphodiesterase inhibition. J Surg Res 2006;133(1):22–8.
38. Scott DW, Miller WH, Griffin CE. Immune-mediated disorders. In: Muller & Kirk's small animal dermatology. 6th edition. Philadelphia: WB Saunders; 2001. p. 742–56.
39. Fernandes JL, de Oliveira RT, Mamoni RL, et al. Pentoxifylline reduces pro-inflammatory and increases anti-inflammatory activity in patients with coronary artery disease-a randomized placebo-controlled study. Atherosclerosis 2008; 196(1):434–42.
40. Duman DG, Ozdemir F, Birben E, et al. Effects of pentoxifylline on TNF-alpha production by peripheral blood mononuclear cells in patients with nonalcoholic steatohepatitis. Dig Dis Sci 2007;52(10):2520–4.
41. Satapathy SK, Sakhuja P, Malhotra V, et al. Beneficial effects of pentoxifylline on hepatic steatosis, fibrosis and necroinflammation in patients with non-alcoholic steatohepatitis. J Gastroenterol Hepatol 2007;22(5):634–8.
42. Maiti R, Agrawai NK, Dash D, et al. Effect of pentoxifylline on inflammatory burden, oxidative stress and platelet aggregability in hypertensive type 2 diabetes mellitus patients. Vascul Pharmacol 2007;47(2–3):118–24.
43. Raffetto JD, Khalil RA. Matrix metalloproteinases and their inhibitors in vascular remoldeling and vascular disease. Biochem Pharmacol 2008;75(2):346–59.
44. Mulivor AW, Lipowsky HH. Inhibition of glycan shedding and leukocyte-endothelial adhesion in postcapillary venules by suppression of matrixmetalloprotease activity with doxycycline. Microcirculation 2009;4:1–10.
45. Liu J, Xiong W, Baca-Regen L, et al. Mechanism of inhibition of matrix metalloproteinase-2 expression by doxycycline in human aortic smooth muscle cells. J Vasc Surg 2003;38(6):1376–83.
46. Hackmann AE, Rubin BG, Sanchez LA, et al. A randomized, placebo-controlled trial of doxycycline after endoluminal aneurysm repair. J Vasc Surg 2008;48(3): 519–26.

47. Iovieno A, Lambiase A, Micera A, et al. In vivo characterization of doxycycline effects on tear metalloproteinases in patients with chronic blepharitis. Eur J Ophthalmol 2009;19(5):708–16.
48. Lee HM, Ciancio SG, Tuter G, et al. Subantimicrobial dose doxycycline efficacy as a matrix metalloproteinase inhibitor in chronic periodontitis patients is enhanced when combined with a non-steroidal anti-inflammatory drug. J Periodontal 2004;75(3):453–63.
49. Gu Y, Lee HM, Sorsa T, et al. Doxycycline inhibits mononuclear cell-mediated connective tissue breakdown. FEMS Immunol Med Microbiol 2010;58(2): 218–25.
50. Lau AC, Duong TT, Ito S, et al. Inhibition of matrix metalloproteinase-9 activity improves coronary outcome in an animal model of Kawasaki disease. Clin Exp Immunol 2009;157(2):300–9.
51. Hori Y, Kunihiro S, Sato S, et al. Doxycycline attenuates isoproterenol-induced myocardial fibrosis and matrix metalloproteinase activity in rats. Biol Pharm Bull 2009;32(10):1678–82.
52. Lewington JH. Diseases of the ferret ear, eye and nose. In: Ferret husbandry, medicine and surgery. 2nd edition. Sydney (Australia): Saunders Elsevier; 2007. p. 311.
53. Watari T, Kaneshima T, Tsujikoto H, et al. Effect of thromboxane synthetase inhibitor on feline infectious peritonitis in cats. J Vet Med Sci 1998;60(5):657–9.
54. Moraes LA, Paul-Clark MJ, Rickman A, et al. Ligand-specific glucocorticoid receptor activation in human platelets. Blood 2005;106(13):4167–75.
55. Debets JM, Ruers TJ, van der Linden MP, et al. Inhibitory effect of corticosteroids on the secretion of tumor necrosis factor (TNF) by monocytes is dependant on the stimulus inducing TNF synthesis. Clin Exp Immunol 1989;78(2):224–9.
56. Williams BH. Therapeutics in ferrets. Vet Clin North Am Exot Anim Pract 2000; 3(1):131–53.
57. Antinoff N, Hahn K. Ferret oncology: diseases, diagnostics, and therapeutics. Vet Clin North Am Exot Anim Pract 2004;7(3):579–625.
58. Bourinbalar AS, Fruhstorfer EC. The effect of histamine type 2 receptor antagonists on human immunodeficiency virus (HIV) replication: identification of a new class of antiviral agents. Life Sci 1996;59(23):365–70.
59. Kabuta H, Yamamoto S, Shingu M. The effect of cimetidine on survival of mice infected with herpes simplex virus type 2, murine encephalomyelitis and vesicular stomatitis virus infections. Kurume Med J 1989;36(3):95–9.
60. Hirai N, Hill NO, Motoo Y, et al. Antiviral and antiproliferative activities of human leukocyte interferon potentiated by cimetidine in vitro. J Interferon Res 1985; 5(3):375–82.
61. Nishiguchi S, Tamori A, Shiomi S, et al. Cimetidine reduces impairment of cellular immunity after transcatheter arterial embolization in patients with hepatocellular carcinoma. Hepatogastroenterology 2003;50(50):460–2.
62. Katoh J, Tauchiya K, Osawa H, et al. Cimetidine reduces impairment of cellular immunity after cardiac operations with cardiopulmonary bypass. J Thorac Cardiovasc Surg 1998;116(2):312–8.
63. Powers LV. Bacterial and parasitic diseases of ferrets. Vet Clin North Am Exot Anim Pract 2009;12(3):531–61.
64. Hoppes S, Xenoulis PG, Berghoff N, et al. Serum cobalamin, folate, and methylmalonic acid concentrations in ferrets (Mustela putorius). In: Proceedings of the 29th Annual AAV Conference & Expo with AEMV. Savannah (GA), August 11–14, 2008. p. 61–3.

65. Reiter RJ, Melchiorri D, Sewerynek E, et al. A review of the evidence supporting melatonin's role as an antioxidant. J Pineal Res 1995;18(1):1–11.
66. Reiter RJ, Tan DX, Gitto E, et al. Pharmacological utility of melatonin in reducing oxidative cellular and molecular damage. Pol J Pharmacol 2004;56(2):158–70.
67. Zararsiz I, Sarsilmaz W, Tas U, et al. Protective effects of melatonin against formaldehyde-induce kidney damage in rats. Toxicol Ind Health 2007;23(10):573–9.
68. Maldonado MD, Mora-Santos M, Naji L, et al. Evidence of melatonin synthesis and release by mast cells. Possible modulatory role on inflammation. Pharmacol Res 2009 Dec 3. [Epub ahead of print].
69. Lahiri S, Singh P, Singh S, et al. Melatonin protects against experimental reflux esophagitis. J Pineal Res 2009;46(2):207–13.
70. Ganguly K, Swamaker S. Induction of matrix metalloproteinase-9 and -3 in nonsteroidal anti-inflammatory drug-induced acute gastric ulcers in mice: regulation by melatonin. J Pineal Res 2009;47(1):43–55.
71. Swamaker S, Mishra A, Ganguly K, et al. Matrix metalloproteinase-9 activity and expression is reduced by melatonin during prevention of ethanol-induced gastric ulcer in mice. J Pineal Res 2007;43(10):56–64.
72. Hung YC, Chen TY, Lee EJ, et al. Melatonin decreases matrix metalloproteinase-9 activation and expression and attenuates reperfusion-induced hemorrhage following transient focal cerebral ischemia in rats. J Pineal Res 2008;45(4):459–67.
73. Esposito E, Mazzon E, Riccardi L, et al. Matrix metalloproteinase-9 and metalloproteinase-2 activity and expression is reduced by melatonin during experimental colitis. J Pineal Res 2008;45(2):166–73.
74. Srinivasan V, Spence DW, Trakht I, et al. Immunomodulation by melatonin: its significance for seasonally occurring diseases. Neuroimmunomodulation 2008;15(2):93–101.
75. Reiter RJ, Calvo JR, Karbownik M, et al. Melatonin and its relation to the immune system and inflammation. Ann N Y Acad Sci 2000;917:376–86.
76. Maestroni GJ. Therapeutic potential of melatonin in immunodeficiency states, viral diseases, and cancer. Adv Exp Med Biol 1999;467:217–26.
77. Bonilla E, Valero N, Chacin-Bonilla L, et al. Melatonin and viral infections. J Pineal Res 2004;36(2):73–9.
78. Huang SH, Cao XJ, Wei W. Melatonin decreases TLR3-mediated inflammatory factor expression via inhibition of NF-kappa B activation in respiratory syncytial virus-infected RAW264.7 macrophages. J Pineal Res 2008;45(1):93–100.
79. Nunes OS, Pereira RS. Regression of herpes viral infection symptoms using melatonin and SB-73: comparison with acyclovir. J Pineal Res 2008;44(4):373–8.
80. Webb CB, Lehman TL, McCord KW. Effects of an oral superoxide dismutase enzyme supplementation on indices of oxidative stress, proviral load, and CD4:CD8 ratios in asymptomatic FIV-infected cats. J Feline Med Surg 2008;10(5):423–30.
81. Webster CR, Cooper J. Therapeutic use of cytoprotective agents in canine and feline hepatobiliary disease. Vet Clin North Am Small Anim Pract 2009;39(3):631–52.
82. Gisselman K, Langston C, Palma D, et al. Calcium oxalate urolithiasis. Compend Contin Educ Pract Vet 2009;31(11):496–500.
83. Osborne CA, Albasan H, Lulich JP, et al. Quantitative analysis of 4468 uroliths retrieved from farm animals, exotic species, and wildlife submitted to the Minnesota Urolith center: 1981–2007. Vet Clin North Am Small Anim Pract 2008;39:65–78.

Disseminated Idiopathic Myofasciitis in Ferrets

Katrina D. Ramsell, PhD, DVM[a],*, Michael M. Garner, DVM, DACVP[b]

KEYWORDS

• Ferrets • Myofasciitis • Polymyositis • Myositis • Neutrophilia

Disseminated idiopathic myofasciitis (DIM) is a recently identified disease in the domestic ferret, *Mustela putorius furo*.[1,2] The disease was first recognized in late 2003, although the earliest possible case this author (K.D.R.) has identified is from 1999. The most recent case, at the time of this writing, was from January 2010. DIM has also been termed "polymyositis" and "myositis" and is a severe inflammatory condition that affects primarily muscles and surrounding connective tissues.[1,2] The authors have approximately 100 suspected cases on file with about half having been confirmed via histopathology.

Inflammatory myopathies are a heterogeneous group of autoimmune or immune-mediated diseases that affect muscles[3–6] and have been studied in a number of species, including humans[3,7,8] and dogs.[4,9,10] Four major types of idiopathic inflammatory myopathy in humans include dermatomyositis (DM), polymyositis (PM), inclusion body myositis (IBM), and immune-mediated necrotizing myopathy (NM).[7,8,11] These myositides appear clinically, histologically, and pathogenically distinct [N]. Canine models for polymyositis and dermatomyositis exist,[9,10,12–15] as does a canine form of immune-mediated masticatory myositis.[4,9,16]

Animal models of inflammatory myopathies have clarified the immunopathogenesis of some of these disorders. Iatragenically induced localized myositis associated with administration of vaccines has been documented in cattle.[17,18] Rats and mice have been used as models for polymyositis, and experimental autoimmune myositis has been induced in rabbits and guinea pigs following immunization of muscle.[19,20] Although research on DIM has been ongoing since it was first described, the etiopathogenesis of this disease in ferrets is still unknown. Advances in the understanding of

The American Ferret Association has established a research fund to study DIM.

[a] Northwest Exotic Pet Vet LLC, 6895 SW 160th Avenue, Beaverton, OR 97007, USA
[b] Northwest ZooPath, 654 West Main, Monroe, WA 98272, USA
* Corresponding author.
E-mail address: exoticpetvet@hotmail.com

doi:10.1016/j.cvex.2010.05.011
1094-9194/10/$ – see front matter © 2010 Elsevier Inc. All rights reserved.

vetexotic.theclinics.com

human and animal inflammatory myopathies may help elucidate the pathogenesis of DIM in ferrets.

This article summarizes clinical and pathologic findings in DIM patients. Recommended diagnostic procedures and clinical management are addressed, and possible etiologies for the disease are discussed.

SIGNALMENT AND HISTORY

DIM generally affects ferrets younger than 18 months old. Age range for early cases was 5 months to 24 months of age with an average age of 10 months,[1] and recently cases of ferrets as old as 4 years have been diagnosed. Both male and female ferrets are susceptible to DIM. There does not appear to be an association between susceptibility of the disease and coat color. Ferrets diagnosed with DIM have been mostly from 2 large breeding facilities, but a few were from private breeders. Almost all ferrets had been neutered and descented at their original breeding facility before shipment. Most ferrets suspected or confirmed to have DIM lived in multiferret households, and some were residing at shelters or rescue facilities. Households were in a number of states throughout the United States. Ferrets diagnosed with DIM have been fed various diets, including ones mostly formulated for ferrets, but also some cat and kitten products.

Vaccine histories were evaluated from cases if the information was available. A number of ferrets received the recommended series of distemper vaccinations. Many ferrets were inoculated with only one canine distemper vaccination, between 4 and 7 weeks of age, at the breeding facility. Some ferret owners have the misconception that young ferrets have been fully vaccinated against canine distemper before being shipped to the pet store.

Early case histories indicated that all confirmed DIM cases had been vaccinated with one particular distemper vaccine, Fervac-D (United Vaccines, Madison, WI, USA), which is no longer being produced. Two other distemper vaccines given to ferrets diagnosed with DIM were Purevax (Merial, Athens, GA, USA) and Galaxy-D (Schering-Plough Animal Health, Omaha, NE, USA). Some DIM ferrets received an approved rabies vaccine (Imrab-3, Merial).

Because Fervac-D is no longer available, large ferret breeding facilities have had to choose an alternative product to vaccinate and protect young ferrets from canine distemper. Recent inquiries to 3 large ferret breeding facilities revealed that Distox-Plus (a modified live mink distemper-virus enteritis vaccine, Clostridium botulinum type-C-Pseudomonas aeruginosa bacterin-toxin) (Schering-Plough Animal Health) is currently being used and is cost effective. Distem-R TC (a modified live mink distemper vaccine) (Schering-Plough Animal Health) was being used in some facilities after Fervac-D was removed from the market, but now it too is no longer available. Although Purevax is the only distemper vaccine currently approved for use in ferrets, many practitioners and shelters use Galaxy-D.

CLINICAL SIGNS

The onset of clinical signs for DIM is usually acute to subacute, often followed by rapid decline over a period of 12 to 36 hours. Clinical signs for DIM are summarized in **Table 1**. Afflicted ferrets usually have multiple, concurrent symptoms. The most common initial clinical signs are a high fever (often 104–108°F), severe lethargy, paresis, and dehydration (**Fig. 1**). Most affected ferrets are depressed but cognizant. Other symptoms observed during the onset of DIM include inappetence, enlarged lymph nodes, subcutaneous masses, and abnormal stools. Greenish, mucoid, and

Table 1
Clinical signs of ferrets with DIM

Most Common Signs	Somewhat Common Signs	Less Common Signs
Fever	Painful (mostly lumbosacral/rear legs)	Serous nasal discharge
Lethargy	Abnormal stools	Pinpoint dermal lesions (often orangish)
Paresis	Enlarged lymph nodes	Ocular discharge
Depression	Subcutaneous masses	Labored/congested breathing; coughing
Inappetence	Weight loss	Panting
Dehydration	Tachycardia	Bruxism
	Tachypnea	Pale gums
	Heart murmur	Edema
		Seizures

dark diarrhea has been observed in several patients. Some ferrets will refuse crunchy food but will eat soft food. A number of suspected and confirmed patients with DIM have developed hyperesthesia or dysesthesia, displaying responses indicative of pain when they are palpated or touched. The greatest sensitivity is usually in the lumbosacral region or hind legs. Tachycardia (heart rate often over 300 beats per minute), tachypnea, and heart murmurs occur somewhat often and seem to become more prominent as the disease progresses.

Other signs that may be observed in ferrets with DIM include serous nasal discharge, ocular discharge, bruxism, pale gums, panting, labored or congested

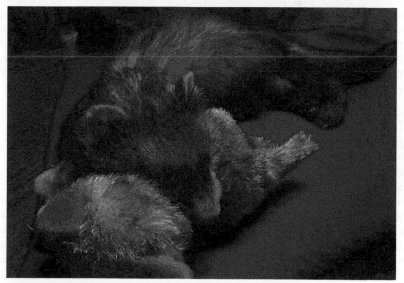

Fig 1. Ferrets with DIM are typically depressed, very lethargic, paretic, and dehydrated. (*Courtesy of* Yvonne DeCarlo; with permission.)

breathing, coughing, and rarely edema or seizures. Some ferrets have had skin lesions such as infected hair follicles, small dermal masses, or pinpoint orangish dots on the trunk or face. Although clinical signs of DIM usually develop quickly, the duration of the illness can be days to weeks, or even months. Most ferrets with DIM have continued to progressively decline until they either died or were humanely euthanized.

DIAGNOSTIC RESULTS
Hematology

Although the white blood cell (WBC) count may initially be in the normal range, most ferrets with DIM eventually exhibit a moderate to marked mature neutrophilia, occasionally with a left shift. The WBC count is less than 50,000/μL in most DIM cases (normal reference range for WBCs in ferrets is 2500–8000/μL; Antech Diagnostics), but the mature neutrophil count has approached 100,000/μL in a few cases. Neutrophils are often slightly to moderately toxic in patients with DIM. Mild to moderate anemia is a common finding in ferrets with DIM. The anemia may be initially nonregenerative and then later become regenerative. Target cells, schistocytes, and Dohle bodies have been identified rarely in patients with DIM.

Serum chemistry values in ferrets with DIM often reveal mild hyperglycemia and hypoalbuminemia. Serum alanine aminotransferase (ALT) has also been mildly to moderately increased in several patients with DIM. Interestingly, creatine kinase (CK), a value typically elevated with severe inflammation and muscle tissue necrosis, is not elevated in ferrets with DIM. As discussed later, this is attributed to the fact that although there is severe inflammation within the muscle bundles and fascil planes between muscles, there is usually minimal muscle necrosis. Ferrets that underwent additional diagnostic testing were negative for canine distemper, Aleutian disease virus, feline infectious peritonitis, *Sarcocystis,* and *Bartonella*.

Additional Diagnostic Procedures

Radiologic and ultrasonographic findings in patients with DIM often reveal an enlarged spleen and/or abdominal lymph nodes, but these nonspecific findings are otherwise not contributory to the diagnosis. Exploratory surgery does not reveal pertinent gross lesions in the abdominal viscera other than splenomegaly or lymphadenomegaly. Aerobic and anaerobic bacterial cultures from various affected tissues have been negative and have not revealed a bacterial etiology for DIM. Urinalysis results from several cases included a slightly elevated pH of approximately 7 to 8 (normal range is 5.5–6.5)[21] and the presence of struvite or amorphous phosphate crystals.

PATHOLOGIC FINDINGS

The gross, histologic, and electron microscopic findings that characterize DIM have been described.[1] Gross and histologic images are illustrated in **Figs. 2–10**. Gross lesions from deceased ferrets with DIM may be inapparent or subtle in acutely affected ferrets, or quite striking in more chronic cases. Gross lesions that may be seen include red and white mottling of the esophagus; white streaks in the diaphragm, lumbar, and leg muscles; and marked atrophy of diaphragm and skeletal muscle in advanced cases.[1] Lymphadenomegaly and splenomegaly are also observed frequently.[1] Histologically, all skeletal muscle as well as heart muscle can be affected. Microscopic lesions typically are multifocal and include mild to severe suppurative to pyogranulomatous inflammation in the fascia between muscle bundles, extending into the perimysium and endomysium, and rarely causing necrosis of muscle fibers. Inflammation often extends into surrounding adipose tissue, and muscle atrophy and fibrosis may

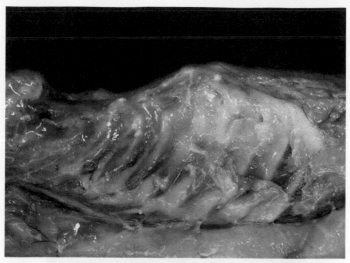

Fig. 2. Ferret, myofasciitis. Note rib cage has adequate fat stores but atrophy of intercostal muscles.

be apparent in ferrets with chronic disease. The circumferential transmural nature of the infiltrate in the muscular tunics along the entire length of the esophagus in advanced cases is possibly a pathognomonic lesion. Electron microscopic examination of the muscle reveals mitochondrial swelling, edema between myofibrils, and myofibril and Z-band disruption. No ultrastructural abnormalities are noted in leukocytes adjacent to affected muscle. All muscle groups appear to be involved in the inflammatory process, and it is likely that the clinical signs observed in patients with DIM are a result of the pain and atrophy that accompany this condition. Nonmuscular organs such as fat, brain, liver, lung, trachea, spleen, and bone marrow may also have mild neutrophilic inflammation in affected ferrets.[1] Extramedullary hematopoiesis is commonly found in the spleen and bone marrow and myeloid left shift without congestion is prominent, which distinguishes the splenic lesion from the mixed extramedullary hematopoiesis and congestion more commonly associated with splenomegaly in old ferrets. Bronchopneumonia is sometimes observed, presumably caused by aspiration associated with force feeding or regurgitation because of the esophageal lesions.

TREATMENT

One consistent characteristic of ferrets with DIM has been a general lack of response to treatment and a high mortality rate. For 3 years after DIM was first recognized, treatment with an array of antibiotics and various medications (glucocorticoids, nonsteroidal anti-inflammatory drugs, antipyretics, analgesics, interferon, and cyclosporine), along with supportive care was ultimately unsuccessful in all patients. One patient received a dose of cyclophosphamide the day before the owners elected euthanasia. Some patients seemed to temporarily respond to treatment with the immune-modulating drugs, but the patients later relapsed and succumbed to the disease. Acupuncture was used as a form of therapy in one confirmed case and one suspected case. Both owners felt that acupuncture was advantageous to their ferrets by providing temporary, palliative relief (**Fig. 11**A and B).

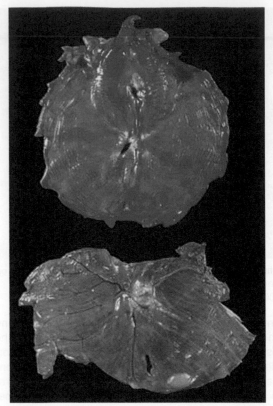

Fig 3. Ferret, myofasciitis. Note normal diaphragm of aged-matched control ferret (*top*), and atrophic muscles of affected diaphragm (*bottom*). (*From* Garner MM, Ramsell K, Schoemaker NJ, et al. Myofasciitis in the domestic ferret. Vet Pathol 2007;44(1):25–38; with permission.)

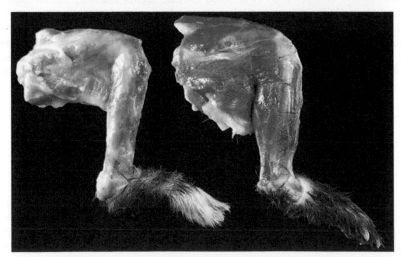

Fig. 4. Ferret, myofasciitis. Note normal hind leg of age-matched control ferret (*right*), and atrophic muscle of affected ferret (*left*). (*From* Garner MM, Ramsell K, Schoemaker NJ, et al. Myofasciitis in the domestic ferret. Vet Pathol 2007;44(1):25–38; with permission.)

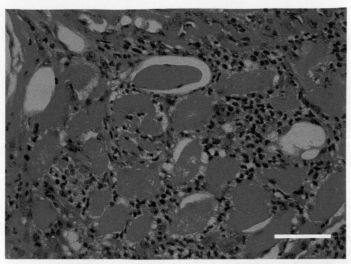

Fig. 5. Ferret, myofasciitis. Biceps femoris. Note infiltrate of neutrophils within and around myofibers, associated with myofiber displacement and necrosis (hematoxylin and eosin [H&E] stain, bar = 80 μm).

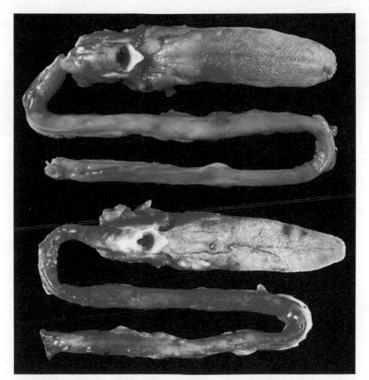

Fig. 6. Ferret, myofasciitis. Note dorsal-ventral flaccid appearance of normal esophagus (*top*) and turgid round red-white mottled appearance of affected esophagus (*bottom*). Also note atrophy of tongue and hyperkeratosis (due to secondary candidiasis) in affected ferret. (*From* Garner MM, Ramsell K, Schoemaker NJ, et al. Myofasciitis in the domestic ferret. Vet Pathol 2007;44(1):25–38; with permission.)

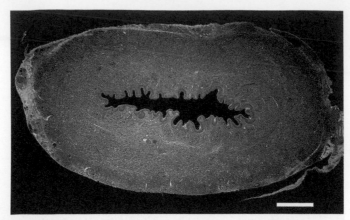

Fig. 7. Ferret, myofasciitis. Transverse section through esophagus. Note transmural circumferential inflammatory cell infiltrate that spares only the mucosa (H&E stain, bar = 270 μm). (*From* Garner MM, Ramsell K, Schoemaker NJ, et al. Myofasciitis in the domestic ferret. Vet Pathol 2007;44(1):25–38; with permission.)

Since the beginning of 2006, a few confirmed cases and several suspected cases have improved and are doing very well after receiving a combination of drugs including cyclophosphamide, prednisolone, and chloramphenicol. The recommended treatment protocol for ferrets with DIM is summarized in **Table 2**. Prednisolone and chloramphenicol without the cyclophosphamide has not resulted in recovery or even significant improvement of ferrets with DIM. Cyclophosphamide, a nitrogen-mustard derivative and chemotherapeutic agent with alkylating metabolites, has marked immunosuppressive activity and causes reduction in WBC and antibody production.[22]

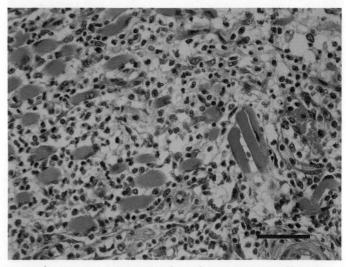

Fig. 8. Ferret, myofasciitis. Muscular tunic of esophagus. Note myofiber disarray owing to infiltrate of large numbers of neutrophils (H&E stain, bar = 160 μm). (*From* Garner MM, Ramsell K, Schoemaker NJ, et al. Myofasciitis in the domestic ferret. Vet Pathol 2007;44(1):25–38; with permission.)

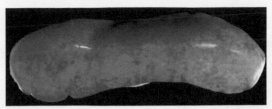

Fig. 9. Ferret, myofasciitis. Note generalized pallor of enlarged spleen. (*From* Garner MM, Ramsell K, Schoemaker NJ, et al. Myofasciitis in the domestic ferret. Vet Pathol 2007;44(1):25–38; with permission.)

In veterinary medicine, it is used both as an antineoplastic agent and as an immuno-suppressant.[22] If DIM is an immune-mediated disease, cyclophosphamide is most likely reversing or suppressing the deleterious effects of DIM via immunosuppression, but the mechanism of action of this drug in this particular disease has not been dis-cerned. Interestingly, treatment for the human myopathies polymyositis and dermato-myositis include primarily glucocorticoids and secondarily glucocorticoid-sparing agents such as azathioprine and methotrexate, but inclusion body myositis is gener-ally refractory to immunosuppressive therapy and intravenous gamma globulins.[23,24]

Three biopsy-confirmed DIM cases recovered after being treated with the recom-mended treatment protocol. One ferret died 3.5 years after onset of DIM from other causes. Two ferrets are still living at the time of this writing, approximately 3.5 years after onset of the disease. Several suspected cases appear to have recovered after receiving presumptive treatment with the DIM treatment protocol, but they were not biopsy-confirmed cases. One confirmed case began treatment for DIM 6 days after onset of signs, improved significantly over a period of a week, then relapsed and was euthanized.

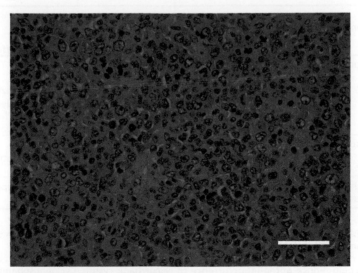

Fig. 10. Ferret, myofasciitis. Note myeloid hyperplasia in red pulp of spleen, which accounts for the splenomegaly and grossly pale appearance of the spleen (H&E stain, bar = 150 μm). (*From* Garner MM, Ramsell K, Schoemaker NJ, et al. Myofasciitis in the domestic ferret. Vet Pathol 2007;44(1):25–38; with permission.)

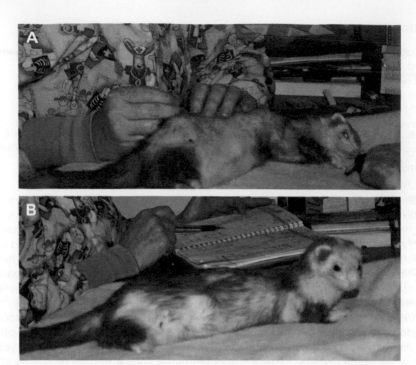

Fig. 11. A DIM-confirmed ferret before and after acupuncture treatment. The ferret is depressed and recumbent at the beginning of the session (*A*). The ferret is more alert and upright at the end of the session (*B*). (*Courtesy of* Nancy Wilson; with permission.)

Table 2
Recommended DIM treatment protocol

Drug	Suggested Dose	Potential Side Effects
Prednisolone[a]	1 mg/kg PO q 12 h for 3 months, then q 24 h until recovery has been achieved (wean off)	GI ulceration Muscle wasting Elevated liver enzymes Abdominal fat deposition Dermatologic effects PU/PD/polyphagia
Cyclophosphamide[b]	10 mg/kg on day 1, day 14, then every 4 weeks for 3 months or until recovery has been achieved	Neutropenia Hemorrhagic cystitis GI toxicity
Chloramphenicol[c] (palmitate)	50 mg/kg PO q 12 h for 6–8 weeks	Bone marrow suppression GI signs

Abbreviations: GI, gastrointestinal; PD, polydipsia; PO, oral; PU, polyuria; q, every.
   [a] Prednisolone can be made up as a "bitter-free" suspension that is more palatable than some human commercial formulations.
   [b] Subcutaneous fluids should be administered in conjunction with administration of cyclophosphamide to help reduce potential occurrence of hemorrhagic cystitis. Cyclophosphamide can be given via a subcutaneous injection. Oral cyclophosphamide is not palatable to ferrets, and partial tablets should not be given as the drug is not evenly distributed throughout the tablet. A complete blood count should be done before each cyclophosphamide treatment.
   [c] Chloramphenicol palmitate oral suspension can be made at a compounding pharmacy.

POTENTIAL ETIOLOGIES

Although bacterial infection was considered initially as a possible etiology for DIM based on the suppurative nature of the lesions, the failure of patients with DIM to respond to a variety of antibacterial drugs and the inability to demonstrate bacteria in the lesions has prompted investigation into other possibilities. Viral infections usually do not evoke such a severe suppurative inflammatory response as that observed with DIM, and no viral agents have been detected to date by electron microscopy. With the recent advent of crystal array molecular testing for the presence of virus nucleic acid in tissue, a viral etiology may be further explored. Protozoa have not been identified histologically in DIM lesions, and immunohistochemical stains have been negative for *Sarcocystis neurona*, *Neospora caninum*, and *Toxoplasma gondii*. Fungal stains and cultures have also been negative, making a fungal infection also unlikely. Affected ferrets have been fed a variety of diets and there is no known exposure to any toxic substances, so food contaminants or environmental toxins are unlikely causes of DIM.

It is noteworthy that a disease histologically indistinguishable in lesion morphology and distribution was inadvertently induced in ferrets during an experimental vaccine trial.[1] The only known commonality among ferrets suspected or confirmed to have DIM is the administration of at least 1 dose of canine distemper vaccine. Vaccines and vaccine aduvants are being investigated as a potential cause for this condition. Adjuvants can cause local tissue reactions, granulomas, or abscesses at injection sites in other species.[25] Polyarthritis, uveitis, myositis, and autoimmune reactions have been documented in vaccinated people.[25–27] Animal vaccines, unlike those produced for humans, are often produced in cell lines of the species for which the vaccine is intended, which makes contamination with potentially pathogenic, latent, or passenger viruses more likely.[25]

Since an apparent peak in suspected and confirmed cases during 2004 to 2005, the number of reported DIM cases has decreased quite dramatically over the past 3 years. Age of onset in ferrets with DIM has ranged from 11 weeks to 4 years. One ferret showed signs 1 day after being vaccinated, and another ferret, which had received only the 1 vaccination routinely given at the breeding facility, showed signs 4 years later. If DIM is vaccine-associated, it is difficult to explain why there is such a variable time interval between administration of the canine distemper vaccine and the onset of clinical signs. There may be a delayed mechanism in the development of the disease, or the disease may exist subclinically for a period of time and then progress rapidly after initial clinical signs develop. It is also not understood why some ferrets decline rapidly over a period of only a few days but others seem to remain in a relatively unchanging poor state of health for weeks or even months with supportive care.

Although ferrets have come from different breeders, it is possible there is a genetic predisposition for DIM. There are reports of a heritable predisposition for some forms of myositis in humans[28] and dogs.[15] A syndrome in closely related Akita dogs has many similarities to DIM and appears to have a genetic link.[29] In addition, vaccines, infections, certain drugs, and other factors are known to serve as triggers in development or exacerbation of autoimmune disease in genetically susceptible humans.[30] Interestingly, one ferret (half European polecat and half New Zealand ferret) that came from a private breeder died from DIM, and his father and half brother died at a young age from an illness with signs very similar to DIM. Although we have the vaccine history for the confirmed case, vaccine histories were incomplete for the related ferrets. Genetic predisposition may serve as an explanation as to why DIM in ferrets is uncommon and has such an apparently idiosyncratic response.

Disseminated idiopathic myofasciitis may be an acquired immune-mediated disease, although such diseases generally are not suppurative in nature. In humans, idiopathic inflammatory myopathies are systemic autoimmune diseases that have predominate mononuclear inflammatory cell infiltrates in the skeletal muscle.[6] Cells typically involved in the pathogenesis of disease are B-lymphocytes, T-lymphocytes, macrophages, dendritic cells, and natural killer cells.[6] References to neutrophilic myositis in humans are uncommon, with 2 case reports associating the disease to inflammatory bowel disease[31] and celiac disease.[32] Interestingly, DIM is a type of neutrophilic myositis, and inflammatory bowel disease is common in ferrets.[33]

A variety of molecular alterations occur in inflammatory myopathies of humans. Recent studies reveal that cytokines and chemokines are critically involved in the initiation and progression of the human inflammatory myopathies.[34] DM is mainly a humoral event, whereas PM and IBM are characterized by invasion of auto-aggressive cytotoxic T cells and macrophages into viable muscle fibers.[3] Although a general increase of specific chemokines occurs in all 3 inflammatory myopathies, chemokine distribution reflects the 2 different immune responses in these diseases.[3] Interleukin-21, a cytokine produced predominately by CD4+ T cells, has been reported to play an important role in tissue-damaging immune response in various organs, and neutralization of IL-21 appears to have beneficial effects of the progression of inflammatory diseases in mice.[35] Myositis-specific antibodies have been detected in humans with PM and DM and are considered useful markers for clinical diagnosis, classification, and predicting prognosis of these inflammatory myopathies.[23,36] Overexpression of the MHC class I heavy chain protein is a common feature in muscle lesions, including idiopathic myositis, and can lead to severe myositis with rapid onset of muscle weakness and pathologic change in young mice.[37] The MHC/CD8 complex is considered a specific immunopathological marker, as it distinguishes antigen-driven inflammatory cells of PM and IBM from nonspecific, secondary inflammation in other disorders such as dytrophies.[38] These are all examples of how research is progressively clarifying the biochemical pathways and processes of inflammatory myopathies. Advances in molecular immunopathology are elucidating the disease processes in human and animal myopathies and the therapeutic strategies that will be most effective in treating individual patients. Hopefully, information from other studies will guide investigations into the etiology and pathogenesis of DIM.

RECOMMENDATIONS

Ferrets suspected of having DIM should have a thorough physical examination and diagnostic tests, including a comprehensive blood panel, urinalysis, and radiographs. When signalment and clinical signs are consistent with those of DIM and a prominent neutrophilic leukocytosis is present, biopsies of skeletal muscles and any masses or enlarged lymph nodes should be surgically obtained. As DIM has a multifocal distribution, 2 to 3 external skeletal muscle biopsies are recommended from lumbar, hind leg, shoulder, or temporal regions. Animals presenting for necropsy should have a comprehensive tissue set collected for histologic examination, including the target tissues of esophagus, skeletal muscle, and heart. Paired tissue samples should be frozen for future reference.

Ferrets suspected of having DIM should receive aggressive supportive care, including supplemental feedings, fluids, and broad-spectrum antibiotics until a definitive diagnosis can be made. If a ferret is definitively diagnosed with DIM, treatment with cyclophosphamide, prednisolone, and chloramphenicol may be effective. The complete blood count should be monitored regularly in ferrets treated for DIM. Biopsy and necropsy samples should be submitted for histologic examination for diagnostic purposes and to facilitate DIM research. The American Ferret Association (www.ferret. org) has a DIM case report form that can be completed for presumptive and confirmed cases. Increased awareness of DIM and submission of accurate case reports with complete histories will contribute to our database and contribute to our investigation of this devastating disease in ferrets.

SUMMARY

DIM in ferrets is a severe inflammatory disease that primarily affects skeletal, smooth, and cardiac muscles and surrounding connective tissues. It affects male and female ferrets and is most common in ferrets younger than 18 months old. Although the disease has distinct clinical features, biopsy of skeletal muscle is the only way to get a definitive antemortem diagnosis. DIM has a high mortality rate, but the current treatment protocol has been effective in some cases. Future studies of DIM in ferrets should include continued investigation of potential infectious and vaccine-induced etiologies as well as identifying molecular pathways in the immune system and muscle lesions.

ACKNOWLEDGMENTS

The authors thank the many practitioners in private practice who contributed cases. We are also grateful to the many owners who provided valuable information about their pets. We appreciate the support of the American Ferret Association. This article is dedicated to all the ferrets that have lost their lives to this devastating disease.

REFERENCES

1. Garner MM, Ramsell K, Schoemaker NJ, et al. Myofasciitis in the domestic ferret. Vet Pathol 2007;44(1):25–38.
2. Garner M, Ramsell K. Myofasciitis: an emerging fatal disease of the domestic ferret. Exotic DVM 2006;8(3):23–5.
3. De Paepe B, Creus KK, De Bleecker JL. Chemokines in idiopathic inflammatory myopathies. Front Biosci 2008;13:2548–77.
4. Wu X, Brooks R, Komives EA, et al. Autoantibodies in canine masticatory muscle myositis recognize a novel myosin binding protein-C family member. J Immunol 2007;179(7):4939–44.
5. Orbach H, Amitai N, Barzilai O, et al. Autoantibody screen in inflammatory myopathies high prevalence of antibodies to gliadin. Ann N Y Acad Sci 2009;1173: 174–9.
6. Reed AM, Ernste F. The inflammatory milieu in idiopathic inflammatory myositis. Curr Rheumatol Rep 2009;11(4):295–301.
7. Cherin P. Inflammatory myopathies. Acta Clin Belg 2004;59:290–9.
8. Mantegazza R, Bernasconi P, Confalonieri P, et al. Inflammatory myopathies and systemic disorders: a review of immunopathogenetic mechanisms and clinical features. J Neurol 1997;244:277–87.
9. Evans J, Levesque D, Shelton GD. Canine inflammatory myopathies: a clinico-pathologic review of 200 cases. J Vet Intern Med 2004;18:679–91.
10. Lewis RM. Immune-mediated muscle disease. Vet Clin North Am Small Anim Pract 1994;24:703–10.
11. Amato AA, Barohn RJ. Evaluation and treatment of inflammatory myopathies. J Neurol Neurosurg Psychiatry 2009;80(10):1060–8.

12. Warman S, Pearson G, Barrett E, et al. Dilation of the right atrium in a dog with polymyositis and myocarditis. J Small Anim Pract 2008;49(6):302–5.

13. Clark LA, Credille KM, Murphy KE, et al. Linkage of dermatomyositis in the Shetland sheepdog to chromosome 35. Vet Dermatol 2005;16(6):392–4.

14. Wahl JM, Clark LA, Skalli O, et al. Analysis of gene transcript profiling and immunobiology in Shetland sheepdogs with dermatomyositis. Vet Dermatol 2008; 19(2):52–8.

15. Hargis AM, Haupt KH, Hegreberg GA, et al. Familial canine dermatomyositis. Initial characterization of the cutaneous and muscular lesions. Am J Pathol 1984;116:234–44.

16. Shelton GD, Cardinet GH 3rd, Bandman E, et al. Fiber type-specific autoantibodies in a dog with eosinophilic myositis. Muscle Nerve 1985;8:783–90.

17. O'Toole D, McAllister MM, Griggs K. Iatrogenic compressive lumbar myelopathy and radiculopathy in adult cattle following injection of an adjuvanted bacterin into loin muscle: histopathology and ultrastructure. J Vet Diagn Invest 1995;7: 237–44.

18. O'Toole D, Steadman L, Raisbeck M, et al. Myositis, lameness, and recumbency after use of water-in-oil adjuvanted vaccines in near term beef cattle. J Vet Diagn Invest 2005;17(1):23–31.

19. Ytterberg SR. Animal models of myopathy. Curr Opin Rheumatol 1991;3:934–40.

20. Gendek-Kubiak H, Gendek EG. Histological pictures of muscles and an evaluation of cellular infiltrations in human polymyositis/dermatomyositis, as compared to the findings in experimental Guinea pig myositis. Cell Mol Biol Lett 2003;8(2): 297–303.

21. Hoeffer HL. Clinical techniques in ferrets. In: Proceedings of the Atlantic Coast Veterinary Conference. Atlantic City, October 9–11, 2001.

22. Plumb DC. Veterinary drug handbook. 5th edition. Ames (IA): Blackwell; 2005. 203–206.

23. Dimachkie MM, Barohn RJ. Idiopathic inflammatory myopathies. Front Neurol Neurosci 2009;26:126–46.

24. Pongratz D. Therapeutic options in autoimmune inflammatory myopathies (dermatomyositis, polymyositis, inclusion body myositis). J Neurol 2006;253(Suppl 5): V64–5.

25. Green CE, Schultz RD. Immunoprophylaxis. In: Infectious diseases of the dog and cat. 3rd edition. Philadelphia: WB Saunders; 2006. p. 1069–119.

26. Hanissian AS, Jaupt KH, Hegreberg GA, et al. Vasculitis and myositis secondary to rubella vaccination. Arch Neurol 1973;3:202–4.

27. Jani FM, Gray JP. Influenza vaccine and dermatomyositis. Vaccine 1994;15:1984.

28. Guis S, Mattei JP, Nicoli F, et al. Identical twins with macrophagic myofasciitis: genetic susceptibility and triggering by aluminic vaccine adjuvants? Arthritis Rheum 2002;47:543–5.

29. Dougherty SA, Center SA, Shaw EE, et al. Juvenile onset polyarthritis in Akitas. J Am Vet Med Assoc 1991;198:849–55.

30. Cohen AD, Schoenfeld Y. Vaccine-induced autoimmunity. J Autoimmun 1996; 9(6):699–703.

31. Qureshi JA, Staugaitis SM, Calabrese LH. Neutrophilic myositis: an extraintestinal manifestation of ulcerative colitis. J Clin Rheumatol 2002;8(2):85–8.

32. Alawneh K, Ashley C, Carlson JA. Neutrophilic myositis as a manifestation of celiac disease: a case report. Clin Rheumatol 2008;27(Suppl 1):S11–3.

33. Burgess M, Garner M. Clinical aspects of inflammatory bowel disease in ferrets. Exotic DVM 2002;4(2):29–34.

34. De Paepe B, Creus KK, De Bleecker JL. Role of cytokines and chemokines in idiopathic inflammatory myopathies. Curr Opin Rheumatol 2009;21(6):610–6.
35. Monteleone G, Sarra M, Pallone F. Interleukin-21 in T cell-mediated diseases. Discov Med 2009;8(42):113–7.
36. Mimori T, Imura Y, Nakashima R, et al. Autoantibodies in idiopathic inflammatory myopathy: an update on clinical and pathophysiological significance. Curr Opin Rheumatol 2007;19(6):523–9.
37. Li CK, Knopp P, Moncrieffe H, et al. Overexpression of MHC class I heavy chain protein in young skeletal muscle leads to sever myositis: implications for juvenile myositis. Am J Pathol 2009;175(3):1030–40.
38. Dalakas MC. Inflammatory disorders of muscle: progress in polymyositis, dermatomyositis and inclusion body myositis. Curr Opin Neurol 2004;17(5):561–7.

Index

Note: Page numbers of article titles are in **boldface** type.

A

Abdominal (coelomic) enlargement, in koi, 340–341
    enlarged ovaries causing, 342
Abdominal (coelomic) neoplasia, in koi, 343–344
Abdominal radiographs, for rabbit gastrointestinal syndrome, 529–531
Abdominocentesis, for internal disorders, of koi, 337–338
    of select species, 459–460
Acupuncture, for disseminated idiopathic myofascitis, in ferrets, 565, 570
Adenocarcinomas, renal disease related to, in avians, 401
Adrenal glands, microscopic lesions of, with proventricular dilatation disease,
    in psittacines, 475–476
Adrenalectomy, for adrenocortical neoplasia, in ferrets, 448
Adrenocortical disease, in ferrets, 439. See also *Adrenocortical neoplasia.*
Adrenocortical neoplasia, in ferrets, **439–452**
    description of, 443
    diagnostics for, 445–446
    histopathology of, 444
    incidence vs. prevalence of, 443–444
        sterilization impact on, 444–445
    insulinoma vs., 439–443
    signs and symptoms of, 445–446
    summary overview of, 439, 449
    therapeutics for, 446–449
        medical therapies as, 446–448
        of conditions secondary to adrenocortical disease, 448–449
Alanine aminotransferase (ALT), disseminated idiopathic myofascitis and, in ferrets, 564
    hepatic disorders and, in avians, 417
    insulinoma and, in ferrets, 440–441
    renal damage and, in avians, 404
Alkaline phosphatase (ALP), hepatic disorders and, in avians, 417
    renal damage and, in avians, 404
Allopurinol, for gout, in avians, 407
Alopecia, with adrenocortical neoplasia, in ferrets, 445
    with hyperthyroidism, in guinea pigs, 510
Amantadine hydrochloride, for proventricular dilatation disease, avian bornavirus and,
    505–506
        in psittacines, 488
Aminoglycoside toxicity, renal disease related to, in avians, 400, 407
Amphibians, metabolic bone diseases in, **375–392**
    calcium homeostasis and, 376–379
    diagnostics for, 376, 381–384
    diet factors of, 386–389

Amphibians (*continued*)
    husbandry factors of, 381, 384–386
    injury prevention for, 389
    pyramiding and, 389
    ramifications of, 381
    summary overview of, 375–376
    types of, 379–381
Amyloidosis, renal disease related to, in avians, 398
Anal tape test, for pin worms, in select species, 458
Analgesia, for rabbit gastrointestinal syndrome, 527, 539–540
Anastrozole (Arimidex), for adrenocortical neoplasia, in ferrets, 448
Androgen overproduction, with adrenocortical neoplasia, in ferrets, 446
    therapeutics for, 448
Anemia, with hepatic disorders, in avians, 423
    with rabbit gastrointestinal syndrome, hypovolemic shock and, 535
Anesthesia, for blood sample collection, of select species, 455–456
    for fecal sample collection, of select species, 458
    for koi, 335–336, 338–339
        monitoring during, 337, 339–340
    for physical examination, of select species, 454–455
    for radiography, of select species, 461
Antibiotics, for coronavirus-associated disease, in ferrets, 554–555
    for disseminated idiopathic myofascitis, in ferrets, 565, 571–572
    for dystocia, in psittacines, 432
    for internal disorders, in koi, 340–341
        of select species, 466–467
    for renal disease, in avians, 407
Antibody tests, for coronavirus-associated diseases, in ferrets, 549–550
    for proventricular dilatation disease, avian bornavirus and, 502
        in psittacines, 473, 477
Antidiarrheals, for coronavirus-associated disease, in ferrets, 554–555
Antigen tests, for internal disorders, of select species, serum, 458
        urine, 459
    for proventricular dilatation disease, in psittacines, 477, 498
Antioxidants, for coronavirus-associated diseases, in ferrets, 555–556
    for proventricular dilatation disease, in psittacines, 489
Antithyroid drugs, for hyperthyroidism, in guinea pigs, 515–516
Antiulcer antibiotics, for coronavirus-associated disease, in ferrets, 555
Antivirals, for proventricular dilatation disease, avian bornavirus and, 505–506
    in psittacines, 488
Aquatic species, metabolic bone disease in, calcium supplementation for, 388–389
Arginine vasotocin, for dystocia, in lizards, 364–365
    in snakes, 369
Ascites, with hepatic disorders, in avians, 423–424
Aspartate aminotransferase (AST), dystocia and, in lizards, 364
    hepatic disorders and, in avians, 417–418
    insulinoma and, in ferrets, 440–441
    renal damage and, in avians, 404
Aspiration, as dystocia therapy, in psittacines, 433
    fine-needle, of thyroid gland, in guinea pigs, 511–512
    of tissue and fluid, for internal disorders, in koi, 334, 341, 344–345

Aspirin (Ascriptin), for coronavirus-associated diseases, in ferrets, 554
Atrophic muscle, with disseminated idiopathic myofascitis, in ferrets, 564–569
Autoimmune diseases, avian bornavirus and, 499–500
    disseminated idiopathic myofascitis as, in ferrets, 561, 572
Avian bornavirus (ABV), proventricular dilatation disease related to, **495–508**
        autoimmunity and, 499–500
        control and prevention of, 505–506
        description of, 473–474
        diagnosis of, 501–502
        DNA studies of, 496–497
        experimental disease examples, 500–501
          evidence for, 500
          in cockatiels, 501
          in mallards, 500
          in Patagonian conures, 501
        immunohistochemistry of, 477–478, 484
        in other avian species, 505
        in psittacine species, 495–505
        in the eye, 499–500
        isolation of, 497–498
        molecular and serology assays of, 482–484
        pathogenesis of, 498–499
        prevention of, 490
        summary overview of, 495–496, 506
        transmission of, 502–505
          ABV shedding and, 503–505
          fecal-oral route for, 503
          respiratory route for, 503
        viral description of, 497
Avian paramyxovirus (APMV), proventricular dilatation disease virus vs., 473
Avians, avian bornavirus in, **495–508**. See also *Avian bornavirus (ABV)*.
        scope of species detected, 495, 505. See also *Psittacines.*
    biopsies of, for proventricular dilatation disease, 482–483, 502
        for therapy monitoring, 490
    hepatic disorders of, **413–427**
        diagnosing dysfunction in, 415–422
          clinical pathologic analysis for, 415–418
          clinical signs and, 415
          hepatic biopsy for, 421–422
          imaging for, 418–421
          patient history and, 415
        liver anatomy review for, 413–414
        liver functions and, 414–415
        medical management of, 422–425
          for anemia, 423
          for ascites, 423–424
          for encephalopathy, 423
          nutraceuticals in, 424
          nutritional support in, 423
          targeted plans for, 422–423
        secondary complications of, 423

Avians (*continued*)
    summary overview of, 424–425
necropsy of, for proventricular dilatation disease, 496, 502
proventricular dilatation disease in, **471–494**. See also *Proventricular dilatation disease (PDD)*.
    avian bornavirus and, **495–508**. See also *Avian bornavirus (ABV)*.
psittacine. See *Psittacines*.
renal diseases of, 395–408
    clinical signs of, 395
    diagnostics for, 402–406
        advanced imaging as, 405
        bloodwork as, 402–403
        murexide test as, 406
        N-acetyl-β-D-glucosaminidase as, 404
        radiographs as, 405
        renal biopsy as, 405–406
        ultrasound as, 405
        urate character as, 403–404
        urinalysis as, 403
        urine enzymes as, 404
    infectious causes of, 396–397
        bacteria as, 396
        fungi as, 396–397
        parasites as, 397
        viruses as, 396
    noninfectious causes of, 397–402
        amyloidosis as, 398
        congenital diseases as, 401
        gout as, 399–400
        lipidosis as, 398–399
        myoglobinuric nephrosis as, 399
        neoplasia as, 401
        nutrition as, 397–398
        toxicity as, 400–401
        urolithiasis as, 402
    summary overview of, 393, 395–396, 408
    treatment of, 406–408
        antibiotics for, 407
        fluid support in, 406
        for gout/hyperuricemia, 407–408
        nutrition in, 407
        principles for, 406
renal system of, **393–411**
    anatomy of, 393–394
    diseases of, 395–408
    injury to, 395, 404
    physiology of, 393–395
    assessment of, 402–403
summary overview of, 393, 408

B

B vitamins, for proventricular dilatation disease, in psittacines, 489
Bacterial infections, internal disorders related to, in koi, 334, 340–341, 344–345
    renal disease related to, in avians, 396
Barium studies, for internal disorders, in koi, 336–337
        in select species, 462
    for proventricular dilatation disease, in psittacines, 480–481
Bicalutamide (Casodex), for adrenocortical neoplasia, in ferrets, 448
Bile acid assays, for hepatic disorders, in avians, 418
Bile pigment nephrosis, in avians, 403–404
Bile/bile salts, in avians, hepatic disorders impact on, 417–418
        normal physiology of, 413–414
Biochemistry tests, for adrenocortical neoplasia, in ferrets, 446
    for coronavirus-associated diseases, in ferrets, 550
    for disseminated idiopathic myofascitis, in ferrets, 564
    for dystocia, in psittacines, 432
    for hepatic disorders, in avians, 415–417
    for internal disorders, in koi, 334
    for metabolic bone disease, in reptiles and amphibians, 381–382
        treatment options based on, 389–390
    for proventricular dilatation disease, in psittacines, 479
        for therapy monitoring, 489
    for rabbit gastrointestinal syndrome, 531
Biopsy(ies), bone, for metabolic bone disease, in reptiles and amphibians, 384
    crop, for proventricular dilatation disease, in psittacines, 482–483
        for therapy monitoring, 490
    endoscopic, for internal disorders, of select species, 465–466
    for proventricular dilatation disease, in birds, 482–483, 502
        for therapy monitoring, 490
    hepatic (liver), for hepatic disorders, in avians, 421–422
        in koi, 342
    internal organ, of koi, 338, 342, 344
    muscle, for disseminated idiopathic myofascitis, in ferrets, 569, 572–573
    pancreatic, for insulinoma, in ferrets, 441
    renal (kidney), for metabolic bone disease, in reptiles and amphibians, 384
        for renal disease, in avians, 405–406
    skin, fin, and gill, for internal disorders, of koi, 334, 337
    thyroid, in guinea pigs, 511–512
Birds. See *Avians.*
Bisphosphonates, for metabolic bone disease, in reptiles and amphibians, 390
Blood pressure, with hypovolemic shock, in rabbits, 533, 537
Blood products, for hypovolemic shock, with rabbit gastrointestinal syndrome, 531, 535
Blood sample collection, for internal disorders, of select species, 455–457
Blood supply, to kidneys, in avians, 393–394
    to liver, in avians, hepatic disorders and, 417–418
        review of normal, 413–414
Body weight, hypothyroidism and, in guinea pigs, 521
    in dehydration assessment, for rabbit gastrointestinal syndrome, 537
    of koi, length relationship to, 342–343

Bone biopsy, for metabolic bone disease, in reptiles and amphibians, 384
Bone density scan, for metabolic bone disease, in reptiles and amphibians, 383, 387
Bone marrow, cytology of, for neoplasia, in select species, 460–461
    disseminated idiopathic myofascitis involvement of, in ferrets, 565
Borna disease virus (BDV), proventricular dilatation disease related to, 474, 497
        control and prevention of, 506
        molecular and serology assays of, 484
Bornaviruses, in avians. See also *Avian bornavirus (ABV)*.
    proventricular dilatation disease related to, 473–474. See also *Proventricular dilatation disease (PDD)*.
        immunohistochemistry of, 477–478, 484
Bradycardia, with hypovolemic shock, in rabbits, 533
Brain lesions, in select species, diagnostic approaches to, 464
    microscopic, with proventricular dilatation disease, in psittacines, 475–477
        immunohistochemistry of, 477–478
    with coronavirus-associated diseases, in ferrets, 547, 549
Breeding behavior, in chelonians, 350, 354
    in lizards, 361
    in snakes, 366

C

Calcidiol, metabolic bone disease and, in reptiles and amphibians, 382
Calcitonin, metabolic bone disease and, in reptiles and amphibians, 376, 378–379
        supplementation with, 390
Calcitriol, metabolic bone disease and, in reptiles and amphibians, 376, 379
        supplementation with, 390
Calcium carbonate, for metabolic bone diseases, in reptiles and amphibians, 387
Calcium citrate, for metabolic bone diseases, in reptiles and amphibians, 387
Calcium EDTA toxicity, renal disease related to, in avians, 400
Calcium homeostasis, metabolic bone disease and, in reptiles and amphibians, 376–379
        depletion factors of, 380–381
        diagnostics for, 381–382
        treatment options based in, 389–390
Calcium phosphate, for metabolic bone diseases, in reptiles and amphibians, 387
Calcium supplementation, for metabolic bone diseases, in reptiles and amphibians,
    IV and/or IM options for, 390
        oral options for, 386–388
        post-excision of parathyroid gland, in guinea pigs, 517–518
Calcium-enhanced water, for metabolic bone disease, in reptiles and amphibians,
    388–389
Carbimazole, for hyperthyroidism, in guinea pigs, 515–516
Cecum, radiographic findings of, with rabbit gastrointestinal syndrome, 529–530
Celecoxib, for proventricular dilatation disease, in psittacines, 487–488
Celiotomy, for dystocia, in snakes, 368–369
    for ovariectomy, in lizards, 362–363
        in snakes, 368
Cerebrospinal fluid analysis, for internal disorders, of select species, 464
Chelonians, reproductive disorders in, 349–359
        dystocia as, 353–356
        follicular stasis as, 353
        imaging of. See *specific pathology*.

infertility as, 350–352
    normal reproduction vs., 349–350
    phallus prolapse as, 357, 359
    yolk coelomitis as, 356–358
Chemical restraint, for blood sample collection, of select species, 455–456
    for gastrointestinal syndrome evaluation, of rabbits, 527–528
    for physical examination, of select species, 454–455
    for radiography, of select species, 461
Chemokines, disseminated idiopathic myofascitis and, in ferrets, 572
Chlorambucil (Leukeran), for coronavirus-associated diseases, in ferrets, 552
    for disseminated idiopathic myofascitis, in ferrets, 568, 570, 572
Cholecalciferol, metabolic bone disease and, in reptiles and amphibians, 375
        calcium homeostasis and, 378–379
        supplementation with, 387–388
Cisapride, for rabbit gastrointestinal syndrome, 538–539
Clearance tests, for hepatic disorders, in avians, 415, 418
Cloaca/cloacal opening, eggs manually milked out of, in snakes, 369
    normal, in chelonians, 350–351
    in lizards, 358
    in snakes, 365–366
Clostridium vaccination, for proventricular dilatation disease, in psittacines, 488
Coagulopathy, with hepatic disorders, in avians, 416, 422
        medical management of, 423
Cockatiels, experimental avian bornavirus disease in, 501, 506
Coelioscopy, for internal disorders, in koi, 338
Coelomic (abdominal) cavity, enlargement of, in koi, 340–341
        enlarged ovaries causing, 342
    hepatic disorders and, in avians, 414, 416, 422–423
    neoplasia of, in koi, 343–344
Coelomitis, yolk, in chelonians, 356–358
    in snakes, 370
Colchicine, for gout, in avians, 408
Collapsed egg, in psittacines, 433
Colloids, for hypovolemic shock, with rabbit gastrointestinal syndrome, 531, 533
Colon, radiographic findings of, with rabbit gastrointestinal syndrome, 529–530
Complete blood counts (CBCs), for adrenocortical neoplasia, in ferrets, 446
    for disseminated idiopathic myofascitis, in ferrets, 564, 572
    for dystocia, in psittacines, 432
    for hepatic disorders, in avians, 415–417
    for internal disorders, of select species, 456, 458
    for metabolic bone disease, in reptiles and amphibians, 381
    for proventricular dilatation disease, in psittacines, 479, 489
Computed tomography (CT), of hepatic disorders, in avians, 419–420
        PET scan with, 421
    of internal disorders, in koi, 340–343
        in select species, 465
    of renal disease, in avians, 405
    of thyroid gland, 511, 514
Congenital diseases, renal disease related to, in avians, 401
Contrast imaging studies, for internal disorders, of koi, 336–337
        of select species, 462–464

Contrast (*continued*)
  for proventricular dilatation disease, in psittacines, 479–481
Copulation, in chelonians, 352
  in lizards, 358, 360–361
Coronavirus-associated diseases, in ferrets, **543–560**
  clinical signs of, 545, 549
  description of, 544–545
  diagnosis of, 549–551
    antibody tests for, 549–550
    biochemical changes and, 550
    ELISA testing, 550
    PCR-based testing, 544, 550
    RT-PCR-based testing, 550–551
    scope of testing for, 549
    serum protein electrophoresis for, 550
  differential diagnosis of, 549, 551
  epizootic catarrhal enteritis as, 543–544
  pathogenesis of, 547–548
  pathology of, 545–549
    brain lesions, 547, 549
    granulomatous lesions, 545–546
      vascular involvement of, 547–549
    histologic lesions, 547–548
    immunohistochemistry findings in, 547, 549–551
    less-specific gross lesions, 546
    pyogranulomatous lesions, 547–548
    transmission electron microscopy in, 547
  prevention of, 556
  summary overview of, 543, 556
  treatment of, 551–556
    antioxidants in, 555–556
    immune modulation in, 552–553
    immune suppression in, 552
    nutritional support in, 555
    symptomatic, 554–555
    vasculitis medications for, 553–554
Cortisol overproduction, in ferrets, 439. See also *Adrenocortical neoplasia.*
Counseling, for psittacines owners, on proventricular dilatation disease, 485–486
COX-1 inhibitors, for proventricular dilatation disease, in psittacines, 486–487
COX-2 inhibitors, for proventricular dilatation disease, in psittacines, 486–488
Cranial vena cava, as venipuncture site, for select species, 457
Creatine kinase, disseminated idiopathic myofascitis and, in ferrets, 564
  renal damage and, in avians, 403–404
Creatinine kinase, hepatic disorders and, in avians, 417–418
Crop biopsy, for proventricular dilatation disease, in psittacines, 482–483
  for therapy monitoring, 490
Crop cytology, for proventricular dilatation disease, in psittacines, 479
Crystalloids, isotonic, for hypovolemic shock, with rabbit gastrointestinal syndrome,
  531, 533–535
Cultures, for disseminated idiopathic myofascitis, in ferrets, 564
  for internal disorders, in koi, 334, 341

of select species, 458–459
    cytologic sampling and, 459–461
for proventricular dilatation disease, in psittacines, 473
    fecal vs. crop, 479
of hepatic samples, in avians, 422, 424
Cyclophosphamide (Cytoxan), for coronavirus-associated diseases, in ferrets, 552
    for disseminated idiopathic myofascitis, in ferrets, 568, 570, 572
Cyprinus carpio. See *Koi.*
Cystocentesis, for urine collection, in select species, 459
Cysts, renal, in avians, 401
Cytokines, disseminated idiopathic myofascitis and, in ferrets, 572
Cytology, crop, for proventricular dilatation disease, in psittacines, 479
    fecal, for internal disorders, of select species, 459–461
        for proventricular dilatation disease, in psittacines, 479
    for internal disorders, in koi, 334
    of abdominal samples, in select species, 459–460
    of bone marrow, in select species, 460–461
    of neoplasia, in select species, 460
    of reproductive tract, in select species, 460
    of respiratory tract, in select species, 459–460
    of thoracic samples, in select species, 459

D

Debulking agents, for adrenocortical neoplasia, in ferrets, 448
Decompensatory phase, of hypovolemic shock, with rabbit gastrointestinal syndrome, 532–533, 535
Dehydration, with rabbit gastrointestinal syndrome, fluid therapy for, 537–538
    based on deficit estimations, 536–537
Dental disease, in select species, cytologic sampling of, 460–461
    endoscopic examination of, 465–466
    imaging of, 465
Deslorelin acetate (Suprelorin), for adrenocortical neoplasia, in ferrets, 447
Diaphragm, gross vs. histologic findings in, with disseminated idiopathic myofascitis, in ferrets, 564, 566
Diarrhea, with coronavirus-associated disease, in ferrets, 554–555
Diazoxide (Proglycem), for insulinoma, in ferrets, 442
Diet factors, of metabolic bone diseases, in reptiles and amphibians, 386–389
    of rabbit gastrointestinal syndrome, 526, 529–530, 534
Diet modification, for insulinoma, in ferrets, 442–443
Diet therapy. See also *Nutritional support.*
    for metabolic bone diseases, in reptiles and amphibians, 386–388, 390
    for proventricular dilatation disease, in psittacines, 489
Digestive system. See also *Gastrointestinal tract (GIT).*
    abnormalities of, in koi, 338, 341
    proventricular dilatation disease and, in psittacines, 475, 478
Disinfectants, for avian bornavirus control, 505
Disseminated idiopathic myofascitis (DIM), in ferrets, **561–575**
        clinical signs of, 562–564
        diagnosis of, 564
            additional procedures for, 564

Disseminated (*continued*)
        hematology results in, 564
        recommendations for, 572
     pathologic findings with, 564–565
        gross and histologic images of, 564–569, 572
     potential etiologies of, 571–572
     signalment and, 562, 572
     summary overview of, 561–562, 573
     treatment of, 565, 568–570
        recommended protocol for, 568, 570
        supportive care in, 565, 572–573
     vaccine histories and, 562, 571
DNA microarrays. See also *Nucleotide sequencing.*
   of proventricular dilatation disease virus, 473, 496
Doppler evaluation, color flow, of adrenocortical neoplasia, in ferrets, 446
   of blood pressure, with hypovolemic shock, in rabbits, 533, 537
Doxorubicin, for insulinoma, in ferrets, 443
Doxycycline (Vibramycin), for coronavirus-associated diseases, in ferrets, 553–554
Drug therapy. See also *specific drug, e.g.,* Celeoxib.
   for internal disorders, of select species, 466–467
Dual energy x-ray absorptiometry (DXA) scan, for metabolic bone disease,
   in reptiles and amphibians, 383, 387
Dusting, calcium, for metabolic bone diseases, in reptiles and amphibians, 388
Dystocia, in chelonians, 353–356
   in lizards, 363–365
   in psittacines, 431
      assessment of, 431
      clinical signs of, 431–432
      description of, 431
      diagnosis of, 431
      therapy of, 431–434
   in select species, ultrasound evaluation of, 465
   in snakes, 367–370

E

Echocardiography, for anesthesia monitoring, of koi, 337–338
Egg binding, in koi, 342–343
   preovulatory. See *Follicular stasis.*
Egg development, failure of, in chelonians, 352
Egg fertilization, in chelonians, 350
Egg incubation, parameters for, of chelonians, 352
Egg production. See also *Folliculogenesis.*
   chronic, in psittacines, 430–431
   failure within normal periods. See *Dystocia.*
   normal, in lizards, 358
      in snakes, 366
Egg retention. See *Dystocia.*
Egg rupture, with dystocia, in psittacines, 433
Electrocardiography (ECG), for anesthesia monitoring, of koi, 339–340
Electrolyte regulation, physiology of, in avians, 394
Electron microscopy (EM), of disseminated idiopathic myofascitis, in ferrets, 564–565

of proventricular dilatation disease virus, 473
Encephalopathy, hepatic, in avians, medical management of, 423
Endoscopy, for internal disorders evaluation, of koi, 338, 341
    of select species, 459, 465–466
  for removal of multiple eggs in oviduct, in psittacines, 433–434
  for renal disease evaluation, in avians, 405–406
Environmental factors, of internal disorders. See *Husbandry.*
Enzyme activity profiles, for hepatic disorders, in avians, 417
Enzyme-linked immunosorbent assay (ELISA), for avian bornavirus, 501–502
  for coronavirus-associated diseases, in ferrets, 550
  for internal disorders, of select species, 458
Epididymis, of psittacines, 437
Epizootic catarrhal enteritis (ECE), in ferrets, 543–544
Esophagus, gross vs. histologic findings in, with disseminated idiopathic myofascitis, in ferrets, 567–568
Ethanol injection, percutaneous, for hyperthyroidism, in guinea pigs, 517
Excision. See *Surgical excision.*
Exploratory surgery, for disseminated idiopathic myofascitis, in ferrets, 564
  for insulinoma, in ferrets, 441
  for internal disorders, in koi, 338, 343–344
Eye, avian bornavirus in, 499–500

F

Fall prevention, for reptiles and amphibians, with metabolic bone disease, 389
Fecal analysis, for internal disorders, of select species, 458
  for proventricular dilatation disease, in psittacines, 479
Fecal-oral transmission, of avian bornavirus, 503
Feline coronavirus (FCoV), in ferrets, 543–544
Feline infectious peritonitis (FIP), in ferrets, 543, 545, 550–551
Femoral pores, as gender-specific trait, in lizards, 359
Ferret enteric coronavirus (FRECV), in ferrets, 543–544, 551
Ferret systemic coronavirus (FRSCV), in ferrets, 543–545
    clinical signs of, 545
    diagnosis of, 549–551
    pathogenesis of, 547–548
    pathology of, 545–549
    treatment of, 551–556
Ferrets, adrenocortical neoplasia in, **439–452**
    description of, 443
    diagnostics for, 445–446
    histopathology of, 444
    incidence vs. prevalence of, 443–444
      sterilization impact on, 444–445
    insulinoma vs., 439–443
    signs and symptoms of, 445–446
    summary overview of, 439, 449
    therapeutics for, 446–449
      medical therapies as, 446–448
      of conditions secondary to adrenocortical disease, 448–449
  coronavirus-associated diseases in, **543–560**

Ferrets (*continued*)
    clinical signs of, 545, 549
    description of, 544–545
    diagnosis of, 549–551
        antibody tests for, 549–550
        biochemical changes and, 550
        ELISA testing, 550
        PCR-based testing, 544, 550
        RT-PCR-based testing, 550–551
        scope of testing for, 549
        serum protein electrophoresis for, 550
    differential diagnosis of, 549, 551
    epizootic catarrhal enteritis as, 543–544
    pathogenesis of, 547–548
    pathology of, 545–549
        brain lesions, 547, 549
        granulomatous lesions, 545–546
            vascular involvement of, 547–549
            histologic lesions, 547–548
            immunohistochemistry findings in, 547, 549–551
            less-specific gross lesions, 546
            pyogranulomatous lesions, 547–548
            transmission electron microscopy in, 547
        prevention of, 556
        summary overview of, 543, 556
        treatment of, 551–556
            antioxidants in, 555–556
            immune modulation in, 552–553
            immune suppression in, 552
            nutritional support in, 555
            symptomatic, 554–555
            vasculitis medications for, 553–554
    disseminated idiopathic myofascitis in, **561–575**
    clinical signs of, 562–564
    diagnosis of, 564
        additional procedures for, 564
        hematology results in, 564
        recommendations for, 572
    pathologic findings with, 564–565
        gross and histologic images of, 564–569, 572
    potential etiologies of, 571–572
    signalment and, 562, 572
    summary overview of, 561–562, 573
    treatment of, 565, 568–570
        recommended protocol for, 568, 570
        supportive care in, 565, 572–573
    vaccine histories and, 562, 571
    insulinoma in, **439–452**
        adrenocortical neoplasia vs., 443–449
        description of, 439–440
        diagnostics for, 440–441

summary overview of, 439, 449
therapeutics for, 441–443
definitive treatment in, 443
diet modification as, 442–443
for hypoglycemic episode management, 441–442
palliative therapy as, 442
Fin biopsy, for internal disorders, of koi, 334, 337
Finasteride (Proscar/Propecia), for adrenocortical neoplasia, in ferrets, 448
Fine-needle aspirate, of thyroid gland, in guinea pigs, 511–512
Fish, ornamental, internal disorders of, **333–347**. See also *Koi.*
Fluid therapy, for dystocia, in psittacines, 432
for internal disorders, of select species, 466
for metabolic bone disease, in reptiles and amphibians, 390
for rabbit gastrointestinal syndrome, 531–537
dehydration as focus of, 537–538
deficit calculations for, 536–537
hypovolemic shock as focus of, 532–536
initial decision-making on, 528
maintenance fluids calculation, 537–538
oral vs. IV, 528–529
phases of, 531–532
plan for, 531
for renal disease, in avians, 406
^{18}F-Fluorodeoxyglucose (FDG) PET scan (FDG-PET), for hepatic disorders, in avians, 421
Fluoroscopy, contrast, for internal disorders, in select species, 462
for proventricular dilatation disease, in psittacines, 481–482
Flutamide (Eulexin), for adrenocortical neoplasia, in ferrets, 448
Follicular stasis, in chelonians, 353
in lizards, 361–363
in snakes, 367–368
Follicules, retained. See *Follicular stasis.*
Folliculogenesis, in chelonians, 350, 352
Foreign body(ies), endoscopic retrieval of, in koi, 341
in select species, 466
rabbit gastrointestinal syndrome related to, 536
Fracture management, with metabolic bone disease, in reptiles and amphibians, 390
Fungal infections, renal disease related to, in avians, 396–397

G

Gallbladder, in avians, 413
Gamma-glutamyltransferase (GGT), hepatic disorders and, in avians, 417–418
Ganglioneuritis, with proventricular dilatation disease, in psittacines, 475–476, 485
Gas accumulation, intestinal, rabbit gastrointestinal syndrome related to, 525, 529–530, 532–533
Gas (swim) bladder, abnormalities of, in koi, 344–345
Gastric repletion, rabbit gastrointestinal syndrome related to, 529–530, 534
Gastroenteritis, rabbit gastrointestinal syndrome related to, 525–526
Gastrointestinal impaction, rabbit gastrointestinal syndrome related to, 525–526, 529
Gastrointestinal obstruction, in koi, 341
rabbit gastrointestinal syndrome related to, 525–526, 529, 531

Gastrointestinal stasis, in rabbits, **525–541**. See also *Rabbit gastrointestinal syndrome (RGIS)*.

Gastrointestinal tract (GIT), coronavirus-associated disease symptoms in, in ferrets, 545, 549

    symptomatic treatment of, 554–555

  disorders of, in koi, 338, 341

    in rabbits. See *Rabbit gastrointestinal syndrome (RGIS)*.

    in select species, abdominocentesis for, 459–460

      radiographs for, 462–464

    metabolic bone diseases and, in reptiles and amphibians, 378, 380

      gut loading and, 387–388

    proventricular dilatation disease signs in, in psittacines, 478–479, 495–496

      medical treatment of, 486, 488–489

      microscopic lesions as, 475–477

Gastroprotectant therapy, for coronavirus-associated disease, in ferrets, 554

Gender identification, for chelonians, 350, 352

  for lizards, 358–359

  for snakes, 366–367

Genetic studies, of adrenocortical neoplasia, in ferrets, 445

  of disseminated idiopathic myofasciitis, in ferrets, 571

  of insulinomas, in ferrets, 440

  of proventricular dilatation disease virus, 473–474

    avian bornavirus and, 497–498

    in psittacines, 482–484

Gill biopsy, for internal disorders, of koi, 334, 337

Gingival mass, biopsy of, in hedgehog, 460–461

Glomerular filtration rate (GFR), in avians, 394

    assessment of, 402

    injury impact on, 395

  in reptiles and amphibians, metabolic bone disease and, 383

Glucocorticoids, for insulinoma, in ferrets, 442

Glucose level, blood, in hypovolemic shock, with rabbit gastrointestinal syndrome, 535

    with insulinoma, in ferrets, emergency management of, 441–442

      fasting blood, 440

Glutamate dehydrogenase, renal damage and, in avians, 404

Glutamyl dehydrogenase (GLDH), hepatic disorders and, in avians, 417–418

Glycogen production, hepatic, in avians, 414

Gonadal neoplasms, surgical excision of, in koi, 338–339

Gonadectomy, adrenocortical neoplasia incidence correlated to, in ferrets, 444–445

Gout, in avians, articular, 399–400

    dehydration and, 399

    nutrition and, 397

    treatment of, 407–408

    visceral, 399–400

Granulomatous lesions, with coronavirus-associated diseases, in ferrets, 545–546

    vascular involvement of, 547–549

Gross lesions, with coronavirus-associated diseases, in ferrets, 546

  with disseminated idiopathic myofasciitis, in ferrets, 564–569

Guinea pigs, internal disorders of. See *Rodents*.

  thyroid pathologies in, **509–523**

    hyperthyroidism as, clinical presentations of, 510

clinical signs of, 510–511
    diagnosis of, algorithm for, 520–521
        gender-specific values for, 511–512
        imaging for, 511–515
    monitoring recommendations for, 518
    prognosis for, 518–519
    therapy for, 515–518
        algorithm for, 520–521
        goal of, 515
        medical treatment as, 515–518
            advantage vs. disadvantage of, 516
        percutaneous ethanol injection as, 517
        radioactive treatment with I-131 as, 517
            advantage vs. disadvantage of, 517–520
        surgical excision as, 516–517
            advantage vs. disadvantage of, 516–517
  hypothyroidism as, 519–521
    description of, 519, 521
    diagnosis of, 521
    therapy for, 521
  summary overview of, 509–510, 521
Gut loading, metabolic bone diseases and, in reptiles and amphibians, 387–388

H

Handling techniques, for examination. See also *Manual restraint.*
  of koi, 334–335
Hedgehogs, internal disorders of, **453–469**
    cytologic sampling for, 459–461
    hematology and immunoassays for, 458
    medication administration techniques for, 466–467
    MRI of, 464
    physical examination for, 454
    radiographs for, 462, 464
    summary overview of, 453–454
    urinalysis for, 459
    venipuncture for, 456–457
Hematology tests. See *Complete blood counts (CBCs).*
Hematuria, in avians, 404
Hemibaculum, as gender-specific trait, in lizards, 359–360
Hemipenes, casts/plugs of, in lizards, 360–361
    in snakes, 367
  infertility examination of, in snakes, 366–367
  normal, in lizards, 358–359
    in snakes, 365–366
  prolapse of, in lizards, 365
    in snakes, 369–370
Hepatic arteries, in avians, 413
Hepatic disorders, in avians, **413–427**
    diagnosing dysfunction in, 415–422
        clinical pathologic analysis for, 415–418

Hepatic (*continued*)
        clinical signs and, 415
        hepatic biopsy for, 421–422
        imaging for, 418–421
        patient history and, 415
     liver anatomy review for, 413–414
     liver functions and, 414–415
     medical management of, 422–425
        for anemia, 423
        for ascites, 423–424
        for encephalopathy, 423
        nutraceuticals in, 424
        nutritional support in, 423
        targeted plans for, 422–423
     secondary complications of, 423
     summary overview of, 424–425
   in koi, 342
Hepatic ducts, in avians, 413
Hepatic portal veins, in avians, 413–414
Hepatobiliary scintigraphy, for hepatic disorders, in avians, 420–421
Hepatoenteric duct, in avians, 413
        hepatic disorders impact on, 417–418
Herbivores, metabolic bone disease in, calcium supplementation for, 388
Hetastarch, for hypovolemic shock, with rabbit gastrointestinal syndrome,
   531, 533–535, 538
Histopathology, of adrenocortical neoplasia, in ferrets, 444
   of coronavirus-associated diseases, in ferrets, 547–548
   of disseminated idiopathic myofascitis, in ferrets, 564–569
   of hepatic samples, in avians, 422, 424
   of insulinomas, in ferrets, 441
   of proventricular dilatation disease, in psittacines, 496–497
     of crop samples, 482–483
       as definitive diagnostic tool, 484–485
History taking, for disseminated idiopathic myofascitis, in ferrets, 562
   for hepatic disorders, in avians, 415
   for internal disorders, in koi, 334
   for metabolic bone disease, in reptiles and amphibians, 381
Holding tank, for koi, water quality in, 335
Hormone production. See *Steroid hormones.*
Hormone therapy, for chronic egg production, in psittacines, 431
Husbandry, as dystocia factor, in chelonians, 354
     in snakes, 367
   as follicular stasis factor, in lizards, 361
   as metabolic bone disease factor, in reptiles and amphibians, 381, 384–386
     current research on, 384
     diet modifications, 386–389
     pyramiding and, 389
     temperature, 384–385
     UV-B radiation, 375, 379–380, 385–386
   management of, for proventricular dilatation disease, in psittacines, 489–490
   reproductive disorders related to, in reptiles, 354, 361, 366–367

Hyperestrogenism, with adrenocortical neoplasia, in ferrets, 446
        pancytopenia secondary to, 449
        therapeutics for, 448
Hyperinsulinism, with insulinoma, in ferrets, 440–441
Hyperthyroidism, in guinea pigs, **509–523**
        clinical presentations of, 510
        clinical signs of, 510–511
        diagnosis of, algorithm for, 520–521
                imaging for, 511–515
        hypothyroidism vs., 519–521
        monitoring recommendations for, 518
        prognosis for, 518–519
        summary overview of, 509–510, 521
        therapy for, 515–518
                algorithm for, 520–521
                goal of, 515
                medical treatment as, 515–518
                        advantage vs. disadvantage of, 516
                percutaneous ethanol injection as, 517
                radioactive treatment with I-131 as, 517
                        advantage vs. disadvantage of, 517–520
                surgical excision as, 516–517
                        advantage vs. disadvantage of, 516–517
Hyperuricemia, in avians. See *Gout.*
Hypoglycemia, in hypovolemic shock, with rabbit gastrointestinal syndrome, 535
        rebound, with insulinoma, in ferrets, 440
Hypoglycemic episode, with insulinoma, management in ferrets, 441–442
Hypothyroidism, in guinea pigs, **509–523,** 519–521
        description of, 519, 521
        diagnosis of, 521
        hyperthyroidism vs., 510–519
        summary overview of, 509–510, 521
        therapy for, 521
Hypovolemic shock, with rabbit gastrointestinal syndrome, 532–536
        characteristics of, 532–533, 535
        nonresponsive, treatment of, 534–535
        treatment of, 533, 535, 537

I

I-131 radioactive injection, for hyperthyroidism, in guinea pigs, 517
        advantage of, 517–520
        disadvantage of, 517
        monitoring recommendations for, 518
Idiopathic myofascitis, in ferrets, **561–575**. See also *Disseminated idiopathic myofascitis (DIM).*
Imaging. See also *specific modality, e.g.,* Radiography.
        of hepatic disorders, in avians, 418–421
        of insulinoma, in ferrets, 441
        of proventricular dilatation disease, in psittacines, 479–482
        of renal disease, in avians, 405

Immune modulation, for coronavirus-associated diseases, in ferrets, 552–553
    for disseminated idiopathic myofascitis, in ferrets, 565, 568–570, 572
Immune suppression, for coronavirus-associated diseases, in ferrets, 552
Immune-mediated diseases, disseminated idiopathic myofascitis as, in ferrets, 561, 572
Immunoassays, for internal disorders, of select species, 458
    of avian bornavirus, 497–498
Immunofluorescent antibody (IFA) tests, for avian bornavirus, 497–498, 501–502
    for internal disorders, of select species, 458
Immunohistochemistry (IHC), of coronavirus-associated diseases, in ferrets, 547,
    549–551
    of cytologic samples for internal disorders, of select species, 459–461
    of insulinomas, in ferrets, 441
    of proventricular dilatation disease, in psittacines, 474, 477–478, 484
        avian bornavirus and, 497–499
Impaction, gastrointestinal, rabbit gastrointestinal syndrome related to, 525–526, 529
    of oviduct, in psittacines, 434–435
Incision closure, for internal surgery, of koi, 340–341
Incubation parameters, for eggs, of chelonians, 352
Infection control, for avian bornavirus, 505–506
Infections/infectious diseases, coronavirus-associated, in ferrets, **543–560**. See also
    Coronavirus-associated diseases.
    disseminated idiopathic myofascitis related to, in ferrets, 564, 571
    hepatic disorders related to, in avians, 422, 424
    internal disorders related to, in koi, 334, 340–341, 344–345
        in select species, 458
    opportunistic, with metabolic bone disease, in reptiles and amphibians, 381
    proventricular dilatation disease related to, avian bornavirus and, **471–484**.
    See also *Avian Bornavirus (ABV).*
        in psittacines, **471–494**. See also *Proventricular dilatation disease (PDD).*
    rabbit gastrointestinal syndrome related to, 525–526
    renal disease related to, in avians, 396–397, 407
Infertility, in chelonians, 350–352
    in lizards, 358–361
    in snakes, 366–367
Inflammatory disorders, in avians, of renal system, 395
    in ferrets, coronavirus-associated diseases as, pathology of, 547–549
            treatment of, 553–554
        epizootic catarrhal enteritis as, 543–544
        feline infectious peritonitis as, 543, 545, 550–551
        myopathies as, **561–575**. See also *Disseminated idiopathic myofascitis (DIM).*
            potential etiologies of, 571–572
            types of, 561
    in psittacines, metritis as, 435–436
        orchitis as, 437
        salpingitis as, 435–436
Inflammatory myopathies, in ferrets, **561–575**. See also *Disseminated idiopathic
    myofascitis (DIM).*
        potential etiologies of, 571–572
        types of, 561
Infundibulum, of psittacines, 429–430
Injury(ies), renal, in avians, 395, 404

with metabolic bone disease, in reptiles and amphibians, prevention of, 389
    treatment of, 390
Insulinoma, in ferrets, **439–452**
    adrenocortical neoplasia vs., 443–449
    description of, 439–440
    diagnostics for, 440–441
    summary overview of, 439, 449
    therapeutics for, 441–443
        definitive treatment in, 443
        diet modification as, 442–443
        for hypoglycemic episode management, 441–442
        palliative therapy as, 442
Interferon, for coronavirus-associated diseases, in ferrets, 552–553
Internal disorders, of koi, **333–347**
    common diseases and treatment, 340–345
        abdominal (coelomic) enlargement as, 340–341
        abdominal (coelomic) neoplasia as, 343–344
        digestive system abnormalities as, 338, 341
        egg binding as, 342–343
        gas (swim) bladder abnormalities as, 344–345
        obesity as, 341–342
        ovary enlargement as, 342–343
    diagnostic techniques for, 334–341
        anesthesia for, 335–336, 338–339
            monitoring during, 337, 339–340
        common tests as, 334
        CT scans as, 340–341
        endoscopy as, 338
        handling of fish for, 334–335
        history taking as, 334
        MRI as, 340
        radiographs as, 336–337
        surgical perspectives of, 338–340
            closure of incisions, 340–341
            monitoring during, 339–340
        ultrasound as, 336–338
        water quality as, 335
    popularity trends of, 333–334
    summary overview of, 333, 345
of select species, **453–469**
    diagnostic procedures for, 455–466
        computed tomography as, 465
        cytologic sampling as, 459–461
        endoscopy as, 465–466
        fecal analysis as, 458
        hematology as, 458
        immunoassay as, 458
        magnetic resonance imaging as, 464
        necropsy as, 466
        radiographs as, 461–463
            with contrast, 462–464

Internal (continued)
    ultrasound as, 465–466
    urinalysis as, 459
    venipuncture as, 455–457
    physical examination for, 454–455
    summary overview of, 453–454
    therapeutics for, 466–467
Internal organ biopsies, of koi, 338, 342, 344
Intestinal gas, accumulation of, rabbit gastrointestinal syndrome related to, 525,
    529–530, 532–533
Intravenous catheter, for fluid therapy, in rabbits, 528
Invasive methods, for dystocia therapy, in psittacines, 433
Iodine therapy, radioactive, for hyperthyroidism, in guinea pigs, 517
    advantage of, 517–520
    disadvantage of, 517
    monitoring recommendations for, 518
Irises, as gender-specific trait, in chelonians, 350, 352
Isoflurane anesthesia, for blood sample collection, of select species, 455–456
    for physical examination, of hedgehog, 454
Isotonic crystalloids, for hypovolemic shock, with rabbit gastrointestinal syndrome,
    531, 533–535
Isthmus, of psittacines, 429–430

K

Kidney biopsy, for metabolic bone disease, in reptiles and amphibians, 384
    for renal disease, in avians, 405–406
Kidney function, in avians. See *Renal function assessment.*
    metabolic bone disease and, in reptiles and amphibians, 375, 379–381
Kidneys, in avians, anatomy of, 393–394
    disease of. See *Renal disease.*
    injury to, 395, 404
    radiography of, 405
Koi, internal disorders of, **333–347**
    common diseases and treatment, 340–345
        abdominal (coelomic) enlargement as, 340–341
        abdominal (coelomic) neoplasia as, 343–344
        digestive system abnormalities as, 338, 341
        egg binding as, 342–343
        gas (swim) bladder abnormalities as, 344–345
        obesity as, 341–342
        ovary enlargement as, 342–343
    diagnostic techniques for, 334–341
    anesthesia for, 335–336, 338–339
        monitoring during, 337, 339–340
    common tests as, 334
    CT scans as, 340–341
    endoscopy as, 338
    handling of fish for, 334–335
    history taking as, 334
    MRI as, 340
    radiographs as, 336–337

surgical perspectives of, 338–340
    closure of incisions, 340–341
    monitoring during, 339–340
  ultrasound as, 336–338
  water quality as, 335
popularity trends of, 333–334
summary overview of, 333, 345

L

Lactate dehydrogenase (LDH), hepatic disorders and, in avians, 417–418
  renal damage and, in avians, 404
Laparotomy, exploratory, for insulinoma, in ferrets, 441
  for internal disorders, in koi, 338, 343–344
Lead toxicity, renal disease related to, in avians, 400
Length, of koi, body weight relationship to, 342–343
Leuprolide acetate (Lupron), for adrenocortical neoplasia, in ferrets, 447–448
Light exposure. See also *UV-B radiation.*
  adrenocortical neoplasia incidence correlated to, in ferrets, 444–445, 447–448
Lipid metabolism, hepatic, in avians, 414
Lipidosis, renal disease related to, in avians, 398–399
  with obesity, in koi, 342
Liver anatomy, of avians, 413–414
Liver biopsy, for hepatic disorders, in avians, 421–422
    in koi, 342
Liver functions, in avians, 414–415
Liver regeneration, capacity for, in avians, 415
Lizards, reproductive disorders in, 358–365
    dystocia as, 363–365
    follicular stasis as, 361–363
    hemipenal prolapse as, 365
    imaging of. See *specific pathology.*
    infertility as, 358–361
    normal reproduction vs., 358
L-thyroxine, for hypothyroidism, in guinea pigs, 521
Lymph system, disseminated idiopathic myofascitis involvement of, in ferrets, 564–565

M

Macaw wasting disease. See *Proventricular dilatation disease (PDD).*
Magnetic resonance imaging (MRI), of hepatic disorders, in avians, 419–421
  of internal disorders, in koi, 340
    in select species, 464
  of renal disease, in avians, 405
  of thyroid gland, 511, 513
Magnum, of psittacines, 429–430
Mallards, experimental avian bornavirus disease in, 500
Malnutrition, rabbit gastrointestinal syndrome related to, 526
Manual restraint, for examination, of koi, 334–335
  for gastrointestinal syndrome evaluation, of rabbits, 526–527
  for radiography, of koi, 336
    of select species, 461

Medetomidine, for dystocia, in chelonians, 355–356

Medication administration techniques, for internal disorders, of select species, 466–467

Melatonin, adrenocortical neoplasia and, in ferrets, 444, 447–448

    for coronavirus-associated diseases, in ferrets, 555

Meloxicam, for proventricular dilatation disease, in psittacines, 487

Metabolic bone diseases (MBDs), in reptiles and amphibians, **375–392**

    calcium homeostasis and, 376–379

    classic presentations in various species, 375–376

    description of, 375

    diagnostic approaches to, 376

    diagnostics for, 381–384

    diet factors of, 386–389

    husbandry factors of, 381, 384–386

    injury prevention for, 389

    pyramiding and, 389

    ramifications of, 381

    types of, 379–381

Methimazole, for hyperthyroidism, in guinea pigs, 515–516

Metoclopramide, for proventricular dilatation disease, in psittacines, 489

Metritis, in psittacines, 435–436

Microscopic lesions, with proventricular dilatation disease, in psittacines, 475–477

Midazolam, rabbit sedation with, for gastrointestinal syndrome evaluation, 527–528

Mineral supplements, for coronavirus-associated diseases, in ferrets, 555

    for metabolic bone diseases, in reptiles and amphibians, 386–388

Mitotane (Lysodren), for adrenocortical neoplasia, in ferrets, 448

Molecular assays/studies, of disseminated idiopathic myofascitis, in ferrets, 572

    of proventricular dilatation disease, in psittacines, 482–484, 496–497

Mucous membranes, in dehydration assessment, with rabbit gastrointestinal
    syndrome, 536–537

Murexide test, for renal disease, in avians, 406

Muscle, disseminated idiopathic myofascitis of, in ferrets, biopsy of, 569, 572–573

    gross vs. histologic findings of, 564–569

Mycotoxins, renal disease related to, in avians, 400–401

Myelography, for internal disorders, of select species, 463–464

Myofascitis, idiopathic, in ferrets, **561–575**. See also *Disseminated idiopathic
    myofascitis (DIM)*.

Myofibers, histologic findings in, with disseminated idiopathic myofascitis,
    in ferrets, 565, 567–568

Myoglobinuric nephrosis, in avians, 399

N

N protein, avian bornavirus and, 497–498, 502, 506

    detection in eye, 499–500

N-Acetyl-β-D-glucosaminidase (NAG), in renal disease assessment, for avians, 404

Nasogastric tube, for nutritional support, in rabbit gastrointestinal syndrome, 538–540

Necropsy, for disseminated idiopathic myofascitis, in ferrets, 572–573

    for internal disorders, of select species, 466

    for proventricular dilatation disease, in birds, 496, 502

Neoplasia, in avians, renal disease related to, 401, 405

    in ferrets, of adrenal cortex, **439–452**. See also *Adrenocortical neoplasia*.

of pancreatic islet beta-cells, 439–440. See also *Insulinoma.*
in koi, abdominal (coelomic), 343–344
    reproductive organs, 338–339
in select species, cytologic evaluation of, 460–461
    imaging of, 465
of psittacine reproductive organs, ovarian, 436
    oviduct, 436
    testicular, 437
Nephritis, in avians, antibiotics for, 407
    nutrition and, 397
Nephrons, in avians, 394
Nephrosis, in avians, bile pigment, 403–404
    myoglobinuric, 399
    necrotizing, 400
Nervous systems, disorders of, in select species, myelography for, 463–464
    proventricular dilatation disease signs in, avian bornavirus and, 496, 499
        in psittacines, 478–479, 486, 496
            microscopic lesions as, 475–477
                immunohistochemistry of, 477–478
Neurologic conditions, in select species, diagnostic approaches to, 464
Newcastle disease (NDV), in avians, 505
Nonsteroidal anti-inflammatory drugs (NSAIDs), for proventricular dilatation disease,
    in psittacines, 486–488
    toxicity of, renal disease related to, in avians, 400
Nuclear medicine scans, for hepatic disorders, in avians, 420–421
    for internal disorders, of select species, 464–465
    for metabolic bone disease, in reptiles and amphibians, 383–384
    for renal disease, in avians, 405
    of thyroid gland, 511–512
Nucleotide sequencing, of proventricular dilatation disease virus, 473–474, 496–497
Nutraceuticals, for hepatic disorders, in avians, 424
Nutrition, renal disease related to, in avians, 397–398
Nutritional secondary hyperparathyroidism (NSHPT), in reptiles and amphibians,
    375, 380–381
    client handout for, 377–378
Nutritional support, for coronavirus-associated diseases, in ferrets, 555
    for hepatic disorders, in avians, 423
    for metabolic bone disease, in reptiles and amphibians, 381, 386–388, 390
    for proventricular dilatation disease, in psittacines, 489
    for rabbit gastrointestinal syndrome, 538
        nasogastric tube placement for, 538–540
    for renal disease, in avians, 407

O

Obesity, in koi, 341–342
Obstruction, gastrointestinal, in koi, 341
    rabbit gastrointestinal syndrome related to, 525–526, 529, 531
    urinary, in ferrets, with adrenocortical neoplasia, 445, 448
        urethral catheterization for, 448–449
Ochratoxin, renal disease related to, in avians, 400

Octreotide, for insulinoma, in ferrets, 442

Omega fatty acids, for proventricular dilatation disease, in psittacines, 489
    for renal disease, in avians, 407

Oosporein toxicity, renal disease related to, in avians, 400–401

Opioids, rabbit sedation with, for gastrointestinal syndrome evaluation, 527–528

Optic lobe, avian bornavirus in, 499–500

Orchitis, in psittacines, 437

Ornamental fish, internal disorders of, **333–347**. See also *Koi*.

Ova. See *Egg entries*.

Ovariectomy, for dystocia, in snakes, 368, 370
    for follicular stasis, in lizards, 362–363
        in snakes, 367

Ovary(ies), of koi, enlargement of, 342–343
    of psittacines, 429
        neoplasia of, 436
    of select species, ultrasound evaluation of, 465–466

Oviduct, eggs retained in. See *Dystocia*.
    of psittacines, endoscopic removal of multiple eggs in, 433–434
        impaction of, 434–435
        neoplasia of, 436
        prolapse of, 434
        rupture of, 435
    of snakes, prolapse of, 370

Oviposition, delayed, in psittacines. See *Dystocia*.
    inducement of, for dystocia, in chelonians, 354–355

Ovocentesis, for dystocia, in chelonians, 356

Ovulation, in chelonians, 350
    induction of, in koi, 342–343
        in lizards, 362

Oxyglobin, for hypovolemic shock, with rabbit gastrointestinal syndrome, 532, 535

Oxytocin, for dystocia, in chelonians, 354–355
        in lizards, 364–365
        in psittacines, 432
        in snakes, 369

Ozagrel (Xanbon), for coronavirus-associated diseases, in ferrets, 554

P

Pain management, for metabolic bone disease, in reptiles and amphibians, 390

Palliative therapy, for insulinoma, in ferrets, 442

Pancreatic biopsy, for insulinoma, in ferrets, 441

Pancreatic islet beta-cell tumors, in ferrets, 439–440. See also *Insulinoma*.

Pancytopenia, secondary to hyperestrogenism, with adrenocortical neoplasia, in ferrets, 449

Parasites, renal disease related to, in avians, 397

Parathyroid gland, surgical excision of, for hyperthyroidism, in guinea pigs, 517–518
        monitoring recommendations for, 518

Parathyroid hormone (PTH) overproduction, in reptiles and amphibians, calcium homeostasis and, 378–379
    client handout for, 377–378
    nutritional vs. renal, 375, 380–381

Patagonian conures, experimental avian bornavirus disease in, 501

Patient history. See History taking.

Pentoxifylline, for coronavirus-associated diseases, in ferrets, 553

Phallus, prolapse of, in chelonians, 357, 359

Phosphorus, metabolic bone disease and, in reptiles and amphibians, 375, 380
    calcium homeostasis and, 376–379
    diagnostics for, 381–382
    supplementation with, 388

Physical examination, for disseminated idiopathic myofascitis, in ferrets, 572
    for internal disorders, of select species, 454–455
    for metabolic bone disease, in reptiles and amphibians, 381
    for rabbit gastrointestinal syndrome, 526, 528

Pin worms, anal tape test for, in select species, 458

Plastron, in chelonians, 350–351

Plastronotomy, for dystocia, in chelonians, 356, 358

Pneumocystocentesis, of gas bladder, in koi, 345

Polymerase chain reaction (PCR) assay, for coronavirus-associated diseases,
    in ferrets, 544, 550
    for internal disorders, in koi, 334
        in select species, 458
    for proventricular dilatation disease, in psittacines, 483–484, 490, 496
    avian bornavirus and, 496–497, 502–503
        in transmission studies, 503–505

Polyostotic hyperostosis, in psittacines, 430

Polyprenyul immunostimulant, for coronavirus-associated diseases, in ferrets, 552–553

Positron emission tomography (PET), for hepatic disorders, in avians, 420–421

Prednisolone (Pediapred), for coronavirus-associated diseases, in ferrets, 552, 554
    for disseminated idiopathic myofascitis, in ferrets, 568, 570, 572
    for insulinoma, in ferrets, 442

Prednisone, for insulinoma, in ferrets, 442

Pregnancy, radiograph confirmation of, in select species, 462

Preventive therapy, for coronavirus-associated diseases, in ferrets, 556
    for injury, with metabolic bone disease, in reptiles and amphibians, 389
    for proventricular dilatation disease, avian bornavirus and, 505–506
        in psittacines, 490

Probiotics, for coronavirus-associated disease, in ferrets, 554–555

Prokinetics, for rabbit gastrointestinal syndrome, 538–539

Prolapse, of hemipenes, in lizards, 365
        in snakes, 369–370
    of oviduct, in psittacines, 434
        in snakes, 370
    of phallus, in chelonians, 357, 359

Promotility drugs, for rabbit gastrointestinal syndrome, 538–539

Propranolol, for dystocia, in chelonians, 355

Propylthiouracil (PTU), for hyperthyroidism, in guinea pigs, 515–516

Prostaglandin $F_{2\alpha}$, for dystocia, in psittacines, 432

Prostaglandins, for dystocia, in chelonians, 355

Prostatomegaly, in ferrets, with adrenocortical neoplasia, 448
            urethral catheterization for, 448–449
            urinary obstruction secondary to, 445, 448

Protein electrophoresis, serum, for coronavirus-associated diseases, in ferrets, 550

Protein intake, renal disease related to, in avians, 397
Proventricular dilatation disease (PDD), avian bornavirus and, **495–508**
    autoimmunity and, 499–500
    control and prevention of, 505–506
    description of, 473–474
    diagnosis of, 501–502
    DNA studies of, 496–497
    experimental disease examples, 500–501
        evidence for, 500
        in cockatiels, 501
        in mallards, 500
        in Patagonian conures, 501
    immunohistochemistry of, 477–478, 484
    in other avian species, 505
    in psittacine species, 495–505
    in the eye, 499–500
    isolation of, 497–498
    molecular and serology assays of, 482–484
    pathogenesis of, 498–499
    summary overview of, 495–496, 506
    transmission of, 502–505
        ABV shedding and, 503–505
        fecal-oral route for, 503
        respiratory route for, 503
    viral description of, 497
  etiologic determinations of, 496–497
  in psittacines, **471–494**
    antemortem diagnosis of, 477–484
        clinical chemistry in, 479
        clinical signs in, 477–479
        crop biopsy for, 482–483, 490
        fecal and crop cytology in, 479
        hematology in, 479
        imaging for, 479–482
        molecular diagnosis in, 482–484
        proposed approach to, 484–485
        serology in, 482, 484
    avian bornavirus and, 495–505
    clinical management of, 484–490
        amantadine hydrochloride for, 488
        decision making for, 484–486
        husbandry considerations for, 489
        monitoring progress of, 489–490
        nonsteroidal anti-inflammatory drugs for, 486–488
        other drugs for, 488–489
        treatment considerations for, 486
    counseling owners on, 485–486
    etiology of, 473–474
    occurrence clusters of, 471–473
    pathology of, 474–477
        immunohistochemistry findings in, 474, 477–478, 484

prevention of, 490
   species diagnosed with, 471–472, 495
   summary overview of, 471, 490–491
Proventriculus (PV), dilatation disease of, in psittacines, 475–476. See also
   Proventricular dilatation disease (PDD).
Psittacines, proventricular dilatation disease in, **471–494**
   antemortem diagnosis of, 477–484
      clinical chemistry in, 479
      clinical signs in, 477–479
      crop biopsy for, 482–483, 490
      fecal and crop cytology in, 479
      hematology in, 479
      imaging for, 479–482
      molecular diagnosis in, 482–484
      proposed approach to, 484–485
      serology in, 482, 484
   avian bornavirus and, 495–505
   clinical management of, 484–490
      amantadine hydrochloride for, 488
      decision making for, 484–486
      husbandry considerations for, 489
      monitoring progress of, 489–490
      nonsteroidal anti-inflammatory drugs for, 486–488
      other drugs for, 488–489
      treatment considerations for, 486
   counseling owners on, 485–486
   etiology of, 473–474
   occurrence clusters of, 471–473
   pathology of, 474–477
      immunohistochemistry findings in, 474, 477–478, 484
   prevention of, 490
   species diagnosed with, 471–472, 495
   summary overview of, 471, 490–491
   renal disease in. See *Renal disease.*
   reproductive disorders in, **429–438**
   female anatomy review, 429–430
   female disorders, 430–436
      chronic egg production as, 430–431
      dystocia as, 431
         assessment of, 431
         clinical signs of, 431–432
         description of, 431
         diagnosis of, 431
         therapy of, 431–434
      metritis as, 435–436
      ovarian neoplasia as, 436
      oviduct neoplasia as, 436
      oviductal impaction as, 434–435
      oviductal prolapse as, 434
      oviductal rupture as, 435
      polyostotic hyperostosis as, 430

Psittacines (*continued*)
        salpingitis as, 435–436
        uterine rupture as, 435
      male anatomy review, 436–437
      male disorders, 437
        orchitis as, 437
        testicular neoplasia as, 437
      summary overview of, 429
Pyogranulomatous lesions, with coronavirus-associated diseases, in ferrets, 547–548
Pyramiding, metabolic bone disease and, in reptiles and amphibians, 389

R

Rabbit gastrointestinal syndrome (RGIS), **525–541**
  causes of, 525–526
  description of, 525
  diagnostic workup for, 529–531
    initial decision-making on, 528
    laboratory tests in, 531
    radiography in, 529–534
  fluid administration for, 531–537
    dehydration as focus of, 537–538
    hypovolemic shock as focus of, 532–536
    initial decision-making on, 528
    maintenance fluids calculation, 537–538
    oral vs. IV, 528–529
    phases of, 531–532
    plan for, 531
  initial presentation and evaluation of, 526–529
    decision 1 - restraint options, 526–528
    decision 2 - fluid support, 528
    decision 3 - diagnostic workup, 528
    decision 4 - medical vs. surgical interventions, 528–529
  medical interventions for, analgesia as, 527, 539–540
    initial decision-making on, 528–529
    nutritional support as, 538
    promotility drugs as, 538–539
  physical examination for, 526, 528
  symptoms of, 526
Rabbits, gastrointestinal stasis in, **525–541**. See also *Rabbit gastrointestinal syndrome (RGIS)*.
Radioactive I-131 injection. See *I-131 radioactive injection; Iodine therapy.*
Radiography, for disseminated idiopathic myofascitis, in ferrets, 564, 572
  for dystocia, in psittacines, 432–433
  for hepatic disorders, in avians, 418–419
  for internal disorders, of koi, 336–337, 342–343, 345
    of select species, 461–463
      contrast, 462–464
  for metabolic bone disease, in reptiles and amphibians, 376, 383
  for neoplasia, in psittacines, 436
  for oviduct disorders, in psittacines, 434–435

for proventricular dilatation disease, in psittacines, contrast, 479–481
    for therapy monitoring, 489–490
    survey, 479–480
for rabbit gastrointestinal syndrome, 529–534
  abdominal, 529–531
  clinical condition correlated to, 530, 535–537
  contrast, 531
  serial, 530, 533
for renal disease, in avians, 405
Radioimmunoassay (RIA), of bile acid, for hepatic disorders, in avians, 418
Radionuclide scans. See also *Technetium-99 entries.*
  for hepatic disorders, in avians, 421
  of thyroid gland, 512–513
Recombinant human TSH (rhTSH), for hypothyroidism, in guinea pigs, 521
Recovery water, for koi, post-anesthesia, 335–336
Red blood count (RBC). See *Complete blood counts (CBCs).*
Renal calcifications, in avians, nutrition and, 397–398
Renal cysts, in avians, 401
Renal disease, in avians, 395–408
  clinical signs of, 395
  diagnostics for, 402–406
    advanced imaging as, 405
    bloodwork as, 402–403
    murexide test as, 406
    N-acetyl-β-D-glucosaminidase as, 404
    radiographs as, 405
    renal biopsy as, 405–406
    ultrasound as, 405
    urate character as, 403–404
    urinalysis as, 403
    urine enzymes as, 404
  infectious causes of, 396–397
    bacteria as, 396
    fungi as, 396–397
    parasites as, 397
    viruses as, 396
  noninfectious causes of, 397–402
    amyloidosis as, 398
    congenital diseases as, 401
    gout as, 399–400
    lipidosis as, 398–399
    myoglobinuric nephrosis as, 399
    neoplasia as, 401
    nutrition as, 397–398
    toxicity as, 400–401
    urolithiasis as, 402
  summary overview of, 393, 395–396, 408
  treatment of, 406–408
    antibiotics for, 407
    fluid support in, 406
    for gout/hyperuricemia, 407–408

Renal (*continued*)
           nutrition in, 407
           principles for, 406
Renal function assessment, in avians, 402–406
    advanced imaging for, 405
    bloodwork for, 402–403
    murexide test in, 406
    N-acetyl-β-D-glucosaminidase and, 404
    radiographs for, 405
    renal biopsy in, 405–406
    ultrasound for, 405
    urate character in, 403–404
    urinalysis for, 403
    urine enzymes in, 404
Renal portal system, in avians, 393–394
Renal secondary hyperparathyroidism (RSHPT), in reptiles and amphibians, 375,
   380–381
    diagnostics for, 383–384
    therapeutic considerations of, 389
Renal system, of avians, **393–411**
    anatomy of, 393–394
    diseases of, 395–408. See also *Renal disease.*
    injury to, 395, 404
    physiology of, 393–395
       assessment of, 402–403
    summary overview of, 393, 408
Reproductive disorders, in chelonians, 349–359
    dystocia as, 353–356
    follicular stasis as, 353
    infertility as, 350–352
    normal reproduction vs., 349–350
    phallus prolapse as, 357, 359
    yolk coelomitis as, 356–358
  in koi, 338–339
  in lizards, 358–365
    dystocia as, 363–365
    follicular stasis as, 361–363
    hemipenal prolapse as, 365
    infertility as, 358–361
    normal reproduction vs., 358
  in psittacines, **429–438**
    female anatomy review, 429–430
    female disorders, 430–436
      chronic egg production as, 430–431
      dystocia as, 431
        assessment of, 431
        clinical signs of, 431–432
        description of, 431
        diagnosis of, 431
        therapy of, 431–434
      metritis as, 435–436

        ovarian neoplasia as, 436
        oviduct neoplasia as, 436
        oviductal impaction as, 434–435
        oviductal prolapse as, 434
        oviductal rupture as, 435
        polyostotic hyperostosis as, 430
        salpingitis as, 435–436
        uterine rupture as, 435
     male anatomy review, 436–437
     male disorders, 437
        orchitis as, 437
        testicular neoplasia as, 437
     summary overview of, 429
  in reptiles, **349–373**
     chelonians, 349–359
     imaging of. See *specific pathology.*
     lizards, 358–365
     snakes, 365–370
     summary overview of, 349
  in select species, 459
     cytologic sampling for, 460
     imaging of, 462–466
  in snakes, 365–370
     dystocia as, 367–370
     follicular stasis as, 367–368
     infertility as, 366–367
     normal reproduction vs., 365–366
     prolapses as, 369–370
Reproductive system, disorders of. See *Reproductive disorders.*
  normal, of chelonians, 349–350
     of lizards, 358
     of snakes, 365–366
Reptiles, metabolic bone diseases in, **375–392**
     calcium homeostasis and, 376–379
     diagnostics for, 376, 381–384
     diet factors of, 386–389
     husbandry factors of, 381, 384–386
     injury prevention for, 389
     pyramiding and, 389
     ramifications of, 381
     summary overview of, 375–376
     types of, 379–381
  reproductive disorders in, **349–373**
     chelonians, 349–359
     imaging of. See *specific pathology.*
     lizards, 358–365
     snakes, 365–370
Respiratory tract disorders, in select species, cytologic sampling of, 459–460
     radiographs of, 462
Respiratory transmission, of avian bornavirus, 503
Restraint. See *Chemical restraint; Manual restraint.*

Reverse transcription PCR (RT-PCR) assay, for coronavirus-associated diseases, in ferrets, 550–551
    for proventricular dilatation disease, in psittacines, 483–484, 490
RNA viruses, avian bornavirus as, 497, 505
    coronavirus as, 550
Rodenticide toxicity, renal disease related to, in avians, 400
Rodents, internal disorders of, **453–469**
        computed tomography of, 465
        cytologic sampling for, 459–461
        hematology and immunoassays for, 458
        MRI of, 464
        physical examination for, 455
        radiographs for, 462–464
        summary overview of, 453–454
        therapeutics for, 466–467
        urinalysis for, 459
        venipuncture for, 456–457
Rupture, as female psittacine reproductive disorder, of eggs, 433
      of oviduct, 435
      of uterus, 435

    S

S-adenosylmethionine (SAMe), for hepatic disorders, in avians, 424
Salpingitis, in psittacines, 435–436
Salpingotomy, for dystocia, in chelonians, 356
Screening, for avian bornavirus, 505–506
Sedation. See *Chemical restraint.*
Seed impactions, with proventricular dilatation disease, in psittacines, 475, 478
Seed-based diets, for renal disease, in avians, 407
Select species, internal disorders of, **453–469**
    diagnostic procedures for, 455–466
        computed tomography as, 465
        cytologic sampling as, 459–461
        endoscopy as, 465–466
        fecal analysis as, 458
        hematology as, 458
        immunoassay as, 458
        magnetic resonance imaging as, 464
        necropsy as, 466
        radiographs as, 461–463
            with contrast, 462–464
        ultrasound as, 465–466
        urinalysis as, 459
        venipuncture as, 455–457
    physical examination for, 454–455
    summary overview of, 453–454
    therapeutics for, 466–467
Seminiferous tubules, of psittacines, 436
Serology assays. See *specific assay, e.g.,* Polymerase chain reaction (PCR) assay.
Sex hormones overproduction. See also *Adrenocortical neoplasia.*

in ferrets, 439, 446
   therapeutics for, 446–448
Sexing, of chelonians, 350, 352
   of lizards, 358–359
   of snakes, 366–367
Sexual dimorphism, in chelonians, 350–351
   in snakes, 366
Shedding sites, avian bornavirus transmission and, 503–505
Signalment, disseminated idiopathic myofascitis and, in ferrets, 562, 572
Silymarin, for hepatic disorders, in avians, 424
Skin biopsy, for internal disorders, of koi, 334, 337
Skin closure, for surgical incisions, of koi, 340–341
Snakes, reproductive disorders in, 365–370
     dystocia as, 367–370
     follicular stasis as, 367–368
     imaging of. See *specific pathology.*
     infertility as, 366–367
     normal reproduction vs., 365–366
     prolapses as, 369–370
Soft- or thin-shelled eggs, with dystocia, in psittacines, 433
Spawning cycle, of koi, 342–343
Sperm production, in chelonians, 349, 352
   in lizards, 358
   in snakes, 365, 367
Spleen, disseminated idiopathic myofascitis involvement of, in ferrets, 564–565
Sterilization, adrenocortical neoplasia incidence correlated to, in ferrets, 444–445
Steroid hormones, overproduction of. See also *Adrenocortical neoplasia.*
   in ferrets, 439
     therapeutics for, 446–448
Stomach, radiographic findings of, with rabbit gastrointestinal syndrome, 529, 531
Sugar gliders, internal disorders of, **453–469**
   cytologic sampling for, 459–461
   hematology and immunoassays for, 458
   MRI of, 464
   physical examination for, 455
   radiographs for, 462, 464
   summary overview of, 453–454
   therapeutics for, 466–467
   urinalysis for, 459
   venipuncture for, 456–457
Superoxide dismutase (SOD), for coronavirus-associated diseases, in ferrets, 555
Supportive care, fluids as. See *Fluid therapy.*
   for disseminated idiopathic myofascitis, in ferrets, 565, 572–573
   nutrition as. See *Nutritional support.*
Surfactants, for proventricular dilatation disease, in psittacines, 488
Surgical excision, of insulinoma, in ferrets, 443
   of thyroid/parathyroid glands, for hyperthyroidism, in guinea pigs, 516–518
     monitoring recommendations for, 516–518
Surgical exploration, for diagnosis. See *Exploratory surgery.*
Surgical intervention, for internal disorders, of koi, closure of incisions, 340–341
     diagnostic applications of, 338–340

Surgical (*continued*)
   monitoring during, 339–340
   for rabbits gastrointestinal syndrome, 529
Swim (gas) bladder, abnormalities of, in koi, 344–345
Symptomatic treatment, of coronavirus-associated diseases, in ferrets, 554–555
   of hepatic disorders, in avians, 423

T

T3 level, gender-specific values for, in guinea pigs, 511
T4 level, gender-specific values for, in guinea pigs, 511
Technetium-99 diethylenetriaminepentacetic acid (DTPA) scan, for metabolic bone
   disease, in reptiles and amphibians, 383–384
   for renal disease, in avians, 405
Technetium-99 dimercaptosuccinic acid (DMSA) scan, for metabolic bone disease,
   in reptiles and amphibians, 383–384
   for renal disease, in avians, 405
Technetium-99 mercaptoacetyltriglycine (MAG3) scan, for metabolic bone disease,
   in reptiles and amphibians, 383–384
Tepoxalin, for proventricular dilatation disease, in psittacines, 487
Testes, of lizards, 358
   of psittacines, 436
      inflammation of, 437
      neoplasia of, 437
Thoracocentesis, for internal disorders, of select species, 459–460
Thyrogen, for hypothyroidism, in guinea pigs, 521
Thyroid gland, in guinea pigs, fine-needle aspirate of, 511–512
   surgical excision of, for hyperthyroidism, 516–517
      monitoring recommendations for, 518
Thyroid hormones, gender-specific values for, in guinea pigs, 511–512
Thyroid pathologies, in guinea pigs, **509–523**
   hyperthyroidism as, clinical presentations of, 510
      clinical signs of, 510–511
      diagnosis of, algorithm for, 520–521
         imaging for, 511–515
      monitoring recommendations for, 518
      prognosis for, 518–519
      therapy for, 515–518
         algorithm for, 520–521
         goal of, 515
         medical treatment as, 515–518
         advantage vs. disadvantage of, 516
      percutaneous ethanol injection as, 517
      radioactive treatment with I-131 as, 517
         advantage vs. disadvantage of, 517–520
      surgical excision as, 516–517
         advantage vs. disadvantage of, 516–517
   hypothyroidism as, 519–521
      description of, 519, 521

diagnosis of, 521
therapy for, 521
summary overview of, 509–510, 521
Thyroid storm, avoiding during diagnostic process, in guinea pigs, 514–515
Thyroidectomy, for hyperthyroidism, in guinea pigs, 516–518
monitoring recommendations for, 518
Thyroid-stimulating hormone (TSH) stimulation test, for hypothyroidism, in guinea pigs, 521
Thyroxine level, in guinea pigs, 519–521
gender-specific values for, 511–512
L-Thyroxine, for hypothyroidism, in guinea pigs, 521
Tissue and fluid aspiration, for internal disorders, in koi, 334, 341, 344–345
Toxins/toxicity(ies), renal disease related to, in avians, 400–401
Tracheal aspiration, endoscopic assisted, for internal disorders, of select species, 459–460
Tracheal intubation, of select species, endoscopy for, 465
Transmission electron microscopy, with coronavirus-associated diseases, in ferrets, 547
Tumors. See *Neoplasia.*

U

Ultrasonography, for adrenocortical neoplasia, in ferrets, 445
for disseminated idiopathic myofascitis, in ferrets, 564
for hepatic disorders, in avians, 418–419
for insulinoma, in ferrets, 441
for internal disorders, of koi, 336–338, 342–343
of select species, 465–466
for metabolic bone disease, in reptiles and amphibians, 383
for rabbit gastrointestinal syndrome, 529
for renal disease, in avians, 405
of thyroid gland, in guinea pigs, 511–514
Undigested food, proventricular dilatation disease and, in psittacines, 475, 478
Urate character, in renal function assessment, for avians, 403–404
Urate oxidase, for gout, in avians, 407–408
Urea, in avians, assessment of, 402
physiology of, 394
Ureteral stones, in avians, 402
Ureters, in avians, 394
pathologic dilation of, 394–395, 402
Urethral catheterization, for secondary urinary obstruction, with adrenocortical neoplasia, in ferrets, 448–449
Uric acid, in avians, assessment of, 402
physiology of, 394–395
Urinalysis, for disseminated idiopathic myofascitis, in ferrets, 564, 572
for internal disorders, of select species, 459
for rabbit gastrointestinal syndrome, 531
for renal function assessment, in avians, 403
Urinary catheterization, for urine collection, in select species, 459
Urinary obstruction, in ferrets, with adrenocortical neoplasia, 445, 448
urethral catheterization for, 448–449
Urinary output, for dehydration assessment, in rabbit gastrointestinal syndrome, 537
Urine enzymes, renal damage and, in avians, 404
Urine specific gravity, in renal function assessment, for avians, 403

Urodeum, in avians, 394
Urogenital tract, disorders of, in select species, endoscopic biopsy for, 466
        imaging of, 462–463, 465
    of avians, 394–395
Urolithiasis, in avians, 402, 405
Uterine rupture, in psittacines, 435
UV-B radiation, metabolic bone disease related to, in reptiles and amphibians, 375, 380
        calcium homeostasis and, 379
        research review of, 385–386

V

Vaccinations, disseminated idiopathic myofascitis and, in ferrets, 562
    for proventricular dilatation disease, in psittacines, 488
Vagina, of psittacines, 429–430
Vaginal sphincter, of psittacines, 430, 432
Vasculitis, with coronavirus-associated diseases, in ferrets, pathology of, 547–549
        treatment of, 553–554
Venipuncture, for internal disorders, of select species, 455–457
Ventral color scintigram, of thyroid gland, 512–513
Ventriculus, proventricular dilatation disease and, in psittacines, 479–481
Viral infections, in avians, bornaviruses as. See also *Avian Bornavirus (ABV)*.
        proventricular dilatation disease related to, **471–484,** 473–474, 497. See also
        Proventricular dilatation disease (PDD).
        immunohistochemistry of, 477–478, 484
        molecular and serology assays of, 484
        renal disease related to, 396
    in ferrets, coronavirus-associated diseases as, **543–560.** See also
    Coronavirus-associated diseases.
        disseminated idiopathic myofascitis related to, 571
Vitamin A deficiency, renal disease related to, in avians, 397, 407
Vitamin D deficiency, renal disease related to, in avians, 397
Vitamin D_3, metabolic bone disease and, in reptiles and amphibians, 375
        calcium homeostasis and, 378–379
        diagnostics for, 382
        supplementation with, 387–388
Vitamin supplements, for coronavirus-associated diseases, in ferrets, 555
    for metabolic bone diseases, in reptiles and amphibians, 387
    for proventricular dilatation disease, in psittacines, 489
    for renal disease, in avians, 407
Vomiting, with coronavirus-associated disease, in ferrets, 554
Vulvar swelling, in ferrets, with adrenocortical neoplasia, 445–447

W

Water, calcium-enhanced, for metabolic bone disease, in reptiles and amphibians,
    388–389
    holding tank, for koi diagnostic procedures, 335
    recovery, for koi, post-anesthesia, 335–336
Water regulation, physiology of, in avians, 394

Western blot analysis, for proventricular dilatation disease, avian bornavirus and, 497, 499, 501–502
    in psittacines, 484
White blood count (WBC). See *Complete blood counts (CBCs).*

Y

Yolk coelomitis, in chelonians, 356–358
    in snakes, 370

Z

Zinc toxicity, renal disease related to, in avians, 400

Printed and bound by CPI Group (UK) Ltd, Croydon, CR0 4YY

14/10/2024

01773702-0001